The
COMPLETE
ELDERCARE
PLANNER

The
COMPLETE
ELDERCARE
PLANNER

REVISED AND UPDATED EDITION

Where to Start, Which Questions to Ask,
and How to Find Help

JOY LOVERDE

THREE RIVERS PRESS • NEW YORK

Three Rivers Press and the Tugboat design are registered trademarks of Random House, Inc.

Previous editions of this work were published by Silvercare Productions, Chicago, in 1992 and 1993. Later published by
Hyperion, New York, in 1997, and by Three Rivers Press, an imprint of the Crown Publishing Group, a division of
Random House, Inc., New York, in 2000.

Grateful acknowledgment is made to the following for permission to reprint previously published material:

Alzheimer's Association: "Ten Warning Signs of Alzheimer's," copyright © 2008 by Alzheimer's Association.
Reprinted by permission of Alzheimer's Association.

Soho Press, Inc.: Excerpt from *The Sixteen Pleasures* by Robert Hellenga,
copyright © 1994 by Robert Hellenga. All rights reserved. Reprinted by permission of Soho Press, Inc.

Library of Congress Cataloging-in-Publication Data

Loverde, Joy.
The complete eldercare planner : where to start, which questions to ask,
and how to find help / Joy Loverde. — Rev. and updated ed.
Includes index.
1. Older people—Home care—United States—Planning. 2. Aging parents—Care—United States—Planning.
3. Caregivers—United States—Life skills guides. I. Title.
HV1461.L6843 2009
362.6—dc22
2008026891

ISBN 978-0-307-40962-1

Printed in the United States of America

Design by Helene Berinsky

10   9   8   7

Revised and Updated Edition

This book celebrates people young and old who have touched my life and have since died, especially Dad, Nonno, Nonna, Graziano, Leo, Guy, Sergio, Frank, Jack, Eloise, Mary, Michelle, Rita, Bob, Ursula, Manny, Ellen . . . I know you're in Heaven watching over me. I also dedicate this book to the person who has taught me the most about successful aging, Martin K. Bayne.

CONTENTS

The
COMPLETE
ELDERCARE
PLANNER

INTRODUCTION

We don't choose eldercare. Eldercare chooses us.

When eldercare comes knocking on the door, many people run in the opposite direction; but not you. Whether you assumed the job, sought it, or inherited the responsibility out of obligation, even guilt, chances are if you are holding this book in your hands, you accepted—willingly or otherwise—your role as caregiver; yet caregiving has been part of your life plan *all along.*

Just as childhood, adolescence, young adulthood, and middle age are developmental phases of life, we acknowledge that someone we care about is going to get old and that someone is going to need care and attention. *And we don't need 24/7 involvement to be considered a caregiver.* We may be living with loved ones and caring for them, or we may be picking up the phone and checking in every once in a while. Whatever the case may be, when there are older people in our lives, and we've increased the amount of attention we give them, and we're starting to be more concerned, we are caregivers.

At first, eldercare may feel as if the rug has been pulled out from under you; you're falling and grabbing for something—anything—steady to hang on to, and there's nothing there. You laugh when things are sad; you cry when things go well. You never quite touch ground, and you soon realize that life is never going to be the same. People who once took care of you or walked by your side are now on another journey. You can walk with them for a while longer, then face the sad fact that they will ultimately leave you.

The caregiving journey will take you to places unimaginable, and in the process you will learn more about yourself than ever before. Each day has the potential to bring to the surface life-altering issues and events that offer you the opportunity to develop skills and talents you never knew you had—resourcefulness, stamina, flexibility, and faith, to name a few. You won't come away from the caregiving experience the same as when you started, nor will you look at life, and death, in the way you did before.

While even the kindest and most gracious older people can be difficult and demanding at times, ideally, you'll find a way to respond to them with empathy and love. Or you may tolerate your elders out of guilt and fear the burdens they represent, but beware of falling into the pity pit. Do not be blinded by the problem-solving elements of eldercare or you'll miss the valuable lessons they have to teach.

The simple truth about elders is this: They want their lives to be validated, and they do not want to die alone. Go to them as best you can and you will be rewarded handsomely. Eldercare wakes up the soul and brings us face-to-face with our own mortality. Eldercare teaches us to live in the present, and is the conduit that serves as a daily reminder of what is ultimately important in our lives. Let your elders lead, because every conversation is a privilege, and the moments we share with them bring us closer to who *we* are and make us wiser in ways that are eventually revealed to us over time.

We become the beneficiaries of these unique gifts the moment we find the courage to talk with our elders. Discussing eldercare issues and keeping the lines of communication open is *never* easy; consequently, many family members do not have the courage or endurance to do so. They may forfeit the chance to hear and say the most healing words of all, which can be spoken only after the hard work is done: *"Thank you for all you have done for me"* and *"I love you."* Knowing how truly difficult the process of talking with older people can be, you will find numerous conversation tips throughout *The Complete Eldercare Planner* giving you every opportunity to engage in meaningful conversations that you will carry in your heart for the rest of your life.

There are no blueprints.

We do many things for our elders in the caregiving years. We rush to the hospital in the middle of the night, and we spend countless hours making telephone calls; we cook and clean up, and we make sure they take their medications; we listen to them complain, and we take them shopping for shoes; we watch television with them for hours, and we sit quietly as they doze. Caregiving is nothing less than a labor of love. We do what we have to do with the understanding that we have no way of knowing what lies ahead and how we'll cope.

Caregiving is full of surprises. There are countless stories of estranged parents who come looking for and expecting their children to care for them long after they abandoned them physically and emotionally. Mothers and fathers who are paying the price for their bad judgment are facing the fact that they now need help. The anger and resentment in this caregiving situation is understandable. The question then becomes, do we abandon caring for parents who abandoned us or do we come to their rescue?

Seasoned family caregivers know all too well about the stresses of eldercare even under the best of circumstances: dwindling financial resources; care receivers who don't acknowledge kind deeds; and siblings and other family members who criticize our efforts and question our motives. And caregiving is not necessarily a short-term commitment. Over time, close relationships, our own health and wealth, and our jobs and careers are at risk if we're not careful.

There are no blueprints in caregiving, and so I offer the following self-assessment questionnaire to guide you. If anything else, the answers to these questions will reveal when it's time for you to supplement your care plans:

Do you get along with your elders and have a fair amount of influence over them?
Perhaps at times your sister gets along with Mom better than you do. People outside the family circle or an "authority figure" may be more influential and able to accomplish what you cannot—perhaps a doctor, a member of the clergy, a geriatric case manager, or an attorney may be able to step in on your behalf.

Do you live far away?
Be realistic about your ability to handle all of the eldercare details from a distance. *Are there some things you simply cannot accomplish from far away? Is it realistic right now for you to pick up and move or ask your elder to do the same? Can you share duties with someone who lives closer?*

Are you willing to ask for and accept help?
There is no getting around this one. If you have trouble delegating tasks or accepting help from others, then it's simply a matter of time before the quality of your own life will begin to crumble.

Do you have strong problem-solving abilities?
Day-to-day eldercare problems are complex, multidimensional, and sure to challenge the brightest of minds. If your confidence in researching options and making difficult decisions is low, you are better off surrounding yourself with professional advisers and, in some cases, letting geriatric case managers assess the situation and supplement the care and decision-making process.

Are you good at learning new things and taking advice?
Everybody—from health-care professionals to the neighbor down the street—will have a strong opinion on how your elder should be cared for. While some of their suggestions may be off target, others may be worth considering. *How flexible and open-minded are you? Can you make changes in midstream?*

Are you a walking time bomb?
Is your life already filled to capacity? Are you currently handling major, time-consuming obligations between parenting, your own career, and other commitments? How much time can you realistically afford to devote to your elders? Eldercare requires patience, and tolerance for this kind of work may not be part of your emotional makeup. For example, if you've never assisted an older adult with bathing and dressing for the day, you may not realize that this seemingly simple activity could eat up the better part of the morning. *What might be your reaction to an elder who asks you the same question over and over again in a matter of minutes?*

Are you thick-skinned?
Disappointment, loneliness, and frustration come with the job of caregiving. Your circle of friends may start to shrink; siblings and relatives will find excuses to keep their distance from you and your elders. *Are you good at deflecting criticism? Can you bounce back after a hard day's*

work? Can you forgive others for their shortcomings? Are you willing to get help if you suspect that you are becoming increasingly depressed?

Are you an effective money manager?

Eldercare is a bottomless pit of ongoing expenses. Beyond health care, there are other eldercare-related costs that will quickly drain the money supply: senior housing, special diets, medications, transportation, and more. *Are you proactive rather than reactive when it comes to managing money? Will you seek financial advice? Will you stick to a budget in order to avoid a family financial crisis? Are you willing to talk to other family members about paying for long-term care?*

Is it possible that you will have to quit your job to perform eldercare duties?

Most people cannot afford to give up their own primary means of support. *Are you willing to research your company's work-life eldercare programs? Will you be risking your job security by being candid with your boss about your eldercare situation? If your employer offers work-life benefits, are you making good use of them now?*

Once you know where the caregiving roller coaster is going, are you still in for the ride?

Millions of us are facing this question. We all have limitations—getting help is the *smart* thing to do. Sometimes love is best served when we do not place ourselves in a position of resentment. We are fortunate now, for unlike the caregivers before us, we have options such as geriatric case managers, assisted-living communities, and adult day services and a host of other alternatives.

From one caregiver to another, I know how emotionally and physically challenging eldercare can be. Being responsible to others unquestionably affects our every waking moment—at home, in the workplace, where and how we live, and how we cope. If eldercare has chosen you, I will be with you every step of the way since I, too, walk in your shoes—even now. Every page, every sentence, and every word in this book is my personal message of support to you, and I have the utmost respect for your decision to accept the role of caregiver.

Joy Loverde

ELDER EMERGENCY INFORMATION CHART

(This worksheet is also available online at www.elderindustry.com)

Today's date_____

Elder's name_____

Address_____

City/State/Zip_____

Telephone (home, work, mobile)_____

Date and place of birth_____

Driver's license number and state issued_____

Auto make, model, and license plate number_____

Social Security number_____

Medicare number_____

Do not resuscitate (DNR) order in effect?_____

Allergies_____

Blood type_____

Current medications_____

Advance directives_____

Religious directives_____

_____

_____

_____

_____

IMPORTANT TELEPHONE NUMBERS

(Call 911 for ambulance, fire, and police emergencies)

HEALTH CARE

Doctor_____

Doctor_____

Dentist_____

Hospital_____

Pharmacy_____

Home care_____

Aging agency_____

_____

Visiting nurse_____

_____

Insurance_____

Insurance_____

Insurance_____

Adult day services_____

_____

_____

_____

_____

_____

_____

_____

_____

_____

_____

NETWORK

Family_____

Family_____

Family_____

Health-care proxy_____

_____

Power of attorney_____

_____

Neighbor_____

Neighbor_____

Friend_____

Community center_____

_____

Social worker_____

_____

Clergy_____

Coworker_____

_____

_____

_____

_____

_____

_____

_____

_____

SERVICES

Electrician_____

Gas co._____

Water co._____

Computer_____

Cable TV_____

Plumber_____

Maintenance_____

House sitter_____

Pet sitter_____

Landlord_____

Banker_____

Attorney_____

Accountant_____

House alarm_____

Locksmith_____

_____

_____

_____

_____

_____

_____

_____

_____

_____

1

Effective Planning

A Place to Start

I work full-time. How am I supposed to take on this responsibility and keep my job, too? Where will the money come from to pay for care? I'm an only child and I can't possibly do this alone. I live miles away from my family, so who can I turn to for help? Why do I feel so guilty all the time? How do I know if I'm doing the right thing?

Most of us are inadequately prepared to face and accept the complex challenges associated with eldercare. And yet the aging of our loved ones is a natural part of life and a predictable phase of human development. The need to care for our elders is also a normal part of life, and something we *can* plan for.

Each caregiving situation is unique and typically involves simultaneous complex physical, emotional, and financial issues. How one family addresses an eldercare situation is not necessarily the right approach for another. What seems to be working one day could change drastically—overnight. How then do we proceed under these seemingly chaotic circumstances? **The answer lies in planning.**

Planning, however, takes on a whole new meaning when it comes to caring for older family members. Historical family decision-making patterns will no longer apply; the question of *"Who's in charge?"* is up for grabs. What was once written in stone regarding family rules and roles will no longer apply. What we *can* plan on when care issues crop up is the never-ending challenge of responding to changes of all kinds. When it comes to eldercare, family life as we once knew it will never be the same.

The true nature of assisting an older loved one includes a roller coaster of emotional upsets; consequently, the process of caregiving requires conscious and continuous management of our attitudes and our decisions. *The Complete Eldercare Planner* is your road map through this unfamiliar and often unsettling territory and is an invaluable tool as you begin to create your customized caregiving strategies.

A PLACE TO START

- Planning and preparation are critical for effective eldercare.
- Experts agree that rule number one in thoughtful planning is to use a planner to write things down.

Whether you are planning for future needs or currently helping a loved one through a crisis situation, **The Complete Eldercare Planner** ***will assist you in pulling it all together.***

OBJECTIVES

After completing **"A Place to Start,"** *you will be able to:*

Create opportunities to open up the lines of communication.

Minimize the number of crisis situations.

Reduce confusion in crisis situations.

Gain greater peace of mind by planning ahead.

PLAN ONE

Don't *read* this book. *Use* it.

We're all busy people who have the need to juggle multiple commitments *and* stay organized, and *The Complete Eldercare Planner* has been designed to help you do just that.

Manage Paperwork

Be sure to make use of the spaces provided for recording telephone numbers, setting goals, and locating documents. Over the years, readers of the first and second editions of this book have offered valuable feedback regarding the worksheets and checklists supplied throughout this book. As a result of readers' insightful suggestions, the forms in this book are now readily accessible online.

To download, customize, and store the documents at your convenience, please go to the Joy Loverde website (www.elderindustry.com). You may choose to store your documents on your desktop, a CD-ROM, or a flash drive. Making the effort to complete the information electronically, then printing and storing paperwork in clearly labeled files, will pay big dividends. Do what you can to keep the information current and accessible.

An important document that you will want to complete and keep handy right away is the **"Elder Emergency Information Chart"** found on page 5. You'll have peace of mind knowing that you have access to immediate assistance when you need it.

Prioritize Caregiving Issues

The **introduction** and **Objectives** sections at the beginning of each chapter offer a quick overview of the chapter contents and help you to prioritize your most pressing caregiving issues. Knowing the basis for what you are reading, and *why*, will be especially helpful when the emotional aspect of caregiving threatens to undermine your ability to do what is needed at the time. Effective planning is specific, realistic, and *written*.

Staying on course with your care plans will be easier with the use of the **"Eldercare Goals Chart"** found on page 25. Tracking your progress with the use of the **action checklists** offered at the end of every chapter will also give you insights on where to focus your attention.

Tap into Professionals

There are knowledgeable and skilled professionals available to help you along the way. Look to the **"Low-Cost and Free Resources"** sections in each chapter and the hundreds of **organizations** and **websites** listed throughout *The Complete Eldercare Planner,* and at the end of every chapter. **Indexes** of the organizations and websites can be found at the end of the book. Resources are listed alphabetically for a faster and easier search.

You now have everything you need to get started.

PLAN TWO

Carve your own caregiving path.

How you approach and implement your care plans will most likely be different from others who are in similar situations. There are no cookie-cutter answers. Your family decision-making patterns, the help you receive from others, eligibility for specialized programs, and the availability of financial resources are some of the reasons why each care plan is customized. Ultimately, your process may include incorporating one plan, several plans, and even a combination of plans in order to solve a particular issue. Decide what method of planning and care works best for *you.*

Since nothing remains the same for very long when it comes to the people we care for, the process of caregiving will require ongoing assessments of the situation at hand. Older people are in constant transition; change is *always* on the horizon. A plan may work one day and not the next. Remaining open-minded and flexible will be one of the keys to your effectiveness as a family caregiver.

Open up the lines of communication *right now* with your elders and family members. Making assumptions about what is happening instead of talking with each other always does more harm than good. Do your best to approach problems and situations from fact, not fiction. Seek the advice of geriatric-care professionals if you need an unbiased opinion.

Keep your eldercare planning and timeline expectations realistic. Ask yourself on a regular basis these three simple questions: *What can happen? What will my elder be able to do about what happens? What can the rest of the family do to help?*

And plan early. When we plan we have choices, and the well-being of the entire family will rest on the quantity and quality of eldercare options, decisions, and plans that were put in place ahead of time. If fears about getting started are keeping you from acting now, *the consequence of doing nothing is far worse.*

PLAN THREE

Implement planning principles.

Follow these six basic planning principles for maximum results.

1. **Set goals.** Know what you are doing and *why*. Make use of the "Eldercare Goals Chart" on page 25.

2. **Create support systems and use them.** Surround yourself and your elders with family members and friends as well as people from the local community as a way to share responsibilities and protect against caregiver stress. Don't turn *anyone* away if they are willing to help you.

3. **Write it down.** Put dates on all of your notes. Record plans, goals, ideas, phone numbers, questions, answers, promises, decisions, tasks, and appointments and keep them in a convenient, accessible location. Make good use of the forms in this planner. Download the forms from the website www.elderindustry.com if it will make it easier for you to write things down.

4. **Organize information.** Create a system using a file or binder that organizes your eldercare information. You'll constantly be digging for paperwork of all kinds. Be sure your system is mobile—you may have to produce documents at a moment's notice. Keep all paperwork in a safe, twenty-four-hour accessible location. Better yet, if you have a computer, download vital information onto a flash drive and keep it on your key chain. Flash drive key chains are available at your local computer outlet and convenience stores.

5. **Allow sufficient time for research.** Gathering information and creating options is critical to thoughtful action. Always research more than one option. You have a better chance of being successful with your elders and family members when you offer choices and options.

6. **Research all costs and who pays.** Create budgets and seek sources of funding eldercare-related expenses early on.

EFFECTIVE PLANNING | 13

PLAN FOUR

⧉ Be prepared for the runaround.

Gathering information, locating resources, making appointments, and putting caregiving services in motion can cause a great deal of stress and anxiety. Detailed application processes, waiting lists, lengthy interviews, endless document searching, being put on hold, outdated telephone numbers, out-of-date websites, and web links that go nowhere are not uncommon. Use the checklist below to help minimize the negative effects of potentially stressful situations.

Quick Eldercare Planning Tips

- When initiating telephone calls, always get the name, title, and the direct telephone number (and cell-phone number if available) of the person on the other end of the phone.
- Take notes during important calls, including the date the call was made.
- Confirm appointments a day in advance with *everyone* involved.
- Repeat the purpose of the appointment to make sure *everyone* is on the same page.
- Arrange to have someone accompany your elder to *every* appointment.
- Attend all meetings with paper and pen in hand. Ask permission to tape-record the conversation if that's easier (and they allow it).
- Distribute copies (*not originals*) of important and legal documents.
- Evaluate the quality of services received and report anyone who treats you or your elder disrespectfully.

Staying in their own home is a popular choice for older adults and with a growing aging population, the number of assisted-living services and options available is also expanding. Assessing and arranging for community and state assisted-living and at-home services, however, is no easy task. Here's why.

- Each person requires a unique combination of eldercare services.
- Caregiving services and eldercare programs are often listed under different names from state to state.
- Programs and services are rarely available from *one* source.
- The process of becoming eligible for state-offered public programs is complicated.

When investigating **in-home eldercare services**, ask the following questions, where applicable, and keep a *written* record of your findings.

What's your name and title?
Are you a staff member or a volunteer? (Ask to speak to a staff member.)
What services are available?

How much do services cost?

What is the average cost for my particular needs?

Are fees or commissions negotiable? Is there a sliding scale?

Are initial consultations available free of charge?

What free services are available?

What other costs should I anticipate?

Are payment plans available?

Does insurance cover costs?

Is the cost of your services tax deductible?

What documents do I need to supply to you? Originals? Copies?

Will you put fees and estimates in writing?

Will you provide written contracts? Regulations?

Will you itemize bills?

Will you provide references? Credentials?

Do you have brochures or literature you can send me?

Are you a member of any professional organizations?

Are you certified? Licensed? Bonded?

Will you put me on your mailing list?

Do you provide pickup and delivery service? Transportation?

Do you have telecommunication access for hearing- or visually impaired people?

PLAN FIVE

Prioritize your caregiving responsibilities.

If you're just getting started and putting a plan in place, and you'd like direction on which eldercare issues should be addressed first, here are the top three issues that you'll most likely encounter—*in this order:*

1. Money matters (see chapter 6)
2. Housing (see chapter 9)
3. Locating documents (see chapter 15)

PLAN SIX

Make good use of eldercare resources.

The eldercare service providers, organizations, and websites listed at the end of every chapter will assist you in a variety of ways. If you're providing family caregiving assistance and are not computer savvy or do not have frequent access to a computer, obtain copies of your elder's local telephone directories—the **White Pages,** the **Blue Pages,** and the **Yellow Pages.** Be sure to update copies of telephone books whenever new editions become available.

Look under the following headings in the **Blue Pages** of the telephone book to obtain government office contact information:

- Area agency on aging/department for the aging
- Department of insurance (Medicare)
- Department of mental health
- Department of public aid (food stamps, Medicaid)
- Department of public health
- Department of rehabilitation services
- Internal Revenue Service (tax relief)
- Department of transportation (reduced fares, taxi coupons)
- U.S. Department of Veterans Affairs

If you plan to use the **Yellow Pages** of the telephone book to locate eldercare resources, here are the headings to research:

- Hospitals (ask for the discharge planner)
- Religious congregations
- Community centers
- Social-service organizations

Call the **local hospital, religious congregations, community centers,** and **social-service organizations** and ask about the availability of the following resources:

- Free community eldercare directories
- Books, tapes, and DVDs on caregiving topics
- Caregiver newsletters
- Websites
- Physician referrals services
- Community education programs
- Prerecorded telephone health information
- Registered nurse telephone advice
- Medication management services
- Hospice services
- Behavioral-health programs

- Home respiratory services
- Visiting nurses
- Chronic disease and pain management
- Personal-care services
- Home medical equipment
- Hotline telephone numbers
- Caregiver support groups
- Parish nurse services
- Volunteer programs
- Benefits eligibility
- Community health fairs
- International eldercare resources
- Foreign language services

Take a look at the eldercare services listed below. Under each service are suggestions about the many different organizations from which you can obtain assistance. Contact them for recommendations on local service providers. There are several ways to search for the organizations listed below. While some people will make use of the local telephone book's Yellow Pages and Blue Pages, others may conduct a keyword search in their Internet browser.

HOMEMAKER SERVICES *(housecleaning, personal and health care, errands, cooking)*
- Area agency on aging
- Church groups
- Civic groups
- Social-service organizations
- Home-health-care agency
- Family and friends' referrals
- Classified newspaper ads

HOME REPAIR/MAINTENANCE SERVICES *(upkeep, installations, improvements)*
- Area agency on aging
- Social-service organizations
- Neighborhood improvement programs
- Church groups

NUTRITION SITES/MEALS PROGRAMS *(home-delivered meals, group meals)*
- Area agency on aging
- Church groups

- Community centers
- Hospital discharge planner

COMPANION SERVICES *(friendly visits to the homebound)*
- Area agency on aging
- Church groups
- Hospital discharge planner
- Neighborhood clubs
- Social-service organizations
- Civic groups
- Volunteer organizations
- YMCA/YWCA
- City recreation department
- Hospice volunteers
- Youth groups

TELEPHONE REASSURANCE PROGRAMS *(people who will make daily phone contact with homebound elders who live alone)*
- Police station (nonemergency)
- Hospital discharge planner
- Community centers
- Social-service organizations
- Civic groups
- Home-health-care agency

OBSERVATION PROGRAMS *(letter carriers and utility workers trained to identify signs that an older person may need help)*
- Public-utility office
- Post office
- Area agency on aging
- Neighborhood watch programs
- Police station (nonemergency)

TRANSPORTATION SERVICES *(van services available to disabled people for medical appointments)*
- Area agency on aging
- Home-health-care agency
- Hospital discharge planner

- Public-transportation office
- Social-service organizations
- Church groups
- Civic groups

SENIOR-HOUSING OPTIONS *(from independent living to skilled nursing care)*
- Active adult communities
- Retirement communities
- Area agency on aging
- State ombudsman
- Community centers
- Hospital discharge planner

IN-HOME HEALTH-CARE SERVICES *(from managing medications to skilled nursing care)*
- Visiting nurses association
- Area agency on aging
- Social-service organizations
- Home-health-care agency
- Family services agency
- Hospital discharge planner
- Continuing-care retirement community
- Skilled-nursing-care facility
- United Way

EMERGENCY RESPONSE SYSTEMS *(transmitters to call for help)*
- Hospital discharge planner
- Area agency on aging
- Fire and police stations (nonemergency)

RESPITE CARE SERVICES *(providing time off for family caregivers)*
- Hospital discharge planner
- Nursing homes
- Community centers
- Social-service organizations
- Home-health-care agency

HOSPICE PROGRAMS *(care and counseling for dying patients and their family members)*
- Hospital discharge planner
- American Cancer Society

- Visiting nurses association
- Physician
- Church groups
- Social-service organizations

Caught Off Guard: Suddenly, You're a Caregiver

The responsibilities associated with eldercare are often initiated in a crisis. At any given time, we can find ourselves on the receiving end of an emergency telephone call informing us that a loved one needs help immediately, momentarily throwing us off balance and leaving us feeling scared and confused as we hang up the phone. *Unquestionably, the emotional climate surrounding an eldercare emergency is highly charged when we suddenly become the appointed family caregiver.*

The advent of an eldercare crisis almost always surfaces intense and sometimes conflicting emotions. It's not uncommon to simultaneously feel extremely loving toward the person who needs care and angry for being put in the situation in the first place. Initially, our emotions can temporarily immobilize us, and we may feel so zapped of energy and mentally drained that instead of kicking into high gear, we head for the comfort of our bed and pull the covers over our eyes.

After the initial shock of an eldercare crisis has worn off, the next course of action involves accepting reality; we will *always* wish we were not in this situation to begin with. However, it is what it is—a person in need of some kind of assistance—and once we accept that fact, we can focus on developing a care plan. This section of *The Complete Eldercare Planner* will help you to quickly gain an understanding of the immediate problem and what can be done to stabilize the situation. The solutions that work best will incorporate *your* needs as well as those of your elder's. Use the **"Decision-Making Worksheet"** on page 23 to guide you.

The keys to surviving an unanticipated crisis are getting a handle on the eldercare responsibilities, researching your options, being resourceful, communicating effectively, and seeking assistance as needed. Most important, don't let anyone rush you; resist the temptation to make quick decisions. Take it one step and one day at a time. *You are in more control of the situation than you think.*

PLAN ONE

Reduce confusion and runaway emotions.

In the absence of eldercare-related plans and discussions, follow these tips to help get you pointed in the right direction.

Get the big picture. Turn to the contents pages of this book to determine which chapter will help you to address the issue at hand. For a quick review of important and legal documents, go to "The Documents Locator" chapter of this book, starting on page 327.

CAUGHT OFF GUARD: SUDDENLY, YOU'RE A CAREGIVER

- Unexpected problems build a caregiver's confidence in mastering the eldercare decision-making process.
- Eldercare is full of surprises. Expect situations (and people) to change.

Even in the absence of planning, family caregivers can quickly get control of the situation at hand.

OBJECTIVES

*After completing **"Caught Off Guard: Suddenly, You're a Caregiver,"** you will be able to:*

Compile eldercare-planning tools.

Accumulate caregiving resources quickly.

Gather an informal network of support.

Tap into expert advice.

Make informed decisions in the event of an emergency.

Get organized. Create a file. You'll want one place to store important papers. Also create word documents on your computer and store the folder on your desktop for quick access. Back up the information on a flash drive and keep the flash drive on your key chain. Keep hard copies of all documents in a convenient, twenty-four-hour accessible location. Maintain access to a copy machine, fax machine, Internet and e-mail, and overnight mail service.

Write everything down. Take notes and record the dates of conversations on all notes. Make lists—names, contact information, who is doing what, doctors' instructions, and so on. Complete the "Elder Emergency Information Chart" on page 5.

Obtain telephone directories. If access to the Internet is limited, obtain copies of your elder's local telephone books. The White Pages, Blue Pages, and Yellow Pages of the telephone directory will list local resources for products and services.

Locate your elder's personal address book. The names and contact information in this address book will be the key to locating friends, service providers, community resources, professional advisers, and much more. Make a copy of the address book and keep it with you at all times.

Create a helpers list. Create a list of people whom you believe would be willing to help you. Write down home, mobile, and work telephone numbers, and mail and e-mail addresses. Make copies of this list and distribute to involved family and friends. Keep the list handy. For additional resources for helpers, contact the organizations and websites listed at the end of each chapter. Here is your starter list:

other family members	friends
neighbors	coworkers
church members	volunteers
advisers	hired help

Make a to-do list. There's plenty to do and many ways for others to be helpful. Make a list of things you and your elder need help with, such as running errands, housekeeping, and shopping. When people ask how they can help, let them choose from your list. If they don't ask, pick up the telephone and solicit their assistance. Be assertive.

Create access to the professionals. Obtain the telephone numbers and e-mail addresses of those professionals who assist your elder—doctor, dentist, social worker, nurse, pharmacist, police, insurance agent, lawyer, accountant, and clergy. Review your elder's personal telephone book for additional names and contact information.

PLAN TWO

Access expert advice.

If your elder is in the hospital or under a doctor's care, due to Health Insurance Portability and Accountability Act (HIPAA) regulations, you may need to establish authority to discuss his or her medical condition with the doctor. Every hospital staffs a hospital discharge planner and/or a patient advocate, so be sure to seek their advice on HIPAA regulations early on. Be proactive in the hospital setting to feel more capable and confident with what is expected before your loved one leaves the hospital.

Also call the **local agency on aging** for information regarding home health care and additional community resources and service providers. Call the local continuing-care retirement community and ask if they have an **outreach program** that provides in-home care to nonresidents. Housing and care resources are listed at the end of the "Creating a Care Team" and "Housing" chapters of *The Complete Eldercare Planner*.

Long-distance caregivers might consider the services of a **geriatric case manager.** These experts will make an on-site visit to your relative, assess the situation at hand, and then make recommendations and any necessary care arrangements. *Be prepared to pay out-of-pocket for their services.* Hourly rates range from $50 to $175 per hour, plus an initial assessment fee that can run as high as $500. In the long run, hiring a geriatric case manager even for a few hours may be worth every penny—especially in an eldercare emergency. You can obtain referrals from the hospital discharge planner and the local agency on aging.

PLAN THREE

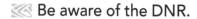 Be aware of the DNR.

Admission into a hospital, medical center, and nursing home will include being served a **do-not-resuscitate** order—more commonly known as a DNR. Accepted by physicians in all fifty states, the DNR is a type of advance health-care directive. In its most simple definition, a DNR is a request that a person *not* be given CPR (cardiopulmonary resuscitation) should his or her heart stop or should he or she stop breathing. Without a DNR order, medical personnel must perform CPR under these circumstances.

While the DNR is a useful tool in some instances, this document should never be signed casually by elders and/or family members. If your elder appears to have mental capacity, the decision to sign the DNR document is ultimately his or hers. Whatever the case may be, seek advice from the doctor before signing on the dotted line, since there are many complex variables to consider. The lesson here is to encourage your elders to assign an agent as a power of attorney for health care *before* anything happens.

PLAN FOUR

Make informed decisions.

Eldercare requires making important decisions, and lots of them. *Do we place Grandma in a nursing home? Should my husband and I move closer to our children now or wait until we retire? Should I give up my job to care for Dad?*

What's right? What's wrong? In today's fast-paced world, deciding one's course of action is difficult. Before radio, television, and computers, important decisions were based on very little information. Today, knowing too much can just as easily cloud our ability to make the right choices. To make matters even more confusing, advisers and well-meaning friends might offer diverse opinions and conflicting information.

Most of us know how to make rational decisions under predictable circumstances, but when confronted with new and unfamiliar issues, and faced with having to make gut-wrenching decisions governing someone else's well-being, we can find ourselves stretched to the limit to stay in control of our emotions.

When you are up against the wall and have to make an important decision, especially one that will directly affect your elder, use the "Decision-Making Worksheet" on the following page as a guide to help you in the process. Being put in the position of caregiver almost always *guarantees* that you will be faced with the dilemma of doing the right thing without really knowing for sure what that right thing is. Remember, no decision is ever final, and you can modify your plans and choices at any time.

DECISION-MAKING WORKSHEET

(This worksheet is also available online at www.elderindustry.com)

WHAT'S RIGHT? WHAT'S WRONG? MAKING INFORMED DECISIONS

Feeling overwhelmed with too many options and choices? Use this worksheet to organize the decision-making process into more manageable parts. Make your best effort to be sure your statements are based on facts, not assumptions or wishful (or fearful) thinking.

First, define the decision you need to make. Then, fill in the pros and cons. Once you see how the benefits and disadvantages stack up, your decision becomes a matter of several smaller key issues.

Today's Date:_____

*The decision I am contemplating is:*_____

The pros are:	The cons are:
_____	_____
_____	_____
_____	_____
_____	_____

Consider these important questions when writing down your pros and cons:

Is *this* the right time for this decision or is it better to wait?

Who else can shed light on this decision (family, friends, doctor, etc.)?

Do I fully understand the answers given by the professionals? (If not, say so and get clarification.)

Do I have all of the information needed to weigh the potential consequences?

What are the needs and wants of those who will be affected by this decision?

What is the extent of my obligations toward the people involved in this decision?

How might this decision negatively affect my physical and emotional health?

Will I put others at risk or hurt anyone with this decision?

How might my personal relationships change for the worse?

What is the best that can happen and what is the worst that can happen?

Have I researched all costs and who pays for what?

The Decision

Review the pros and cons. Does one list outweigh the other? If the potential decision involves legalities such as contracts and considerable costs, get professional advice. If the decision will directly impact your elders, involve them in the decision-making process. Insist on family meetings and discussions as a way to keep everyone involved and accountable.

The two most important facts in the pros column are: _____

_____

_____

_____

The two most important facts in the cons column are: _____

_____

_____

_____

Based on the pros and cons, the decision is: _____

_____

_____

_____

_____

_____

_____

_____

_____

Eldercare Goals Chart
(This worksheet is also available online at www.elderindustry.com)

The most effective goal setting is specific, realistic, and written.

Today's date:_____

GOALS	GOAL ACHIEVED
1. _____	❑
2. _____	❑
3. _____	❑
4. _____	❑

Prioritize and list what you need to do to accomplish each goal.

GOAL 1.	COMPLETED
Call _____	❑
_____	❑
_____	❑
Write _____	❑
_____	❑
_____	❑
Meet _____	❑
_____	❑
_____	❑
Buy _____	❑
_____	❑
_____	❑
Read _____	❑
_____	❑
_____	❑

GOAL 2.   **COMPLETED**

Call _____ ❏

_____ ❏

_____ ❏

Write _____ ❏

_____ ❏

_____ ❏

Meet _____ ❏

_____ ❏

_____ ❏

Buy _____ ❏

_____ ❏

_____ ❏

Read _____ ❏

_____ ❏

_____ ❏

GOAL 3.   **COMPLETED**

Call _____ ❏

_____ ❏

_____ ❏

Write _____ ❏

_____ ❏

_____ ❏

Meet _____ ❏

_____ ❏

_____ ❏

Buy _____ ❑

_____ ❑

_____ ❑

Read _____ ❑

_____ ❑

_____ ❑

GOAL 4.   COMPLETED

Call _____ ❑

_____ ❑

_____ ❑

Write _____ ❑

_____ ❑

_____ ❑

Meet _____ ❑

_____ ❑

_____ ❑

Buy _____ ❑

_____ ❑

_____ ❑

Read _____ ❑

_____ ❑

_____ ❑

Low-Cost and Free Resources

The local telephone directory is a valuable source of information. As described previously, the **Blue Pages, Yellow Pages,** and **White Pages** of the local telephone directory can be very helpful. Be sure to replace directories every year when new editions become available.

Hospital discharge planners offer current information and referrals on local eldercare services. Ask for a free copy of local service-provider lists.

The **public library** is stocked with books on related subjects. Get to know the librarians at the reference desk. Rent **videos** or **DVDs** on related subjects. Research websites on the **Internet,** under the keywords "eldercare," "aging parents," "caregivers," and "aging."

Newspapers and radio and television stations often advertise **free local programs** sponsored by law firms, insurance agencies, financial planners, hospitals, retirement communities, and social-service organizations.

Masonic orders, Rotary Clubs, Lions Clubs, Odd Fellows lodges, veterans' organizations, unions, business clubs, religious groups, and teachers' associations provide special services and volunteers to members and nonmembers alike. Look up **"Associations"** and **"Religious Organizations"** in the Yellow Pages of the local telephone directory or online.

Colleges, universities, adult education centers, and trade schools are a valuable source of information, volunteers, resources, and training programs. See **"Schools"** in the Yellow Pages.

Community action commissions (CACs) and **family service agencies** offer services for low-income, minority, frail, and homebound persons, including social, educational, and recreational activities.

Local **community centers** provide a multitude of services and activities to older adults, including recreation, social gatherings, meals, transportation, and education.

Look to your elder's former **employer** as well as *your* employer for workplace eldercare initiatives and benefits offered to employed and retired family members.

ORGANIZATIONS AND WEB RESOURCES

AARP
601 E Street, NW
Washington, DC 20049
(888) 687-2277
Website: www.aarp.org

Access America for Seniors
Website: www.seniors.gov

Administration on Aging
One Massachusetts Avenue, Suites 4100
    and 5100
Washington, DC 20201
(202) 619-0724; fax: (202) 357-3555
Website: www.aoa.gov

ElderWeb
Website: www.elderweb.com

Global Action on Aging
777 UN Plaza, Suite 6J
New York, NY 11017
(212) 557-3163
Website: www.globalaging.org

**National Advisory Council on Aging—
    Canada**
Website: www.naca.ca

**National Association of Area Agencies on
    Aging**
1730 Rhode Island Ave., NW, Suite 1200
Washington, DC 20036
(202) 872-0888; fax: (202) 872-0057
Website: www.n4a.org

SAGE
(Serving the GLBT community)
305 7th Avenue, 16th Floor
New York, NY 10001
(212) 741-2247
Website: www.sageusa.org

EFFECTIVE PLANNING ACTION CHECKLIST

(This worksheet is also available online at www.elderindustry.com)

A PLACE TO START	To Do By	Completed

Set planning goals

short-term _____ ☐
long-term _____ ☐

Create a system for duplicating and filing

eldercare information _____ ☐
notes _____ ☐
questions _____ ☐
goals _____ ☐
lists _____ ☐
documents _____ ☐
phone numbers _____ ☐
agreements _____ ☐

Have access to

telephone _____ ☐
transportation _____ ☐
copy machine _____ ☐
fax _____ ☐
Internet _____ ☐
e-mail _____ ☐
post office _____ ☐
public library _____ ☐

Review "Communicaring"
  chapter

review eldercare resources _____ ☐
create a backup plan _____ ☐
attend community eldercare programs _____ ☐

CAUGHT OFF GUARD: SUDDENLY, YOU'RE A CAREGIVER

Get organized

review contents pages _____ ☐
prioritize issues _____ ☐
start a file on elder _____ ☐
locate documents _____ ☐
store originals in safe place _____ ☐

Take notes

names and addresses _____ ☐
telephone numbers _____ ☐
plans _____ ☐
instructions _____ ☐
directions _____ ☐
decisions _____ ☐
promises _____ ☐

Get community telephone books

Blue Pages _____ ☐
White Pages _____ ☐
Yellow Pages _____ ☐

Create a helpers list

family _____ ☐
friends _____ ☐
neighbors _____ ☐
coworkers _____ ☐
church members _____ ☐
volunteers _____ ☐

Make a list of help needed _____ ☐

Request and accept help _____ ☐

Create a list of eldercare advisers _____ ☐

Access eldercare experts

hospital discharge planner _____ ☐
agency on aging _____ ☐
geriatric case manager _____ ☐

Make informed decisions

questions answered to satisfaction   _____   ❑

time allowed for research   _____   ❑

costs investigated   _____   ❑

references checked   _____   ❑

legal counsel sought for contracts,
    signatures, financial investments   _____   ❑

family discussions ongoing   _____   ❑

elder involved in decisions   _____   ❑

**Use the "Decision-Making Worksheet"
to help in the process**   _____   ❑

2

Creating a Care Team

How to Tell When Your Elder Needs Help

Contrary to the way older people are typically portrayed in advertisements and movies, the process of aging does not automatically mean that a person will become increasingly incompetent and helpless. Even the use of the words *senior moments* implies that losing one's memory comes with the territory of growing older. Unnecessary problems in the caregiving process arise when we equate a person's chronological age with decline and pathology, and when we readily accept myths, assumptions, and prejudices about getting older. Media portrayals of older adults can be so convincing that even our own elders accept the stereotypes at face value.

Aging people are people in transition, and the need for eldercare is defined by their *ability*, not their age. The loss of beloved family members and friends, a sudden change in health, relocation to retirement housing, budget restrictions, the loss of driving privileges, and even the death of a pet are some of the normal life transitions of an older adult, and consequently may require our attention as situations unfold. *Ideally, our elders will ask for help during times like these; but far too often requests for help never come.* A spouse could easily "cover" for the other, and a physically ailing person may decline assistance as a result of feeling ashamed and powerless. Problems that could have been attended to and even averted are compounded when no one has the courage or willingness to speak up and ask for help.

Most people savor their personal freedom and independence, and want to stay in control of their own lives for as long as possible. However, without the willingness to ask for assistance *when help is clearly needed*, a person's independent lifestyle can be placed in jeopardy. This chapter of *The Complete Eldercare Planner* offers evidence that attention and assistance do not negate our elders' independence. At the same time, we must be willing to face the fact that things may have changed; our role as family caregiver is about to be taken up a notch. Suggestions in this section include making astute observations, asking revealing questions, and paying attention to the telltale signs that indicate our loved ones may need assistance right now.

HOW TO TELL WHEN YOUR ELDER NEEDS HELP

- Unless we know what to look for, problems can go undetected for years.
- Depression among caregivers taking care of family members with Alzheimer's disease can be greatly reduced through counseling and support.

Everyone can expect to assume the role of caregiver at some time in his or her life—spouses, children, family, and friends. None of us ages in a void.

OBJECTIVES

After completing "How to Tell When Your Elder Needs Help," you will be able to:

Detect clues that your elders need help now.

Address dementia issues early on.

PLAN ONE

 Know what's normal and what's not.

Things may look like business as usual on the outside, and some physical and mental changes are barely noticeable. Once in a while, we all forget details and put things off until later; but when a *pattern* of neglect develops, it may be that a more serious situation is at hand. Remember, dementia (mental deterioration) is *not* a normal part of aging and should not be approached as such.

Now is the time to make the effort to sharpen your observational skills and proactively look for patterns of neglect that will surely help to avert more complications later on. Watch for these telltale signs next time you're together.

BASIC TASKS. While seeing elders rocking back and forth to get momentum to stand up from a low sofa or taking more time to get dressed should not alarm you, elders who are having difficulty chewing and swallowing food, making fewer trips to the grocery store, cooking less and less, or failing to follow instructions for taking medications are giving off clues that something's not right and needs your immediate attention.

HYGIENE. Infrequent bathing; unusually sloppy appearance; foul body and/or mouth odor.

RESPONSIBILITIES. Fails to take in mail or leaves mail unopened (bills go unpaid); mountains of papers are scattered on tabletops and floors; checkbook is unreadable and outdated; bank account overdraft notices are accumulating; prescriptions are unfilled; phone calls aren't returned; laundry is piling up; the bottom of cooking pots and pans are burned; refrigerator interior has foul odor; food supply is low; home interior is in disarray; exterior home maintenance is ignored; automobile exterior is scratched and dented.

HEALTH. Weight gain or loss; dizziness; loss or increase in appetite; excessive daytime sleepiness and napping; skin burns; black-and-blue marks (possible signs of falling); speaks loudly, plays television and radio loudly, seems withdrawn (possible signs of hearing loss); takes numerous medications (possibly requires a medication management plan); bed-wetting (incontinence); trembling hands; spilling and dropping things (check carpet for stains); "bumping" into things; insomnia; constant thirst.

ISOLATION. Lacks an interest in friendships and staying active; keeps curtains drawn day and night; has little access to transportation; lives in another city or state and lives alone; speaks of staying home and "not getting out like I used to."

ATTITUDE. Sadness; verbal and/or physical abuse to others; speaks of being depressed and feelings of despair; abuse of alcohol and/or medications; paranoia; refusal to communicate; unusually argumentative; a recent emotional or medical crisis.

If some of these warning signs are present and you're beginning to question his or her ability to function safely, it's time to take action. Often a physical examination will reveal a medical condition that can be treated.

PLAN TWO

Look for specific warning signs of dementia.

There are numerous kinds of dementia—Alzheimer's is just one type. Statistically, families (and doctors who are not dementia specialists) ignore the *early* warning signs, because they incorrectly identify intermittently odd behaviors as a normal part of aging and untreatable senility.

The Alzheimer's Association has developed a **checklist of common symptoms** to help family members recognize the difference between normal age-related memory changes and possible warning signs of Alzheimer's disease.

Ten Warning Signs of Alzheimer's
1. **Memory loss.** Forgetting recently learned information is one of the most common early signs of dementia. A person begins to forget more often and is unable to recall the information later. He or she forgets to attend medical appointments, for example.
2. **Difficulty performing familiar tasks.** People with dementia often find it hard to plan or complete everyday tasks. Individuals may lose track of the steps involved with preparing a meal, placing a telephone call, or playing a game.
3. **Problems with language.** People with Alzheimer's disease often forget simple words or substitute unusual words, making their speech or handwriting hard to

understand. They may be unable to find the toothbrush, for example, and instead ask for "that thing for my mouth."

4. **Disorientation to time and place.** People with Alzheimer's disease can become lost in their own neighborhood, forget where they are and how they got there, and may not know how to get back home.

5. **Poor or decreased judgment.** Those with Alzheimer's may dress inappropriately for weather, wearing several layers on a warm day or little clothing in the cold. They may show poor judgment, like giving away large sums of money to strangers.

6. **Problems with abstract thinking.** Someone with Alzheimer's disease may have unusual difficulty performing complex mental tasks, like forgetting what numbers are for and how they should be used.

7. **Misplacing things.** A person with Alzheimer's disease may put things in unusual places: for example, an iron in the freezer or a wristwatch in the sugar bowl.

8. **Changes in mood or behavior.** Someone with Alzheimer's disease may show rapid mood swings—from calm to tears to anger—for no apparent reason.

9. **Changes in personality.** The personalities of people with dementia can change dramatically. They may become extremely confused, suspicious, fearful, or dependent on a family member.

10. **Loss of initiative.** A person with Alzheimer's disease may become very passive, sitting in front of the TV for hours, sleeping more than usual, or not wanting to partake in normal activities.

It is important to note that many treatable health conditions have the same signs as dementia and Alzheimer's disease. Prescription drug interactions, dehydration, alcohol abuse, depression, heart problems, physical pain, poor vision, and loss of hearing may also impair cognitive functions. The earlier you detect and discuss your observations with your elders, the better. Seeking help *early* can save families heartache and money.

PLAN THREE

Open up the dialogue with your elders.

When eldercare issues demand immediate attention, the next step is to talk about them. But beware. You are about to enter a potential communication minefield. Without knowing the most effective ways to initiate these extremely sensitive conversations with your elders, the probability of them telling you to mind your own business or saying "everything is fine" *when it's not* is almost guaranteed.

Before you begin any eldercare discussions, turn to chapter 4, "Communicaring," in this book. Review the conversation tips and talking points. Make a plan to employ a series of probing yet respectful questions to get this delicate communication process started.

Share the Care

The American family has changed. With people living longer, it's possible for families to consist of more adult members than children. Busier people and dual-career couples also means fewer people are staying home during the day and into the night. We spend most of our time at work, at school, and at play. Out of necessity, and as a way to stay connected, we've created extended families through our association with hospitals, schools, and churches. We also look to where we work for help when we need it. Corporate America more and more is offering work-life programs in an attempt to help fill in the gaps of what used to take place within the confines of our homes—concierge-type services, child care, and everything in-between. There's more physical distance between family members, with many of us living hundreds of miles apart from each other. Undoubtedly, the family unit of decades ago has evolved into something very different than it was in the past.

An important goal of this section of *The Complete Eldercare Planner* is to expand your definition of what it means to "care" for older loved ones. Too often, family caregivers have rigid beliefs on who does the care and how it should be implemented. Making hasty statements such as "My mother will never go to a nursing home!" and taking pride in not asking others to pitch in will surely get the best of you. Unrealistic goals and unhealthy attitudes can sabotage the caregiving process. When we come face-to-face with our own limitations and can't provide the kind of care we wish we could, we feel it's our own fault. The truth is, we may *not* be the most qualified person to take on all of the caregiving responsibilities all of the time. Limitations of relationships, time, stamina, and skill dictate how much help we can *realistically* offer.

SHARE THE CARE

- You cannot assist your elder alone; you will need help.
- If you're providing care from a distance, there's only so much you can do.
- Dealing with our elders from a distance may be the same as dealing with strangers; there is so much we do not know.

One of the most important caregiving tasks is creating formal and informal support networks made up of family, friends, volunteers, and professionals.

OBJECTIVES

After completing "Share the Care," you will be able to:

Create a network of people and community resources.

Consider cost-effective eldercare options.

Balance eldercare needs and your own needs.

PLAN ONE

⚐ Make a list of the tasks you can do and those you can't do or simply don't want to do.

If medical problems are present, find out what specific levels of care will be required short and long term. Classes on patient care for family caregivers are available at most hospitals. Interacting with service providers as well as professional and eldercare advisers should be included on your task list. Here is a list of some of the caregiving activities you can expect to encounter.

HOMEMAKER SERVICES. Household maintenance and repairs, housecleaning, laundry, errands, grocery shopping, cooking, transportation, paying bills.

PERSONAL CARE. Bathing, dressing, feeding, toileting, shaving, grooming, bed and chair transferring.

HOME HEALTH CARE. Skilled nursing care, hospice aid, medications management, patient instruction, physical therapy, nutrition counseling.

QUALITY OF LIFE. Companionship, checking in, social activities, religious and spiritual activities, senior advocacy.

PLAN TWO

⚐ Identify potential helpers and tasks.

The help family caregivers receive from our informal network of support—family members, friends, and volunteers—may be more readily available, reliable, and affordable than paid care providers. **Create a list of people who can help.** Write down names, addresses, home and work telephone numbers, cell-phone numbers, fax numbers, pager numbers, and e-mail addresses, and be honest with people about the potential for being on call day and night. Distribute copies of this list to all family members and explain the importance of calling upon others when and if you are unavailable. Post copies of this list in several convenient locations: near the telephone and on the refrigerator. If you are computer savvy, download this information to a flash drive and keep it on your key chain.

Suggested helpers include the following:

children and stepchildren	mother
cousins	neighbors
coworkers	nephews and nieces
father	siblings
friends	spouse
grandchildren	uncles and aunts

You can secure volunteers and low-cost services by contacting these community organizations:

advocacy groups
agencies on aging
business groups
charities
community centers
community colleges
department stores
family services
fraternal orders
government agencies
grade school/high school
health-care providers
hospice services
hospitals

neighborhood groups
public libraries
recreation groups
religious groups
retirement groups
seniors' organizations
support groups
transportation agencies
universities
veterans' organizations
volunteer organizations
women's groups
youth groups

Now that you know who can help you, define *how* they can help. Make a list of the kinds of services that are needed—for you and your elder. The next time someone asks, "What can I do?" let them pick from your list. Update your list regularly, since what help is needed will change. Here are some of the ways people can be helpful to you:

attending appointments
checking in
child care
cleaning
cooking
dining out
errands
ironing
laundry
letter writing
managing family website
movies and entertainment
paying bills
paying for services
personal grooming

pet care
phone calling
plant care
reading
religious or spiritual interests
repairs
research
sewing
shopping
temporary housing
transporting
visiting
walking
yard work

When eldercare responsibilities involve caring for aging parents, siblings know all too well that caregiving tasks are rarely distributed equally or fairly, nor are they necessarily viewed as a family affair. Denial, sibling rivalry, limited finances, living far away, and being an only child, among other circumstances, tend to place the bulk of the physical and financial responsibilities and decision making on one or maybe two siblings at best.

If you are carrying the bulk of your elder's care, get in the habit of speaking to siblings and other family members and making requests of them on a regular basis. Compare notes and try to listen with an open mind. When siblings are reluctant to help or cannot assist with hands-on tasks, ask them to contribute financially; then you can decide how to make the best use of the money. Review chapter 4, "Communicaring," before you begin any conversations so you'll be better prepared to respond if other family members initially refuse to lend a hand.

PLAN THREE

Establish a network of professional care providers.

Specialized care providers, such as visiting nurses and social workers, can make home care an alternative to institutionalized care. If you're unsure as to the best course of action, this would be a good time to employ a **geriatric case manager** as a way to assess the situation. The questions to ask the care manager will include:

> *What kind of help is needed?*
> *Who can provide the kind of help that is needed?*
> *What are the costs?*
> *Which community programs are available to supplement the kind of in-home care that is needed?*

Geriatric case managers are highly trained social workers and nurses who have extensive experience working with older adults and can also help bridge the geographical gulf, especially if you are assisting your elder from far away. Be aware that for the most part private geriatric case management services are not covered by Medicare; however, some states may offer care management services without cost to the elder through the local area agency on aging. Contact the local aging office or the local hospital discharge planner for referrals. Ask the questions listed on the following page to determine whether a case manager candidate is a qualified professional.

To find other types of reliable, competent in-home helpers, **ask for referrals** from people you trust who may have had successful dealings with service providers. Also ask for recommendations from the doctor; licensed homemaker agencies; home-health-care agencies; the area agency on aging; the hospital discharge planner; social-service agencies; licensed nurse agencies; social workers; clergy; and an employment agency.

An **Internet search** will also turn up scores of local resources that can send qualified helpers to your elder's house. Keywords include "senior citizen services," "home health care," "private nurse," "social services," "caregiver services," "agency on aging," and "homemaker services." Type the name of the city where your elder resides in each search.

These days, more and more neighborhood **senior-housing communities** are offering in-home care as part of their extended services to nonresidents. Contact the local

GERIATRIC CASE MANAGER CHECKLIST

(This worksheet is also available online at www.elderindustry.com)

- What is your educational background?
- What medical and/or educational degrees do you hold?
- Where did you work prior to entering private practice? For how many years?
- How long have you been in business?
- Is this a full-time or a part-time practice?
- Are you certified by the state?
- What are your hours and availability in an emergency?
- What are your emergency backup plans if you're unavailable?
- Who supervises your work?
- How much do you charge for an initial assessment?
- What is your hourly fee?
- What can I expect to pay? What is your billing cycle?
- Which services are arranged outside of your care?
- What is your role once a referral is made?
- How, and how often, will you update me?
- May I have the name of three references who have used your service?

continuing-care retirement community and the local assisted-living and skilled-nursing-care facilities, and ask if they offer in-home care services.

Another resource for in-home care would be the "Situations Wanted" section of the **classified ads**. Private, self-employed home-care workers may be advertising their availability in the local newspaper. Independent in-home caregivers may charge even less than an agency *and* have a network of family and friends who can cover for them if they become unavailable.

If none of the above leads proves successful, **place an ad** in the local newspaper. Rent a post office box as a way to retain privacy and keep unwanted inquiries at bay. Request that résumés and references are sent directly to the post office box address.

PLAN FOUR

Be prepared with specific questions when hiring in-home helpers.

Before beginning the interview process, think about what specific services you may need from the helper. When a job applicant calls, give a short job description, time and day-shift expectations, salary, and benefits. Grant interviews only to those being considered for the position. Ask other family members or a friend to be present during interviews for feedback and support. *Check all references before hiring.*

HIRING IN-HOME HELPERS CHECKLIST

(This worksheet is also available online at www.elderindustry.com)

Today's Date: _____

Applicant's Name: _____

Address/City/State/Zip: _____

Contact Information: _____

Referring Agency: _____

Agency Contact Information: _____

Ask the applicant:

- What makes you interested in this kind of work?
- Tell me about your past home-care work experience.
- Why did you leave your last position?
- Are you in this country legally? (Ask for proof.)
- Have you received any special training?
- Do you have any problems that might hinder you in this job?
- How do you feel about alcohol, drugs, and smoking?
- Is there anything about this job that you would not be willing to do? (Laundry, cooking, etc.)
- What is your time commitment to this position?
- Are you willing to do household chores, such as cooking and light housekeeping?
- How flexible is your schedule?
- Do you have a current driver's license?
- Do you have a car at your disposal? Are you willing and able to drive my car?
- How would you cover your shift if you were ill and could not come to work?
- How would you handle an emergency situation?

Ask the agency:

- Are you licensed and accredited? By whom?
- Is your agency bonded? Is your worker bonded?
- Who pays insurance and taxes and handles employer responsibilities?
- How long have you been in business?
- Do you accept Medicare?
- Do you offer sliding-scale fees?

- What are the fees for services provided by your worker?
- What costs are not covered?
- Who pays the worker, you or me?
- What are the minimum and maximum hours of service?
- Are there limits to services provided?
- What is your screening process when hiring workers?
- How do you supervise your workers?
- Is the worker specially trained to work with older adults?
- Do you find a replacement if your worker is ill or on vacation?
- Do I continue to pay your worker while my elder is in the hospital?
- Can your agency provide me with references for you and your worker?
- What is the process when a worker does not show up for work?
- How soon can a worker begin?

Ask the reference:

- How long have you known this applicant?
- What was the applicant's position and job description?
- Why did the applicant leave your employment?
- How well did the applicant get along with others?
- What were the applicant's strengths? Weaknesses?
- Did you find the applicant trustworthy?
- Were you aware of any substance abuse? Smoking?
- Would you rehire the applicant?
- (Describe the job you have in mind.) Is the applicant well suited for the job?

Ask yourself:

- Do I *really* believe this person is right for the job?
- Will this person take charge and respond quickly in an emergency?
- Is this person organized? Neat? Flexible? Energetic? Pleasant?
- Does this person have the proper training and experience for this job?
- Will this person get along with my elder? Family? Others?
- Will this person know when to consult the family?
- Will this person be sensitive to family traditions?
- Does this person do okay with pets if one is in the household?
- Do family members like and trust this person?
- Do family members believe this person can handle this job?

PLAN FIVE

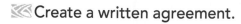Create a written agreement.

You may wish to clarify responsibilities and expectations with hired in-home helpers by creating a written agreement. An attorney can help you draw up a formal job contract, or you can take a more casual approach and simply put your expectations in writing. Putting employment terms in writing is never a bad idea. Modify agreements as needed. Do what you can to keep the information current and accessible. Have your employee sign the agreement *before* work begins.

PAID-CARE-PROVIDER WORK AGREEMENT

(This worksheet is also available online at www.elderindustry.com)

Incorporate the following information in a written agreement.

- Employer name, address, telephone number
- Employee name, address, telephone number
- Employee Social Security number
- Salary, payment method, terms of payment (weekly, bimonthly)
- Benefits (meals, entertainment allowance, vacation, insurance)
- Expenses, transportation fees, reimbursement procedures
- Record keeping/taxes
- Work schedule and timekeeping methods
- Length of service
- Personal days and sick days
- Holidays/makeup time
- Job description
- Emergency procedures
- Worker's emergency contacts (names, day and evening telephone numbers)
- House rules (include policies on smoking, drinking, foul language, tardiness, absence without notice, visitors and guests, property territorial limits/restrictions if any)
- Termination of employment (two weeks, two warnings)
- Reasons for termination (theft, carelessness, failure to carry out duties, violation of house rules, physical or verbal abuse)
- Job exit strategy
- Employee signature and date
- Employer signature and date

PLAN SIX

Take steps to ensure quality service from care providers.

If you plan to employ a full-time in-home care professional, financial and legal considerations such as Social Security contributions (FICA), federal unemployment tax (FUTA), state unemployment tax, and state workmen's compensation contributions are the responsibility of the employer. **Review employment regulations by contacting the Social Security office or the IRS office.** Seeking advice from an accountant or lawyer will also be helpful. Keep careful records. Ask your home insurance agent about proper coverage while employing someone in the home.

The salary range for services begins at minimum wage and depends on the amount of training and experience the worker has and whether an employment agency is involved. Transportation expenses to and from the job site may be an extra cost.

Hiring a worker from an agency does not guarantee quality of services provided by the employee. In fact, while new eldercare service providers seem to surface on a daily basis, there continues to be a lack of government regulation regarding businesses that serve older adults. **Only hire workers who are licensed, insured, and bonded, and look to the state long-term-care ombudsman office and the area agency on aging as reliable resources for conducting a background check on care providers.**

At the same time, it is important for you to continuously monitor the quantity and quality of services rendered by anyone you bring into your elder's home. Here is a checklist of suggestions.

Caregiver Quality-Control Checklist

- Be in contact with in-home care providers on a regular basis—by phone, mail, or, better yet, in person.
- Exchange telephone numbers and let workers know that they can call you collect if they need you.
- Give care providers a list of emergency telephone numbers should something happen to your elder. Also post the emergency contact information near the telephone and on the refrigerator.
- Ask care providers about their emergency contact information should something happen to them while they are on the job, including information about their health insurance carrier.
- After every visit to the doctor, keep the care providers updated on your elder's health condition and medications, and, in turn, have them contact you if they notice any changes.
- Speak up immediately if you sense that something's not right: The day's work isn't done; workers don't keep track of spending money; ongoing complaints about the worker's attitude or the quality of care; clothes, food, and household items are missing from the home; workers arrive late and leave early; or you feel as though you aren't getting important information.

- Be aware that if the care provider is from a different cultural background, communication styles may vary from yours: Care providers may have been taught that asking personal questions and saying no to an authority figure is not acceptable behavior; or they may say yes out of politeness when in fact they don't understand what is being said or asked of them. To get around this, demonstrate tasks and ask them to repeat your actions.
- Print legibly or type special instructions.
- Provide encouragement and support, and let care providers know how much they are appreciated. Thank-you notes, gift certificates, and favorable reports can really make a difference.

PLAN SEVEN

Take formal action if you are dissatisfied with the quality of care.

If your elder is being cared for in a hospital, an assisted-living facility, or a nursing home and is dissatisfied with the quality of care or has other concerns, such as treatment options and confidentiality, ask to speak to the **patient representative** on staff.

An **ombudsman** monitors nursing and board-and-care facilities. Call this advocate if you suspect your family member is being ill-treated. The ombudsman will investigate and refer the case to the state licensing agent. To locate a local ombudsman, look online or refer to the telephone directory White or Blue Pages under "Long-term Care Ombudsman" or call the local agency on aging.

Complaints about hospitals, long-term-care facilities, and residential-care facilities can be directed to the **state department of social services, the department of health services,** and **county licensing offices.** Licensing and certification reports are public information.

PLAN EIGHT

Bridge the gap in eldercare by using community programs.

Assisted-living programs and in-home services help keep homebound older adults independent and in contact with others who can monitor their health and safety. Here are some typical programs.

HOME-DELIVERED MEALS (ALSO KNOWN AS MOBILE MEALS OR MEALS-ON-WHEELS). Meals delivered to homebound older adults offer nutritious meals and also provide opportunities to interact with the volunteers who bring the food.

EMERGENCY RESPONSE DEVICE. The homebound person wears a device (typically, a bracelet or a necklace) that is equipped with a radio transmitter that's activated by pushing a button. An emergency message is then transmitted to the hospital, the police, or another emergency contact.

TELEPHONE MONITORING SERVICE. Daily phone calls ensure peace of mind for the home-bound person. If no one answers the phone at a predetermined time, a visit from a volunteer or paid service provider is the next course of action.

CARRIER ALERT (ALSO KNOWN AS POSTAL ALERT). A mail carrier who notices an unusual accumulation of mail will alert a postal supervisor to designate a person to check on the resident.

IN-HOME HEALTH AND ASSISTED-LIVING SERVICES. Local continuing-care retirement communities (CCRCs) and assisted-living and skilled-nursing facilities may have an outreach program that assists nonresidents. Contact these resources directly.

ADULT DAY SERVICES. Supervised-care centers for adults who cannot be left home alone during the day include comprehensive services ranging from health assessment and nursing care to social and recreational activities. Participation in these programs usually requires a physician's prescription. While adult day services are not necessarily federally licensed, members of the staff must include a director with a professional degree in the field of health and human services, a social worker, and a registered nurse (RN) or licensed practical nurse (LPN) supervised by an RN.

Adult Day Services Checklist

- Request a *written* target-enrollment policy statement.
- Ask about its policy regarding disruptive participants or those who are abusing alcohol or drugs.
- Ask if the care center requests updates on a participant's medical records.
- Find out how the care center provides reports to you on the elder's activities.
- Review the staff-participant ratio. One staff member for every eight participants is typical. In cases where participants are severely mentally and physically impaired, one in five is an acceptable ratio.
- Ask about transportation options.

RESPITE. Primary family caregivers need backup plans. If you're suddenly called out of town, for example, a respite center can provide temporary care in your absence. You might also take advantage of respite care when you are unsure of decisions regarding where your elder will live after a hospitalization. Respite care is available for as little as a few hours at a time. A day, a weekend, and even a month or more can also be arranged. Local nursing homes, assisted-living facilities, and senior retirement-housing campuses are good resources for respite for family caregivers. For additional information and referrals regarding community assisted-living programs, call the local department on aging, a social-service agency, a family service agency, or the hospital discharge planner.

To gain local access to these programs, look in the Yellow Pages under "Nurses" and "Nurses' Registries," "Home Health Agencies," "Senior Citizens' Service Organizations," and "Senior Services." If you are employed, contact your human resources department and find out what arrangements, if any, may be available through your employer's work-life benefits program.

PLAN NINE

Identify volunteer resources.

There are numerous community resources to locate volunteers. Tap into the organizations listed below and find out what they have to offer in terms of people who assist with caregiving-related tasks as well as offer companionship and emotional support:

advocacy groups	public libraries
agencies on aging	religious groups
charities	seniors' organizations
colleges/universities	specialized illness organizations
community centers	support groups
family recreation centers	veterans' organizations
family service agencies	volunteer organizations
grade school/high school	women's clubs
hospice	youth groups
hospital	

Low-Cost and Free Resources

Technology continues to greatly improve the aging experience in the United States by providing unique ways to supplement a variety of care responsibilities. See chapter 10, "Safe and Secure," for resources.

Call the local chapters of **Easter Seals,** the **Red Cross,** and the **United Way** for a variety of services available for older adults. Look in the White Pages of the telephone directory or conduct a keyword search on the Internet for local contact information.

The **Eldercare Locator** refers callers to an extensive network of organizations serving older people. Call the toll-free number: (800) 677-1116. Be prepared to provide the name and address of your elder and a brief description of the problem or the kind of assistance you are seeking.

The **National Family Caregiver Support Program** was authorized by the Older Act of

2000. Under the Department of Health and Human Services and the Administration on Aging, the program is a work in progress. Type the following keyword search on your Internet browser: *National Family Caregiver Support Program.*

Each state offers an **assisted-living program** for people more then sixty years of age who need help with some tasks and can remain safely in their own homes. To qualify, participants must have assets of $12,500 or less, not including a house, a car, or furniture. Contact the local agency on aging.

If you're interested in taking **caregiver classes** that will sharpen your skills when providing direct care, log on to the Internet and type the following keywords in your browser search box: "training for caregivers," "caregiver seminars," and "caregiver training."

Faith in Action
Wake Forest University School of Medicine
Medical Center Boulevard
Winston-Salem, NC 27157
(877) 324-8411, (336) 716-0101; fax: (336)
    777-3284
Website: www.fiavolunteers.org

**National Association for Home Care &
    Hospice**
228 7th Street, SE
Washington, DC 20003
(202) 547-7424; fax: (202) 547-3540
Website: www.nahc.org

**National Association of Private Geriatric
    Care Managers**
1604 N. Country Club Road
Tucson, AZ 85716
(520) 881-8008; fax: (520) 325-7925
Website: www.caremanager.org

National Private Duty Association
941 E. 86th Street, Suite 270
Indianapolis, IN 46240
(317) 663-3637
Website: www.privatedutyhomecare.org

National Respite Locator
Website: www.respitelocator.org

Rural Assistance Center
501 N. Columbia Road, Stop 9037
Grand Forks, ND 58202
Toll-free: (800) 270-1898
Website: www.raconline.org

Rural Information Center
National Agricultural Library
10301 Baltimore Avenue
Beltsville, MD 20705-2351
Toll-free: (800) 633-7701

ShareTheCare
551 Fifth Avenue, 28th Floor
New York, NY 10176
(646) 467-8097
Website: www.sharethecare.org

Society of Certified Senior Advisors
1777 S. Bellaire Street, Suite 230
Denver, CO 80222
Toll-free: (800) 653-1785
Website: www.society-csa.com

Volunteers of America
1660 Duke Street
Alexandria, VA 22314
(703) 341-5000; toll-free: (800)
    899-0089
Website: www.voa.org

Dementia Care and Mental Health

**Alzheimer's Association 24/7
Helpline**
Toll-free: (800) 272-3900; TDD: (866)
403-3073
Website: www.alz.org

**Alzheimer's Disease Education and
Referral Center**
Website: www.alzheimers.org

**Alzheimer's Research
Foundation**
Website: www.alzheimers-research.org

American Association for Geriatric Psychiatry
7910 Woodmont Avenue, Suite 1050
Bethesda, MD 20814-3004
(301) 654-7850; fax: (301) 654-4137
Website: www.aagpgpa.org

ElderCare Online
Website: www.ec-online.net

National Adult Day Services Association
2519 Connecticut Avenue, NW
Washington, DC 20008
Toll-free: (800) 558-5301
Website: www.nadsa.org

CREATING A CARE TEAM ACTION CHECKLIST

(This worksheet is also available online at www.elderindustry.com)

HOW TO TELL WHEN YOUR ELDER NEEDS HELP	To Do By	Completed
Observe your elder		
performing tasks	_____	☐
physical conditions	_____	☐
environment	_____	☐
mental health	_____	☐
Review "Communicaring" chapter	_____	☐
SHARE THE CARE		
List eldercare tasks		
homemaking	_____	☐
personal care	_____	☐
home health care	_____	☐
quality of life	_____	☐
Set caregiver goals		
short-term	_____	☐
long-term	_____	☐
Create a list of helpers	_____	☐
Make a list of help needed		
short-term	_____	☐
long-term	_____	☐
Hire caregivers		
create a list of questions	_____	☐
check all references and licenses	_____	☐
create and sign job contract	_____	☐
have proper insurance	_____	☐
look into Social Security taxes	_____	☐

Have a plan to

    oversee quality of care   _____   ❑

    request reports   _____   ❑

Review community assisted-living programs

    home-delivered meals   _____   ❑

    emergency response devices   _____   ❑

    telephone-monitoring services   _____   ❑

    carrier alert   _____   ❑

    social outlets   _____   ❑

    adult day services   _____   ❑

    respite care   _____   ❑

Consider volunteers   _____   ❑

Obtain a copy of elder's

    telephone directory   _____   ❑

    personal address book   _____   ❑

    community senior directory   _____   ❑

Record emergency telephone
numbers   _____   ❑

Know phone numbers of

    hospital social services   _____   ❑

    family service agency   _____   ❑

    area agency on aging   _____   ❑

    family members   _____   ❑

    friends and neighbors   _____   ❑

    hired caregivers   _____   ❑

    geriatric case manager   _____   ❑

    social worker   _____   ❑

Make sure your elder has
access to a telephone   _____   ❑

**Duplicate and post phone numbers;
keep copies**

    at home   _____   ❑

    at work   _____   ❑

    in car   _____   ❑

    in wallet/purse _____   ❑

    flash drive   _____   ❑

**Duplicate and distribute phone
   numbers to designated persons**   _____   ❑

3

Be Kind to Yourself

Take Care of *You*

Your sister is critical of your caregiving decisions; your husband resents the amount of time you spend away from home; you missed your daughter's piano recital—again; your boss is slowly losing patience waiting for overdue reports.

When you take on the role of family caregiver, you'll be pulled in a hundred different directions—family relationships, job responsibilities, friends and coworkers, personal commitments, and the person who is relying on you for assistance. Someone and something is always vying for your attention.

The first order of business as family caregivers is to safeguard your *own* physical and emotional well-being. That's a tall order. Some days it feels as though the world is crumbling below you, and other days the help you thought was coming never arrives. Feeling depressed and lonely cuts like a knife, and guilt can be your constant companion. *Am I doing enough? Am I doing a good job? Will I be a bad person if I say no to my elder's request?*

Your own health, the quality of your professional and personal lives, and your relationships outside of the one you have with your elders should not suffer as a consequence of providing care. What it takes is a leap of faith. Review this chapter as often as needed as a reminder of the many ways you can be kinder to yourself in the caregiving process. The suggestions in this section of *The Complete Eldercare Planner* will help you assess whether you are on the brink of burnout, and if you have already crossed that line, it will help guide you to a well-deserved balanced lifestyle.

TAKE CARE OF *YOU*

- Unfortunately, many caregivers see themselves only as extensions of the person they are caring for, and they fail to take good care of *themselves.*
- One of today's all-too-silent health crises is caregiver depression.
- Eldercare can affect the workplace—employees arriving late, leaving early, and not showing up for work at all.

As you become an advocate for your elders, who is advocating for you? If you are not your best friend during the caregiving years, who is?

OBJECTIVES

After completing **"Take Care of You,"** *you will be able to:*

Recognize the symptoms of burnout.

Take necessary precautions to relieve caregiver stress.

Address the angry side of caregiving.

Integrate work-life responsibilities.

PLAN ONE

Take an honest look at yourself.

Ask yourself the following questions to monitor your current caregiver stress level.

Caregiver Burnout Checklist

DO I . . .

- Resent the person I am caring for?
- Resent other family members?
- Feel angry most of the time?
- Find little satisfaction in caregiving?
- Feel trapped and burdened?
- Feel like the rest of the family is not doing their fair share?
- Feel guilty most of the time?
- Have the urge to physically and verbally abuse my elder at times?
- Have bouts of feeling inadequate and helpless?
- Often feel enraged?
- Think I could and should be doing a better job of caregiving?

- Feel out of control?
- Have difficulty saying no?
- Tend to please people at my expense?
- Resist asking and accepting help from others?

AM I . . .
- Overeating or eating the wrong kinds of food?
- Abusing alcohol or drugs?
- Not getting any physical exercise?
- Crying frequently?
- Lacking fun and laughter in my life?
- Depleting my own financial resources?
- Late for work or missing work?
- Letting my job performance slip?
- Sleep deprived?
- Experiencing chronic health issues like headaches and lingering colds?

PLAN TWO

Avert burnout.

There are many reasons why you may feel compelled to shoulder too much responsibility and become overly involved in your elders' lives. Feeling needed and useful is a positive life-enhancing experience. However, doing more than is necessary creates problems. Too much assistance and too much attention are equally harmful for the caregiver and the care receiver.

Although strong support of loved ones can, at first, result in a positive, tangible boost to the quality of their lives, when you go overboard and do too much for them, you stand the chance of eroding their sense of dignity and competence.

Nice to do or have to do?

Family caregivers in the burnout stage will exhibit a variety of symptoms, including chronic physical illnesses, ongoing feelings of helplessness, and disillusionment. One of the keys to averting caregiver stress and burnout is to become more in tune with the time-management concept of **"nice to do"** versus **"have to do,"** *especially* when there is evidence that our elders are reasonably capable of making their own decisions and able to safely perform day-to-day tasks for themselves.

There's only so much time and energy to give to others, and the key component to managing your day is knowing the difference between doing what is required, when to defer to others, and when to let go of unnecessary tasks. Formulating responsibilities into a list of what *must* be done (have to do) makes it easier to visualize what you realistically have on your plate. Anything else that you offer (nice to do) is icing on the cake. Prioritization is critical to ensuring that the most important caregiving tasks are completed first. In today's caregiver world, the ability to prioritize must be included in your bag of tricks.

Refer to the following self-assessment questions as often as needed as a way to maintain a healthy balance between family caregiving responsibilities and the *real* needs of your elders.

When it comes to my role as family caregiver, I . . .
- evaluate their strengths and resources, not limitations and weaknesses.
- keep them involved in their own decision-making process.
- facilitate dialogues rather than try to solve their problems for them.
- let them do what they can for themselves, as long as their safety is not at risk.
- adhere to their decision-making time frame, rather than my own.
- accept and deal with what is, rather than what I'd like things to be.
- do not waste energy worrying about people and circumstances that I cannot control.
- am aware that change can occur for better or for worse at any time.
- ask for and accept help from others.
- do not deplete my own financial resources.
- seek financial advice from professionals.
- do not make ironclad promises to anyone about anything, and stay flexible.
- accept that today somebody is likely to be mad at me for something.
- continue to satisfy my own personal, professional, recreational, spiritual, and social needs.
- accept that it is okay not to have all the answers.
- talk about my real feelings to a trusted friend or professional about what is happening.

PLAN THREE

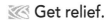 Get relief.

There are people who will help you with eldercare tasks, and there are people who will care for *you*. Ask for help and be sure to accept it when others make the offer, even when you're able and available to perform all of the caregiving tasks. Get used to making ongoing requests for assistance and get other family members used to the idea that you need and deserve their help.

You and your elders need breathing room. You may need a break from caregiving responsibilities, and your elder may need a break from you. If he or she resents having someone else take your place temporarily, resist the temptation to cancel your plans. The following is a potential network of people and organizations you may want to recruit.

FAMILY. Asking for help from family members may seem like a deceptively simple plan, and yet it can be nothing less than stepping into an emotional abyss. Some family members cooperate without any hesitation or difficulty; others run in the opposite direction. Keep asking for their help, but do not rely on them 100 percent if you think they will let you down. Bring in a professional who can mediate and perhaps work out an acceptable division of labor.

FRIENDS, NEIGHBORS, VOLUNTEERS. Let your needs be known to people outside of the family circle. Be precise when defining "help," since what you may need can come in many forms. Make a list of big and little things that are demanding your attention, including getting temporary relief from caregiving responsibilities. Review the "Share the Care" section in chapter 2, "Creating a Care Team," for suggestions on specific ways other people can be helpful to *you.*

EMPLOYERS. Eldercare responsibilities at home can affect you in the workplace, since missing work or not showing up at all can happen at any time. See Plan Six in this section (page 62) for suggestions on keeping a healthy balance of work-life responsibilities.

PERSONAL ASSISTANT. If you are time-crunched and drowning in unfinished tasks, household projects, and errands, the services of a personal assistant or a personal organizer are a telephone call away. Look in the Yellow Pages and the Internet under the keywords "Concierge," "Home Helpers," and "Personal Organizers."

SUPPORT GROUPS. You'll feel less isolated when you share with others who are in the same situation. The professionals don't have all the answers. You and the others you will share with are the ones who live these experiences day in and day out. Group participation helps manage stress and improves skills as a caregiver. Some problems have no solutions, and being with other caregivers affirms the reality of the situation. Contact the local agency on aging, hospital, and community center for locations of support groups.

CYBER COMMUNITY. Talk in real time, leave a note on the message board, or respond to a blogger's website. The Internet offers caregivers chat rooms, discussion forums, and links to online support groups. Internet resources are listed at the end of this chapter.

SPECIFIC ILLNESS ASSOCIATIONS. Organizations dealing with specific illnesses such as cancer, diabetes, heart disease, arthritis, and Alzheimer's often have programs and support groups for family members as well as patients.

PLAN FOUR

Quiet the storm of anger.

Anger is expensive. It can cost you your close relationships, your job, and your self-respect. When we are provoked to anger, our adult judgment often flies out the window. We often regret our thoughtless verbal comeback, and sometimes it's too late to retract the words and the hurt that anger can cause.

Getting angry in the caregiver's world often feels like an everyday experience.

Why isn't the doctor calling me back? Who does my sister think she is talking to me like that? If I get into one more shouting match with my husband, I'm going to file for divorce. Why does Mom insist on walking without her cane?

Suppressed anger is even more destructive. Caregivers hold back their anger completely until it builds up out of control and explodes. The headlines are full of these events: elder abuse, domestic violence, homicide, and even suicide.

We keep repeating the same mistakes when we don't know what our options are. Managing and controlling your anger, even expressing your anger, *does not necessarily free you of it.* After doing these things, our anger is still repressed and waits for something else to trigger our emotions.

Anger management clinics provide on-the-spot "emotional first aid" and can teach us new ways to cope with anger, including:

- using an anger situation to strengthen your relationship with yourself
- facing your fears about being angry in the first place
- seeing negative situations as opportunities to do something productive and constructive
- ending feeling like a victim of the circumstance and out of control
- replacing worthlessness with feelings of self-respect and competence
- learning when anger is justified and a legitimate grievance

Feelings of anger and the guilt for having those feelings carry a heavy emotional toll. If you are discouraged and unable to cope, you have choices. **Don't wait.** Resources for managing anger are listed at the end of this chapter and in "The Reading Room" section of *The Complete Eldercare Planner.*

PLAN FIVE

Get a good night's sleep.

A good laugh and a long sleep are the two best cures.   —Irish proverb

Imagine a full night's sleep with no interruptions, just peace and quiet. Typically, our sleeping patterns in the caregiving years are anything but peaceful. When our elders can't sleep and are prone to nocturnal wandering and activity, we worry about their falling and other mishaps. **You can't be expected to be on call 24/7.**

Here are a few suggestions when dealing with the challenges of an elderly night owl.

Seek medical advice. If your elder is experiencing a pattern of sleepless nights, your first plan of action is to contact the doctor to determine the cause and make treatment suggestions. Sleeplessness can be due to:

> depression
> medication usage and dosage
> drinking liquids too close to bedtime
> incontinence
> changes in bladder function
> urinary tract infection
> hyperthyroidism
> dementia

Exercise during the day. Even if your elder is bedridden, ask a physical therapist about exercise programs. Rent fitness videos or DVDs that target older adults. Get out of the house and get some fresh air. Take daily walks (in bad weather, head for the shopping mall).

Increase day and evening activities. Consider adult day services. Play music, sing songs, and dance together. Play catch with beach balls and balloons. Try shuffleboard or miniature golf.

Give your elder a job. Offer physical activities that help him or her stretch, bend, grasp, carry, and walk—including setting the table, washing the dishes, folding the laundry, shredding unwanted documents, sweeping the porch, brushing the dog, rearranging the contents of drawers, and other activities that keep her or him moving.

Introduce relaxation techniques. Practice deep breathing exercises together and suggest a warm bath at bedtime.

Limit drinking liquids before bedtime. Set limits to unreasonable—and sometimes manipulative—requests, such as having to fetch a glass of water several times during the night.

Hire a relief person. One night a week, hire someone to relieve you of your nightly duties so you can go to your own room, close the door, and get a good night's sleep.

See your own doctor. Be sure your health is in good order.

Eliminate potential household hazards if your elder has a tendency to wander around the house at night.

- Keep certain rooms of the home locked and off-limits at night.
- Set up an activity table or desk near the bed.
- Place a comfortable reading chair in the bedroom.
- Make good use of night-lights, especially in hallways and bathrooms.
- Keep a light on in your elder's favorite room and well-traveled hallways.
- Clear away potentially dangerous items, especially items stored on stairways.

- Remove small portable furniture, such as ottomans, low tables, and area rugs.
- Label rooms with signs on the doors.
- Rent a bedside commode.
- Provide a call button in the bathroom.
- Install locks and latches on doors, cabinets, and gates.

PLAN SIX

Care or career?

Many family caregivers are employed outside the home, and are constantly attempting to achieve a life of balance among different but equally important priorities—namely, **the demands of work and home**. This isn't an easy thing to do; but it is your responsibility to integrate your personal and professional lives, which includes taking advantage of work-life programs that may be available to you at work.

The work-home gap is narrowing. Today, we lunch with children at the company daycare center, pick up laundry at the employee store, work out at the corporate gym, and make arrangements to have our car washed and serviced in the company parking lot. Obtaining eldercare advice and services from our employer is becoming more possible.

It is estimated that 40 percent of all employees who are caring for an aging family member are missing work on a regular basis. Clearly, the caregiving phenomenon is an employer problem, not just an employee problem. Companies understand that sustaining a highly functioning workforce means offering family caregiver programs and benefits to employees. The consequences of avoiding eldercare issues in the workplace translate into employees' loss of concentration, higher use of health benefits, lost work time, increased absenteeism, and a higher employee turnover rate. The resultant disruption at work is significant—so implementing eldercare work-life benefits is critical in maintaining workforce productivity and commitment.

Eldercare issues typically surface in two stages: **the planning stage** and **the crisis stage**. At times, there will be opportunities to plan for the future needs of older family members and times when a crisis will be front and center, and often when you least expect it. Either way, you'd be wise to learn more about your company's flextime policy and about the Family and Medical Leave Act now.

If you're in the midst of a crisis right now and need immediate guidance, turn to chapter 1, "Effective Planning," and review the "Caught Off Guard: Suddenly, You're a Caregiver" section. If your company does not have an eldercare program in place, or you are unable to find the resources you need within your company benefits, look for additional support by reviewing the work-life resources listed at the end of this chapter.

Eldercare-friendly work-life programs include:
   eldercare resource and referral services
   flextime policies

telecommuting

compressed workweeks

job sharing

eldercare seminars and brown-bag lunch workshops

on-site work-life expos to meet local-services providers

long-term care insurance plans

group legal plans

employee assistance programs

geriatric case managers

adult day services

dependent-care spending accounts

contingency care vouchers

subsidized emergency backup

employee store (eldercare books and videos)

employee newsletter articles

caregiver support groups

cosponsored community eldercare events

global relocation assistance

unpaid leave policy

bereavement support

Employees who are **successfully juggling work and eldercare responsibilities** are finding that managing their role of caregiver is very much like managing a small company. The "work" of caregiving can be broken down into a series of tasks, and the employee manages and delegates responsibilities that can be performed by others. The time-consuming tasks of arranging for and supervising the services from afar can not be underestimated. With the willingness to continuously ask for help, employed family members may find that caring for loved ones and continuing to make a living are not mutually exclusive after all.

If you are at all concerned about staying productive on the job while balancing family eldercare responsibilities, become proactive and explore the eldercare work-life policies and programs your company has to offer. If your company does not currently offer any eldercare benefits, ask management to consider doing so. In the meantime, *The Complete Eldercare Planner* will guide you throughout the caregiving process.

Is relocation in your future?

Moving up in our careers can be a wonderful, exciting adventure; but sometimes moving up means moving away. And what about elderly family members—*do we leave them behind or take them with us?* A company transfer is stressful and demanding, and including elders in the mix requires forethought and planning. If they decide to go with you to the new location, be sure that they are included in the decision-making process every step of the way. For helpful tips, refer to the checklist below.

EMPLOYEE ELDERCARE RELOCATION CHECKLIST

(This worksheet is also available online at www.elderindustry.com)

- Ask your employer for the assistance of a professional relocation company. You will need help selling the existing home and learning more about the new location. Do not attempt to move without professional assistance.
- Consider hiring the services of a senior move management company. Check out the National Association of Senior Move Managers website (www.nasmm.com) to locate local service providers. The time is now to sort through and downsize after years of accumulating.
- Before the move, order a telephone directory for your new city. Search the Internet for caregiving services, in-home services, hospitals, and houses of worship.
- Assess your elders' long-term housing and assisted-living needs. Will they live with *you* or is another senior-housing option more desirable?
- If your elders choose to live independently and in their own home, will in-home services be readily available if needed? Review chapter 9, "Housing," in *The Complete Eldercare Planner* for additional senior-friendly housing tips.
- How will your elders get around town while you're at work? Are they able to drive? Is public transportation accessible?
- Discuss long-term health issues and the need to find a doctor in the new location. If relocating overseas, how will health-care expenses be covered?
- Create a plan for staying in touch with friends and family members.
- Discuss the costs associated with living in this new location and create a budget you can live with.
- Will the neighborhood offer easy access to medical care, church, friends, personal services, and shopping? Is it safe for your elders to take a walk or sit outside?
- Will pets be allowed where they live?
- Is the climate and altitude suitable all year round?
- What's the backup plan if your elders decide the move is not right for them?

Do not consider any senior-housing arrangement if . . .

- there are stairs (interior and exterior) to negotiate
- building codes will not allow outdoor ramps or first-floor bathrooms
- a spare room for a first-floor bedroom is unavailable
- there are no community in-home care or in-home medical services available

- transportation services are not available
- installing a first-floor washer and dryer is not allowed or possible
- the bathtub cannot be removed to install a step-in shower

Caregiving: The Spiritual Journey

Where can you find wisdom when there are no rational answers for what's happening in the moment? Where do you turn for strength when your world is falling apart? Why is this happening, and why me?

When we ask these questions, what we are trying to do is find meaning in our suffering, and even with a whole life of experiences behind us nothing quite prepares us for the unpredictable world of family caregiving.

Spirituality may be one of the ways to cope from day to day, including witnessing the decline of loved ones' abilities and accepting losses of every kind. As spiritual human beings, there are places within us that need to be touched and are important to our holistic health and well-being. As much as we treat the physical aspects of aging, we also need to **pay attention to our spiritual side.**

CAREGIVING: THE SPIRITUAL JOURNEY

- Spiritual beliefs have the power to transform and change one's perceptions, values, and behaviors.
- What matters most is the *attitude* taken toward suffering and surviving crises.
- If you get the feeling there must be "something more" than what you are currently experiencing, and you can't get the Peggy Lee song "Is That All There Is?" out of your head, your "spiritual" side may be trying to tell you something.

As caregivers, our first instinct is to make things right; but much of what happens is simply out of our control.

OBJECTIVES

After completing "Caregiving: The Spiritual Journey," you will be able to:

Navigate the emotional wilderness of caregiving.

Tap into spiritual tools and strategies.

Gain access to spiritual resources.

Experts define *spirituality* as the act of looking for meaning in the deepest sense, and looking for it in ways that are authentically yours. While not everyone is religious, in the sense of sharing a communal faith system, everyone is spiritual. There are numerous ways to receive spiritual nourishment, whether you seek it in a faith community, in nature, in art and music, in gardening, or wherever it finds you. Seeking spirituality refreshes and renews us so that we may continue to give.

In attempting to find hope and love in a truly difficult situation, this section of *The Complete Eldercare Planner* offers guidelines on the spiritual side of caregiving. In the midst of life's countless mysteries and letdowns, spirituality can be our anchor and support when the meaning of what is happening in the moment escapes us.

PLAN ONE

You're *not* crazy.

Family caregivers cross an invisible threshold into the unknown. When you are overreacting at times, and almost always taking things personally, the caregiving experience is as frightening as it is healing. Seasoned family caregivers often describe the **emotional roller coaster** of family caregiving as bewildering and dislodging. A steady diet of being with older people and attending to their needs and demands can make even the most experienced of caregivers question their sanity. Coping, as well as simultaneous feelings of compassion and grief are experiences that come early in the caregiving process.

One of the most devastating (and typical) aspects of family caregiving is **isolation**. It's not unusual to constantly worry that family and friends will abandon you if you talk too much about your eldercare problems. Anger and grief may swell up and overcome you, and there's no one to talk to about your fears and anxieties. You may be receiving fewer social invitations, and you may be feeling sad that no one really understands (or seems to care) what you are going through.

While these unfortunate experiences ring true for many family caregivers, lifting the cloud of isolation is critical to your well-being. One way to accomplish this is to seek out the benefits of leading a more spiritual caregiving life.

PLAN TWO

Nurture spirituality.

Tapping into your spiritual self may be helpful when eldercare situations seem unbearable. Here are a few ways to pursue a more satisfying spiritual life. Do what feels natural to *you*.

PRAY. Many people use prayer and other spiritual practices to improve the quality of their lives.[1] Rejoin a faith community, participate in a prayer group, or simply pray on your own.

Learn ways to dialogue with yourself and with your higher power (whatever you conceive *It* to be).

LEARN MEDITATION. Meditation will allow your racing mind to find a calmer and more positive connection with yourself and get control of excessive thinking. Regular meditators report leading healthier and more productive lives. There are many different ways to meditate, and the "best" style of meditation is the one that feels right for you.

TAKE TIME FOR JOY. Does making homemade bread make you happy? How about painting a picture, gardening, taking photographs, or knitting a sweater? A good laugh, a break in the weather, or the realization that things could be worse may also lighten your load. Identify activities that make you feel good and let little bursts of happiness seep into your daily life.

LISTEN TO THE MUSIC. Songs are the sound tracks to our lives. Some take us back to childhood memories, while others are the perfect vehicles to express ourselves today. Songs make us smile and dance, and can also make us weepy. Let the music sing to your soul.

WALK A LABYRINTH. Labyrinths are designed to help quiet the mind and release intuitions. There is no right or wrong way to walk a labyrinth. Labyrinths can be found at churches, at retreat centers, and in parks.

SEEK SPIRITUAL COUNSELING. Hire a spiritual director or speak with a member of the clergy.

WRITE ABOUT IT. A personal journal is a confidante, a creativity tool, and a way of finding clarity. Sorting things out in writing may help prepare you for talking things out with someone else. Journals also provide a safe place to express yourself and offer the most authentic evidence of your point of view at the various stages of your caregiving life. Proprioceptive writing (a technique for exploring the mind through writing) facilitates emotional health, spiritual awakening, creative breakthroughs, and better writing. Courses in proprioceptive writing are available. For more information on this writing technique, conduct an Internet search by typing "proprioceptive writing" in your search engine browser.

ENJOY NATURE. Walking in the park, hearing birds sing, planting flowers, watching fish swim in an aquarium, visiting flower gardens, and listening to the sound of waves can be comforting.

VISIT SPIRITUAL PLACES. Throughout the world, there are shrines, churches, synagogues, and other places that speak to being united with the divine.

LET YOUR BODY MOVE YOU. Body work and a practice of purposeful movements, such as tai chi, massage, yoga, reflexology, and others, contribute to healing in soulful ways.

PLAN THREE

Practice spirituality daily.

Experts tell us that daily spiritual practice holds the key to strengthening whatever we want to improve in our life. Caregiving will give you many opportunities to practice forgiveness, patience, and compassion.

All of the ideas listed in Plan Two will fail to serve you until they become habits in your life. Create a personal wellness calendar and add a spiritual practice to your daily activities.

Self-Talk: Finding Peace of Mind

Over the years, studies about people in the caregiver role have revealed a vast difference in how they respond to their care responsibilities. In other words, some caregivers proved to be less vulnerable to the emotional stresses associated with eldercare than others. Beyond surviving, less-stressed and healthier caregivers had specific strategies for coping with the issues at hand; they were more apt to ask for different things from different people; they sought ways to replenish their inner resources; and they maintained realistic expectations.

Whether it's learning the art of self-talk, taking control of caregiver guilt, being more assertive with nonresponsive siblings, and conducting a family meeting, refer to this section

---

SELF-TALK: FINDING PEACE OF MIND

- The stresses and hardships of caregiving are undeniable.
- We are natural-born self-talkers. As children, we talked to ourselves instinctively, and we can use the same process of self-talk to help get us back on track.
- Caregivers are subject to a whole set of expectations, with the greatest of expectations coming from within ourselves.

Much of how you manage your role as caregivers has to do with your personal point of view and expectations.

OBJECTIVES

After completing "Self-Talk: Finding Peace of Mind," you will be able to:

Establish a self-respecting caregiving environment.

Help loosen the grip of caregiver guilt.

Speak your mind with uncooperative siblings.

Conduct a family meeting.

---

of *The Complete Eldercare Planner* when you need to be reminded that everything you need to carry out your responsibilities effectively (and be kinder to yourself in the long run) is already within your reach.

PLAN ONE

Start with the truth.

We are not born caregivers; we inherit the role. Caregiving is unfair, and usually one person does most of the work. Caregiving is hard work and exhausting; feelings of anger, love, sadness, helplessness, and guilt can overwhelm the caregiver in a matter of seconds. Caregiving is emotionally painful—we know how this story ends.

Every elder is unique, and so is every caregiving situation. We have never been down *this* particular road before. We don't know what's around the corner or what may happen one day to the next. We live in a world of unknowns and have little control over what happens.

Along the way, we meet other caregivers and share stories about the good times, the sad times, and of course, the fearful times. Caregivers love to tell their stories, and in the course of doing so, the differences in experience are hard to miss. While some caregivers speak in terms of having a good handle on their responsibilities and expectations, others talk of falling apart at the seams and barely coping from day to day.

What can account for such varying experiences? **Attitude is everything**. Whether problems and expectations turn out to be difficult or easy depends a great deal on how we see them and how we respond. Caregivers who are not compromising the quality of their own lives share similar values. They see the situation for what it is. They see their elder for who he or she is. They assess eldercare issues from where they are today rather than how they wish it could be. They are flexible. They never expect perfection, and their best is good enough. They also have something in common with the language they use to describe their situations. You may overhear successful caregivers say things like:

The only person I have control over is me.
I deserve respect.
I let others know when I'm angry.
I have limits.
I need all the help I can get.
I don't have all the answers.
I am resourceful.
I have the right to change my mind.
I have choices.
My best is good enough.

PLAN TWO

Protect important relationships.

Friends say that you've become completely consumed with your elder's care; your children don't ask when you're coming home anymore; your husband is angry about money you are spending. *They just don't get it.* You love taking care of your elders; but do the other important people in your life have a legitimate gripe? Are they being shortchanged?

Caring for our elders doesn't replace other close relationships, it adds to them, and being blindsided to being overextended could have serious consequences. On the other hand, family members and friends may be jealous of the many things you do for your elders. It's difficult to know the roots of their complaints, so give them the benefit of the doubt.

The following simple exercise will help you to see things from their perspective. If you find they're right and your life *is* out of balance, you have some decisions to make regarding your approach to family caregiving.

KEEPING LIFE IN BALANCE WORKSHEET

(This worksheet is also available online at www.elderindustry.com)

1. With pencil in hand, draw lines to divide a piece of paper into three columns.
2. Write the name of your elder at the top of the first column; then write the words *Family* and *Personal Interests* above the other two columns.
3. For the next two weeks, keep a list of all of the things you do for yourself and others, and record your actions in the appropriate columns. For example, if you took Mom grocery shopping, put the activity in her column. If you went to the gym, put the activity in the Personal Interest column, and so on.
4. At the end of the two weeks, count the number of activities in each column.
5. Ask yourself: *Is my elder column out of balance with the others? Are my family members' and friends' complaints justified?*

PLAN THREE

Acknowledge special needs.

If you are a caregiver to a person who has Alzheimer's disease, *you* have special needs. You have the responsibility of making numerous decisions for your elder throughout the day—what to wear, when to go to bed, when to bathe. Every decision is yours. **Dementia care** is exhausting; choosing to take on this level of care requires major lifestyle changes for you. Sadly, friends and family may drop out of sight, and you may spend most of your time going it alone. If you have decided that you are up to the task, you are choosing to join the ranks of thousands of family caregivers who are in a similar situation. If you're feeling overwhelmed and isolated, you may want to join a support group (there are plenty online if you can't leave the house for an extended period of time) and consider adult day services a few days a week.

PLAN FOUR

Realize it's not about you.

Most of us take criticism very personally. And when our elders say things like *"You're stupid. Can't you do anything right?"* we may take it as truth. Ornery, rude, and downright mean at times, elderly people have been known to lash out with the nastiest one-liners.

Successful caregivers have learned not to take criticisms from their elders personally. They do so by keeping the following thoughts in mind.

> *It's not about me; it's a reflection of what's going on inside of them.*
>
> *I'm the target of the moment.*
>
> *They're somehow trying to get their power needs met by pulling me down a few pegs.*
>
> *Their impatience is out of proportion.*
>
> *They are angry and taking it out on me.*
>
> *Am I doing the best I can in this situation?*
>
> *Is there an opportunity for me to improve the way I'm doing something for them?*
>
> *Is there a good laugh in all this?*

An adult's abusive behavior has many roots. Fear and depression may be masked by expressions of hostility, impatience, and aggression. A medical examination may reveal a condition that can be treated. Ask yourself the following questions. If the answer to any of them is yes, call the doctor.

Is this person . . .

> *in physical discomfort or pain?*
>
> *forgetful?*
>
> *recovering from a recent fall?*
>
> *grieving over the loss of a close friend or family member?*
>
> *abusing drugs or alcohol?*
>
> *eating properly?*
>
> *having trouble seeing or hearing?*
>
> *mismanaging or reacting to medications?*

PLAN FIVE

⧉ Put self-respecting practices in motion.

While you are trying to be a concerned caregiver, others may be acting out their pains and frustrations on you. **If situations get out of hand, seek professional counseling**.

Here are a few ways to handle explosive caregiving environments.

Self-respecting caregivers get angry.

Caregiving and anger go hand in hand, and the root of *our* anger comes from a variety of sources, including unresolved family conflicts, our elders' irritating habits and personality traits, differences in opinion about what is needed, and degrees of difficulty in caregiving, to name a few. When we admit to ourselves that we are angry, and acknowledge the right to be angry, we don't compromise our self-worth.

Self-respecting caregivers express their anger in ways that teach others how we want them to treat us. Suffering in silence implies our consent for others to treat us badly. We cannot change the basic personalities of people, but we must try to put a stop to any inappropriate behavior toward us. Expressing our anger may include statements such as:

> *What you just did (said) makes me angry. I do not deserve that.*
>
> *It makes me angry when you . . . Please stop it.*
>
> *My bedroom is private, and it makes me angry when you walk in without knocking.*
>
> *I'm angry that you didn't keep your commitment. I rearranged my schedule.*
>
> *We're all adults here, and your criticism is not appropriate.*

Self-respecting caregivers set boundaries.

Verbally abusive people pick on certain people because they are easy targets. Don't make yourself available. There is no disgrace in walking out of a situation that is intolerable or beyond your power to handle; in fact, it is the smart thing to do when you recognize your own limitations.

Before you enter into a conversation, make a decision ahead of time on what you can and cannot realistically accomplish. Set limits. Screen your calls, and let the answering machine pick up every once in a while. Stick to your plans. Limit your contact. Stay at a hotel rather than at your elder's place. Make visits short. You are not obligated to tell your elder everything you do. If you need time away, tell him or her you're not feeling very well and cannot come over today.

Self-respecting caregivers say no.

We may think that the more we say yes, the more we will be loved and appreciated. The truth is that when someone close to us loves us, love doesn't stop because we've said no. Saying yes when we need to say no causes burnout.

People around us will always make requests. They have the right to ask, and we have the right to refuse. You owe it to yourself (eventually, you'll believe this), to turn down requests. Sure, you might feel guilty afterward, but don't let that stop you. Practice these techniques:

No; but I could do this . . .

Yes, I'll help, and here's how [when] I'll help . . .

Yes, I can; however, this is how I plan to do it.

Yes; but all I can spare is an hour of my time. I hope you understand.

No, I can't help now; but maybe I can do it another time.

I'm sorry. I already have plans. If only I had known.

I'm really sorry I can't help; but let me suggest [name another person].

Mom, it would help me a lot if you would ask [sibling] to take you shopping.

I know I'm going to disappoint you, but I've decided to . . .

I enjoyed doing that with you the past few times, but I can't do it this time.

Self-respecting caregivers allow others to be angry.

As caregivers, we must be prepared for the fact that people will get angry at us for some of the things we say and do. There's no getting around this, so allow them the opportunity to express their anger. Don't defend; don't interrupt; let them vent. This may sound strange, but we might even ask for forgiveness. Asking for forgiveness is not an admission of guilt; it can be an effective way to calm the waters in the moment. Here are the words to say:

I'm really sorry I disappointed you.

I know you're upset, and I'm sorry.

I realize you're angry, and I'm really sorry.

Self-respecting caregivers have emotional outlets.

As discussed elsewhere in this chapter, telephone calls to friends, support groups, keeping a journal, writing angry letters (and not mailing them), physical activity, exercise, respite care, and therapy sessions are a few of the techniques that caregivers can draw upon to express their emotions honestly, and without fear of retaliation.

PLAN SIX

Loosen the grip of caregiver guilt.

I know how busy you are at work; don't bother about me. This calculated comment is an example of a manipulative technique that elders may use when they are scared, lonely, depressed, in pain, or angry, and it can send family caregivers into an instant frenzy of guilt, hurt, blame, and resentment. **Erroneous self-talk:** *I'm worthless; I don't do enough.*

If I had taken Mom to the doctor sooner, she wouldn't be so sick now. Total care is unrealistic and unattainable, and when situations fall short of our expectations, we see ourselves as failures. **Erroneous self-talk:** *I'm not good enough.*

I'm being torn apart. When we're at the gym, we're not with our children. When we're out with friends, we're not at the side of our elder. When we're with our elder, we're not with our spouse or partner. When we're on vacation, we're away from it all. **Erroneous self-talk:** *I'm a bad person.*

Guilt is our constant companion. No matter what we do, no matter how much we give, no matter what happens, no matter how much we know, no matter where we are—the guilt remains. And it's painful. But when we're in physical pain, we don't just sit there, do we? Chances are good that we take action to relieve our physical pain. The good news is we can do the same for the negative impact of psychological pain. Make a conscious choice to manage the stirring guilt and its negative impact on the quality of life by heeding these suggestions.

Praise yourself.

Erroneous self-talk: *I'm a real jerk for getting mad at Aunt Mary.* When we make a statement like this, we are overidentifying with our perceived shortcomings. Over time, self-attack will wear you down. Step back and ask yourself, "Am I feeling bad about something I *did*, or about *myself?*" **Focus on what you *did*, rather than who you are, and give yourself full recognition for all that you do for others.**

Eliminate "musts," "shoulds," "ought to's," and "have to's."

Erroneous self-talk: *I should be doing more; after all, Mom took care of me.* Take a hard look at everything you've done so far to make this person or situation change. Has spending more time, energy, or money made a difference? Has anything worked? Perhaps it has, but you're still feeling tormented by your perception that it's not enough. Many caregivers engage in fantasies by wishing or imagining things were different.

Nothing you do will ever be enough in this situation. Under this layer of guilt is grief. We cannot hide from the fact that we will soon live in a world without our loved one—that is the ultimate reality, and we are powerless to avoid this end. **Staying "in the moment"— focusing on maximizing the quality of the time spent together—may be the best you can realistically strive for**.

Feel regretful, rather than guilty.

Erroneous self-talk: *I feel so bad about not visiting Mom.* When you feel guilty for things you *aren't* doing, shift the focus from feeling bad to taking action. Ask yourself, "Am I doing the best that I can right now?" If the answer is no, take one small step toward doing something.

Don't take the bait.

An effective response to someone using manipulative behavior is "Are you trying to make me feel guilty?"

Restate your objective.

Self-talk: Do I *have* to do this, or am I *choosing* to do this? There may be several ways to address a situation. Free yourself to explore all the alternatives.

Acknowledge hurt feelings.

In the process of caregiving, we are bound to make somebody mad at us for something. It goes with the territory. Guilt is our conscience's way of letting us know we should make amends after we do something hurtful. Accept responsibility for misdeeds, and say you're sorry.

Learn from your mistakes.

We cannot always undo harm we may have unknowingly caused; but we can vow to treat others more thoughtfully in the future. Learn to forgive yourself again and again and again.

In the Future . . .

Watch what you say.

Resist the temptation to make open-ended promises. Some caregivers believe that making promises to their elders is a loving, thoughtful thing to do; but this is usually self-destructive in the long run. For example, imagine how guilty you might feel if you promised to visit your aunt every weekend, but last-minute job assignments render your scheduled visits impossible. Or perhaps Mom once asked you to promise never to put her in a nursing home, yet today skilled nursing care happens to be the best care alternative for her well-being. Too many promises serve as a quick fix to uncomfortable feelings and can raise our guilt sky-high later on.

To avoid generating this kind of guilt, **offer commitments rather than promises**. When you speak in terms of commitments, you're giving assurances that you'll be there for the long haul. Here are some words to say when promises cannot, and should not, be offered.

> *When the time comes, I hope I will be able to do what you wish.*
> *I will always be here to talk with you about solutions to problems.*
> *You're not alone. I'm here for you.*
> *I'll always care about you, and together we'll figure this out.*

Prepare, anticipate.

Clear your conscience ahead of time. Do your homework, research options, talk things over, and you'll rest comfortably knowing your decisions were based on the best information available to you at the time.

PLAN SEVEN

⟩⟩ Put up a good fight—don't let siblings off the hook.

One unfortunate truth about caregiving is that the responsibilities within the family are often unevenly and unfairly distributed. The amount of assistance we receive from siblings is largely dependent on our willingness and ability to *demand* it. Ask for help from time to time, but move on to something more productive if other family members refuse. Keep this thought in the back of your mind: When you put your head down on your pillow each night knowing that you have done all you can, the rest will fall into place.

Why siblings don't do their share of eldercare is a more complicated issue than you may think. *Everyone* contributes to the problem.

THE PARENT . . .
wants only this child to care for him or her
lets sons off the hook and instructs daughters that it's their "duty"
drives wedges between children and plays favorites

THE FAMILY CAREGIVER . . .
doesn't ask for help; rather, he or she hints or complains
isn't willing to share the parent's attention with other family members
wants to prove that he or she is the good, always-giving child
feels only he or she can do the best job
thinks it takes too much time to explain what is needed
accepts without question that caregiving is "woman's work"
doesn't have any energy left to argue

THE SIBLING . . .
denies what's happening and chooses to ignore the situation
lives far away
has his or her own major problems and is incapable of being helpful at this time
wants to get back at you for any number of reasons
is focused on after-death issues, including inheritance

Here are a variety of tips to encourage siblings to pitch in. Try several, or just one, but just do something.

Speak up.
Are you *assuming* your siblings know what's going on and *why* you need their help? They may have no idea or understanding of the gravity of a particular situation. Be specific and share details.

Don't complain; request.

Discuss schedules. Set limits on the time and effort you can put in. Give specific assignments. Instead of "You never help out . . . ," say, "I know you have a lot going on at work and it's hard for you, it's hard for me, too, and I need help with [bill paying, grocery shopping, cooking]," or "Which one works better with your schedule? Mom needs a ride to the doctor and needs help grocery shopping."

Fill the distance gap.

Be specific with siblings who live far away. Chances are they don't know *how* to help. Ask them to call your parents on a regular basis; do research on options and services; make service arrangements; send money as a way of being helpful; suggest that parents stay with them once in a while.

Consult your siblings.

When important decisions need to be made, don't accept "You do what's best" as an answer. The decision-making burden is not entirely yours. Ask for specific involvement on your siblings' part. Instead of saying, "What should we do?" try "Do you think we should hire a home-care nurse or look into an assisted-living facility?"

Call their bluff.

When siblings criticize, don't argue or defend your position about how you're handling your elder's affairs. When they say, "You should take Mom to the doctor more often," agree with them (that lets the air out of their argument), and say, "You may be right, and much better at this than me. Why don't you take over this responsibility?" If the bullying persists, bring in a heavyweight. Ask a geriatric case manager or a lawyer to join the next family discussion.

Stay flexible.

There is more than one single or simple answer to every eldercare problem. People are unique and bring to the caregiving situation different life experiences, values, abilities, preferences, relationships, and needs. When your siblings do things differently from you, let them do it their way. Give some of their suggestions a try, and let them know when things work for the better.

Stay on them.

When siblings drop the ball, get on the phone immediately and say, "Three weeks ago, we agreed that you would help Dad with his laundry, and you have not done so. What will help you keep this commitment?" Make them as accountable as you.

Refuse to be anyone's middleman.

Train parents and siblings to talk with each other directly. You are not a messenger. When parents want another child to call, they may say *to you,* "I haven't heard from Linda. Is she all right?" Or a sibling may ask you, "How's Dad feeling?" Take yourself out of the middle by saying,

"I really can't answer for Dad; it's best if you ask him yourself. Why don't you give him a call?" At the same time, remember that you're not in charge of their relationships. Avoid telling siblings how to act and what to do by not saying things like "Don't upset Mom by talking about moving."

Cut loose.

Don't allow yourself to be drawn back into childhood stereotypes. Be the responsible adult you are in all of your other relationships. When fighting erupts, focus on issues, not people. Don't react when someone else brings up ancient family history; it's not worth your energy. Stop apologizing for having a different opinion.

Let your parents do the talking.

Next time Mom asks you to drive her somewhere, tell her you'd love to but already have plans with your family. Suggest that she asks [name other sibling] to drive her. Don't make the call for her; let her do it herself. Siblings may have a tougher time rejecting a parent's direct request for help.

Consider mediation.

Decisions about parent care revive conflicts in adult siblings. If all else fails, eldercare mediation is a type of dispute resolution process that is effective when family members have a difficult time reaching a decision among themselves on what is needed and resolving differences. Resources for mediation services are listed at the end of the "Communicaring" chapter.

PLAN EIGHT

Conduct a family meeting.

Do your siblings assume that because you are single you have all the time in the world to care for aging parents? Are your sisters and brothers better off financially yet never contribute to eldercare expenses? Do you fear for your parents' future well-being and don't know where to start?

Parent care is complex and time-consuming, and family meetings can be an efficient and effective way to deal with family caregiving issues.

There are many benefits to family meetings. Perhaps you're worried about a parent's situation and looking to brainstorm caregiving ideas. Or you may be feeling overwhelmed and a meeting will create an opportunity to invite others to share the care. Whatever the case may be, all sorts of family issues come up—old ones and new ones—and family squabbles are common.

Who should attend?

Limit the meeting to people who are directly affected by the situation. If your spouse expresses a desire to be included, then by all means extend an invitation to him or her. If you suspect that the topic is going to be heated, invite a neutral moderator, such as a long-time family friend or a professional mediator or social worker who specializes in older-adult issues.

Should parents be invited?
The first meeting usually takes place without parents present. The goal is to create a plan of action to work together as a team, or, if nothing else, call a temporary truce to a family feud.

Before the Meeting

Decide together when and where to hold meetings. Whether you choose an office, a restaurant, or someone's home, decide on a setting that presents few distractions. Families often find that meeting after sharing a meal together is conducive to a congenial atmosphere. Create a plan to include those who are unable to attend—a speakerphone, conference calling, and computer conferencing are a few options.

Agree to a specific timetable. What time will the meeting begin and end? Often a series of shorter meetings are more productive than one long meeting.

Decide on a goal for each meeting. A narrow focus works best. Prioritizing issues up front ensures that critical matters are given full attention.

Acquire current factual information. For example, if you plan to discuss long-term care, have on hand financial, insurance, and legal data, obtain medical and psychiatric prognosis information, and know the costs of eldercare-related services.

Working Together

Establish meeting ground rules. Everyone deserves respect. Here are some ways to ensure that no one feels slighted.

- Establish a policy regarding interruptions, including cell-phone usage.
- Allow everyone no more than ten minutes to state concerns and points of view—use a timer, if need be. No interrupting.
- There should also be no insults or derogatory remarks, and absolutely no yelling.
- Stick to the agreed-upon timetable.

Agree on a facilitator to lead the meeting, and designate someone to take notes. Open the meeting by restating the agreed-upon agenda. As people consent to specific actions, record what they have agreed to do. Keep in mind that agreements can be made on a time-limited basis. Summarize plans and options and reach consensus before moving on to the next topic.

A productive meeting ends with a recap of the issues and any decisions made. Set a date for the next meeting, if needed.

Establish a plan to stay in touch. Exchange phone numbers and e-mail. Perhaps the family computer wizard will create a family website in order to make it easy to coordinate schedules and keep everyone updated.

Low-Cost and Free Resources

Type the following keywords in your Internet search browser for information and resources on **anger issues:** "anger management," "anger clinics," "anger and caregiving," and "anger and eldercare."

A keyword search on your Internet browser will unearth a multitude of websites on the topic of spirituality and offer many ideas on pursuing a more **spiritual caregiving life:** retreat centers, spiritual directors, holistic wellness, spiritual places, spirituality and aging, and proprioceptive writing.

ORGANIZATIONS AND WEB RESOURCES

Anger Clinic
29 S. La Salle Street
Chicago, IL 60603-1507
(312) 263-0035
Website: www.angerclinic.com

ElderCare Online
Website: www.ec-online.net

Families for Depression Awareness
Website: www.familyaware.org

Caregiving and Spirituality

Beliefnet
Website: www.beliefnet.com

Sacred Art of Living
Website: www.sacredartofliving.org

Veriditas
(To find labyrinth locations)
Website: www.veriditas.org

Wayne E. Oates Institute
1733 Bardstown Road
Louisville, KY 40205
(502) 459-2370
Website: http://oates.org/institute

Support Groups

CareCommunity
(Support for caregivers who are caring for
someone with a severe or life-limiting
illness)
Website: www.mycarecommunity.org

Caregiver's Home Companion
Website: www.caregivershome.com

Caregiving.com
Website: www.caregiving.com

Children of Aging Parents
PO Box 167
Richboro, PA 18954
Toll-free: (800) 227-7294
Website: www.caps4caregivers.org

**Family Caregiver Alliance / LGBT Caregiver
  Discussion Group**
Website: www.caregiver.org

National Hopeline Network
Website: www.hopeline.com

Rosalynn Carter Institute for Caregiving
800 GSW Drive
Georgia Southwestern State University
Americus, GA 31709-4379
(229) 928-1234
Website: www.rosalynncarter.org

Work-Life Resources

BenefitsLink
1298 Minnesota Avenue, Suite H
Winter Park, FL 32789
(407) 644-4146
Website: www.benefitslink.com

BR Anchor
(Promoting the welfare of relocating
families)

4596 Capital Dome Drive
Jacksonville, FL 32246
(904) 641-1140
Website: www.branchor.com

Families and Work Institute
267 5th Avenue, Floor 2
New York, NY 10016
(212) 465-2044
Website: www.familiesandwork.org

**International Association of Workforce
    Professionals**
1801 Louisville Road
Frankfort, KY 40601
Toll-free: (888) 898-9960
(502) 223-4459
Website: www.iawponline.org

Managing Work & Family
Website: www.mwfam.com

**National Working Caregivers Resource
    Center**
Website: www.americanbusinesscares.net

Joy Loverde Website
Website: www.elderindustry.com

WFC Resources
5197 Beachside Drive
Minnetonka, MN 55343
(952) 936-7898; toll-free: (800)
    487-7898
Website: www.workfamily.com

Working Caregiver
Website: www.workingcaregiver.com

WorkLife Law
Website: www.worklifelaw.org

BE KIND TO YOURSELF ACTION CHECKLIST

(This worksheet is also available online at www.elderindustry.com)

TAKE CARE OF YOU	To Do By	Completed
Create self-care goals		
short-term	_____	☐
long-term	_____	☐
Monitor caregiver stress	_____	☐
Assess caregiver involvement to avoid burnout	_____	☐
Plan for caregiver relief		
schedule days off	_____	☐
join a support group	_____	☐
take a vacation	_____	☐
maintain personal interests	_____	☐
use community respite programs	_____	☐
Monitor sleeping patterns	_____	☐
Explore company work-life programs	_____	☐

CAREGIVING: THE SPIRITUAL JOURNEY

	To Do By	Completed
Acknowledge the emotional wilderness of caregiving	_____	☐
Tap into spiritual tools and strategies		
prayer	_____	☐
meditation	_____	☐
joy	_____	☐
music	_____	☐
labyrinth	_____	☐
counseling	_____	☐
journaling	_____	☐
nature	_____	☐
spiritual places	_____	☐

body work ☐
body movement ☐

Practice spirituality daily _____ ☐

SELF-TALK: FINDING PEACE OF MIND

Learn from other caregivers _____ ☐

Protect important relationships _____ ☐

**Acknowledge the special needs
  of dementia caregiving** _____ ☐

**Establish a self-respecting
  caregiving environment** _____ ☐

Review probability of

physical pain _____ ☐
psychological issues _____ ☐
alcohol and drug abuse _____ ☐
depression _____ ☐
nutrition _____ ☐
grief _____ ☐
visual or hearing impairments _____ ☐
reactions to medications _____ ☐

Put self-respecting practices in motion

acknowledge and express anger _____ ☐
set boundaries _____ ☐
say no _____ ☐
allow others to be angry _____ ☐
create healthy emotional outlets _____ ☐

Loosen the grip of caregiver guilt

self-praise _____ ☐
eliminate self-pressures _____ ☐
regret rather than guilt _____ ☐
resist taking the bait _____ ☐
state caregiving objectives _____ ☐

acknowledge hurt feelings   _____   ❑
learn and move on   _____   ❑

**Speak your mind with
  uncooperative siblings**   _____   ❑

Consider family mediator   _____   ❑

Conduct a family meeting   _____   ❑

4

Communicaring

Take a Deep Breath and Jump In

Talking about eldercare issues and planning for the future isn't easy. Who wants to hash over such unpleasant topics as illness and funeral arrangements when older family members seem perfectly fine? You may have been avoiding talking altogether, afraid that the conversation will be upsetting for you and for them. And you're right. However, taking the easy road now and avoiding eldercare discussions will eventually backfire when complex problems reveal themselves and the emotional (and financial) stability of the entire family is on shaky ground.

When is the best time to initiate eldercare planning conversations? *Right now*—especially if your elders are mentally competent and have the ability to make choices and decisions, and crises aren't raining down on everyone. People don't realize that many of the "emergencies" they end up confronting could have been avoided by *planning*. Devising an effective caregiving plan requires ongoing, thoughtful communication among all parties.

Whether you realize it or not, you already have many of the skills needed for handling eldercare conversations effectively. For example, if you've ever held a job and had to manage others, if you've ever parented a child, or if you've negotiated with someone to get them to do things your way, you used the same techniques that will now help get your point across as you talk about sensitive subjects with others.

Proactive conversations, initiated early on, are easier on everybody. This section of *The Complete Eldercare Planner* will help you take that first communication step—paying attention to *how* we talk with each other will not only save time and energy, it also may result in strengthening family ties.

TAKE A DEEP BREATH AND JUMP IN

- If you're waiting for your elders to announce, "Now's the time to talk about making plans for the future," forget it.
- No matter how much love and trust exists, there will be communication pitfalls and obstacles.
- A little empathy goes a long way during eldercare conversations.
- Caregiver guilt is such a powerful force that you may feel guilty about not feeling guilty.

Older adults think about the future more than you may realize.

OBJECTIVES

*After completing **"Take a Deep Breath and Jump In,"** you will be able to:*

Gain a better understanding of underlying issues such as loss and the need for control and independence.

Maintain a healthy balance of caregiver-elder responsibilities.

Encourage elders to be accountable for their actions.

Use timing to your advantage.

PLAN ONE

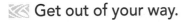 Get out of your way.

What do older adults worry about? The following issues keep people up at night:

1. Running out of money or being scammed
2. Having no purpose in life
3. Loneliness
4. Elder abuse and neglect
5. Burdening someone else with a chronic illness
6. Moving out of the family home

While we may personally know people who fear the day their money well runs dry, the psychological struggles associated with living a nonpurposeful life may not be as well known or understood. Feeling unwanted and unneeded in society is one of the greatest losses someone can experience on a day-to-day basis, and consequently is one of the root causes of illness and depression. Fear of becoming a crime victim has its effect on an elder's willingness to ask for or accept help from people outside the family, or even to venture outdoors. The onset of a chronic illness may be a turning point for elders because their ability to sustain an independent lifestyle may be compromised. Meeting the demands of home ownership may ultimately force an unwanted move.

Surveys consistently confirm that **people want to be in control of their own lives** for as long as possible. The more we family caregivers remain sensitive to our elders' basic needs and wants, the better the odds of keeping the lines of communication open.

The issue is loss.

With aging comes a loss of one kind or another. As older people face dwindling abilities, we, too, deal with our own version of loss. This is especially true when we find ourselves managing the care of parents who once took care and parented us. Acknowledging the complex issues of loss and initiating conversations early on can avert many a crisis down the road.

The word *independence* covers a lot of ground. On a personal level, older adults want to manage their own basic activities of living, such as cooking, personal grooming, and driving a car. Problems fester the moment the ability to handle basic functions begins to decline and they refuse to ask others for assistance.

While some people accept the loss of their abilities and make necessary adjustments, others may struggle with a vengeance. Denial and resistance in the face of loss is *your* challenge as a communicator and caregiver. Every eldercare-related conversation *you* initiate—regardless of the subject matter or our apparent motivation—may be interpreted by the other person as a threat to his or her already perceived sense of dwindling independence.

Preserve autonomy.

Basic personality patterns and traits don't change over time; they may in fact intensify and become exaggerated in later years. As time passes, our elders become more the person they already are. There's no generalizing when it comes to the average older adult. Genetics, life experiences, diet, exercise, fundamental beliefs, and living environments are contributing factors on how people age.

Eldercare is defined by *ability*, not age. Everybody ages differently. Grandpa may be adept at ninety-five while seventy-year-old Aunt Alice requires round-the-clock care. The most effective family discussions focus on what elders *can* do, rather than what they *can't* do. Empowering them to make good use of the abilities they have lessens caregiving demands on you.

Assuming that we already know what's in the minds of our elders will also put undue strains on relationships. When we listen to them, we hear their life history, including every choice and every decision they've made, and we have no way of realistically plugging into that history. The more we listen to what our elders tell us they need and want and the more we can assure them of our respect for their autonomy, the goal of getting them to do what's best for the entire family becomes more attainable.

Establish trust every time.

Every eldercare conversation is subject to a communication breakdown. Conversations can come to a screeching halt at any time and when you least expect it. Every conversation is tainted with the underlying theme of our elders' need for independence; keeping the trust factor high requires us to assure them time after time that our motive is not to "take away" what is rightfully theirs. To better accomplish this goal, listen more than you speak, and ask more questions. You can be a better communicator when you resist the temptation to offer unsolicited advice. When circumstances dictate that the caregiving situation requires a more aggressive communication approach, you will likely know when the timing is right to do so.

Quit scaring yourself.

It's best not to jump to conclusions about dementia if Mom forgets your birthday and Uncle Charlie tells the same joke over and over again. Momentary forgetfulness can at times be a manifestation of other issues, such as mismanagement of medications or a symptom of depression. A medical exam and formal diagnosis from a health-care professional is the only true way to separate fact from fears of what *could* be happening. Make no assumptions when it comes to your elder's physical and mental status.

Do your homework.

Before initiating any conversations, get the facts and gather resources. The more you know about the family's options, community services, and related costs, the more depth you can add to important discussions. Being informed increases your effectiveness as a communicator.

PLAN TWO

≪ Honor thy father and thy mother.

When discussions between a parent and an adult child take place, each person enters the conversation from a distinctly different point of view. Being sensitive to existing parent-child roles and the natural differences between these two relationships will help make interactions with parents go more smoothly.

Conflicting Understanding of Responsibilities

Watching a parent age is a poignant experience and can suddenly trigger irrational fears that decline, or even death, may be right around the corner. We may one day realize that Dad's hair is pure white, for example, or we may observe from a distance that Mom is having difficulty climbing the stairs to her second-floor bedroom. The more fearful we become about our parents' future well-being, the more we make our best attempts to hold back time and make statements such as, "Mom, if you sell the house and move closer to me, we can spend more time together," or "Dad, are you sure you're feeling up to mowing the lawn?" Below the surface, however, we may be struggling with their mortality and having thoughts such as, "When did you get to be so old?" and "You're the parent; you're supposed to take care of *me*," and "I don't want anything to happen to you."

The fact that we will live life without our parents may race through our minds, and at the same time we don't want to believe it is true. Consequently we may believe that our perceived role as the adult child is to shelter and protect our parents from harm of all kinds.

Parents, on the other hand, may operate from a completely different set of attitudes. When they tell us they "don't want to be a burden," they sincerely believe that staying out of our way is the *right* thing to do. Unfortunately, they are also unaware of the serious consequences of being extremely independent-minded. Maintaining independence at an advanced age often requires some level of assistance from others, and resistance to help of any kind can carve a destructive path.

Partnering, Not Parenting

We've been raised to prize independence and individualism, yet in a fundamental way we *are* dependent—on others. We're better together, and need each other in order to meet our needs. The objective of parent-adult child eldercare conversations is to encourage mutually responsible partnerships. *Partnering with,* rather than *parenting,* our parents is the desired approach.

As long as our parents remain mentally able to make their own decisions, we must appreciate the limits of the parent-child relationship. Many adult children have learned the hard way that attempts to impose their opinions, values, and authority on their parents will begin a downward spiral in the communication process, leading to a breakdown in the relationship as a whole.

When we focus our conversation style on influencing parents to seek and accept help from others, and keep them accountable for their own choices, they can remain true to their independent ideals.

PLAN THREE

Try these for openers.

There's no better time than right now to open up a dialogue. If you're feeling scared and apprehensive, that's normal. In time, you'll get the hang of it.

Seize the moment.
Your elders may not be accustomed to asking for help directly and may mask problems by dropping hints. For instance, worries about the cost of medications may be referenced in statements such as "My neighbor is paying close to one thousand dollars a month for prescriptions!" Or they may insist that they are financially sound but complain constantly about the price of tomatoes.

Any conversations *they* initiate—especially when it comes to the subject of their money—present an opening for you to start talking. The best approach to creating a real dialogue in a nonthreatening fashion is to speak in questions. Here are some examples:

How do you suppose your neighbor is coming up with the money to pay for medications?

How can anyone afford prescription drugs these days?

How would you handle the situation if you were in her shoes?

The cost of groceries has me on a pretty tight budget, too. How do you handle it?

Also take advantage of family situations that come up naturally—a death in the family, the onset of an illness, a relative's divorce. During these times, people are more inclined to be thinking about their own mortality and financial issues and, consequently, such occasions provide a natural opportunity to ask what they are doing, *if anything*, about the particular situations under discussion.

Similarly, an approaching birthday or holiday may be the perfect time to offer gifts of service. You might say, *"Dad, I'd love to get you a year's worth of housekeeping for your birthday. May I?"*

Plant the seed.

If the opportunity to start an eldercare conversation doesn't present itself, and you want to get things started, create your own. Clip a current newspaper article that reports a growing eldercare issue, like long-term care. Read the article and highlight important sentences. Mail the article with a personal note, or next time you visit your elder hand him or her the article and say, *"I didn't realize that in-home services are not covered by Medicare. Did you? What are your thoughts on this?"* Clipping articles works especially well if the person you want to talk with is your parent. Remember, in your parents' eyes, you're still "their child," and news articles can well serve as an authority figure when you, by yourself, are not considered as such.

Ask for advice.

Soliciting advice from our elders is an effective way to open up a dialogue. It makes them feel needed and appreciated for their years of experience, rather than threatened. You can say, *"Dad, I'm just beginning to think about planning for my own retirement, and it looks like you're doing pretty well. Do you have any tips for me?"* Here are a few more openers:

I'm getting around to creating my will. How did you go about doing yours?

I've always admired the way you . . . Do you have any suggestions for me?

I've been clearing out my basement. Is donating items to charity a good idea?

Do you think buying life insurance is right for me?

I want to get your opinion about . . .

How would you do this if you were me?

Fish for information.

Gradually losing the ability to perform basic tasks and functions such as buttoning a shirt or climbing stairs would make anyone feel anxious. In fact, spouses may even cover for each other, and you may never *really* know what's going on behind the scenes.

Greeting your elders with a mindless "How are you?" will almost guarantee a knee-jerk response. To dig a little deeper on issues or problems they may be confronting, try this:

Hello. It's so good to hear from you [see you]. What's new in your neck of the woods?
What have you been up to lately?
How's the world treating you?

Turn the tables.

Relationships between children and parents are not static. We adult children may vacillate between a desire to be treated as adults and yet long for the time of innocence when we were sheltered by parents. On the other hand, our parents may see us in one context as advisers, and, in another, as naive children who still rely on their wisdom and experience.

Instead of getting defensive when Mom attempts to nurture you in her old familiar ways by saying, "Honey, are you sure you're eating right?" or "You work too much," think again. Take advantage of this natural bond by asking them to help *you*. You can say:

Dad, there may come a time when I will need to know where you keep your important papers. Just in case something happens, can you help me with this now?

Mom, I don't need to know the details of your life savings, but I should know what you would want me to do in case anything ever happened to you. Can you help me with this?

I'm exhausted after working all day, and coming here after work is wearing me out. I'd like to hire someone to help me out with some of these chores, so we can spend more time doing the fun things we used to do together. What do you think?

Give them an assignment.

Maybe Dad doesn't see the need to purchase long-term care insurance, yet you're convinced that an insurance policy will protect his financial stability. One way to encourage him to consider this option is to ask him to investigate it on your behalf. Tell him you're swamped at work and ask if he would go to the library or explore the Internet to research insurance carriers and policies on your behalf. When he presents you with his findings, ask him what he would do if he were in your shoes. You're both bound to learn a lot.

Ask a favor.

If you're concerned that Mom is letting the yard work slide, and she won't let anybody help her, you can say, *"Mom, I need a favor. Will you let Billy rake the leaves so he'll learn some responsibility?"*

Asking elders to help *us* accomplishes two important goals. It gives them a sense of purpose within the family and helps them feel needed and important; it also creates a nonthreatening approach to talking about potentially explosive subjects. Who knows, you might actually enjoy letting them parent *you* for a change—and sometimes that's *exactly* what you'll need.

PLAN FOUR

❧ Use surefire talking tips.

Adjust your communication approach to fit the current situation, but your objective should always be the same: **Keep your elders involved in their own decisions and account-able for words and actions**. Timing is everything. Consider the important factors in the following checklist before initiating any conversation.

Setting the Stage: Talking Tips Checklist

- Am I overtired or stressed out right now? (Be sure you've had a good night's sleep.)
- Is it better to approach my parents together, or am I likely to accomplish more talking with each of them one-on-one?
- Is my elder a morning person or a night owl? Is *this* the best time to approach him or her?
- Do I have time *now* to get involved in a long and possibly serious discussion?
- Should I have *this* conversation in person rather than over the phone?
- Do I have enough information on this issue to discuss it intelligently, or do I need to do more homework?

Maintain control of the place and time to talk.

When the time is not right, you know it. Nothing you say is well received and nothing you suggest is accepted. You're on the defensive and silently asking yourself, "How can I get out of this situation fast?"

As a rule, when families get together to celebrate occasions such as weddings, anniversaries, birthday parties, and seasonal holidays, it is not an ideal time to talk about eldercare. Family gatherings revive old family patterns, and uninterrupted conversations are practically impossible. Worse yet, siblings who are not on the same page as you regarding parent care may purposely sabotage your intentions. Instead, use your time together to look proactively for warning signs that problems may exist, without expecting to *resolve* them. Review "How to Tell When Your Elder Needs Help" in chapter 2 of *The Complete Eldercare Planner,* starting on page 33.

If your elder approaches *you,* and you know the timing isn't right, postpone the conversation. Listen for a minute, then say, *"I'm really glad you're telling me this, and it's important to me, too. Can we continue this when we both have uninterrupted time to talk?"* or *"I want to give this my full attention. Can we talk about this very soon?"* Then set a date so you won't put it off.

Ease into conversations.

Your being ready to talk about eldercare issues doesn't mean that your elder is. The problems he or she may be facing may be too threatening to confront right now. It may take several attempts before you're able to engage in a meaningful eldercare-related conversation. Be patient. If he or she says everything is fine when you know it's not, let that be okay for a little while. Sit on it for a week or two, and try again. Here are some gentle opening lines when probing for information:

> *You sound upset. Is something bothering you?*
>
> *There's something you'd like to talk about, isn't there?*
>
> *Please tell me more about what you just said. I'm not sure I understand completely.*

Give them your full attention.

If your elders respond positively to your line of questioning, listen patiently. Silence, as Winston Churchill once said, "enhances one's authority." When they start talking, resist interrupting. If they feel that you're really listening, and understanding what they have to say, they will most likely tell you more. Don't rush to fill in gaps of silence when your elder pauses. **Silence is a powerful communications tool**.

To get into specifics, ask specific questions.

When conversations are in full swing, you'll hear statements that seem impractical, senseless, and even perilous. They may tell you about their plans to drive cross country alone or that they're thinking about buying a bigger house. During such conversations, you may feel a strong urge to argue and give suggestions, opinions, and unsolicited advice.

A word of warning: Offer your opinion and you're likely to hear the words "You're trying to run my life." If you attempt to talk them out of their plans, they may turn their back on you. Also, well-intended advice may backfire if they take you up on *your* ideas and then things don't work out as you had hoped. The trust established between you can disappear in a flash.

A steady stream of suggestions and unsolicited advice makes people feel judged and foolish. And once they've had enough of being told what to do, they may build up enough defenses to cut off any further discussions. Trying to steer conversations your way is not a good use of time.

Asking questions *facilitates* conversations and also helps avert relationship breakdowns. The objective of this approach is not to resolve problems but to open up an area of inquiry that keeps the other person accountable. Here are a few questions that will help elders to think things through more thoroughly:

> *Can you tell me more about your plans?*
>
> *How do you plan to accomplish what you want?*
>
> *Have you thought about other options if your plans don't work out?*
>
> *How do you think your plans are going to affect the rest of the family?*
>
> *What makes you think that?*
>
> *How did you come to this conclusion?*

Offer limited assistance.

Some people never ask for help, while others may ask for too much assistance as a way to get attention. Going overboard by being too helpful can establish an unhealthy dependence. Keep your elders in the driver's seat as much and as long as possible, and encourage them to make decisions and solve their own problems along the way. Here are some sample questions that can prompt capable elders to take more responsibility for their own well-being:

What do you plan to do to solve this problem?

Given what you know now, what do you think is your next step?

Do you know someone you can talk to about this?

Communicate caring.

Answers are not always what are needed during eldercare conversations—empathy is. If you can communicate love and concern, your conversations have a better chance of going smoothly. This approach requires time and patience on your part. Take time to listen when your elders speak, and your nonverbal message will communicate compassion—eye contact, speaking slowly and in a soft voice, and a relaxed body posture are all helpful. Walking in the door with a bouquet of fresh-cut flowers might also instantly warm up your elder's heart. Let your elders know you care about their well-being by saying:

I worry that something may happen to you when you [drive at night, are home alone].

I've been thinking about you lately.

I love you, and want you to be happy.

You're very special to me.

Turning Conflict into Cooperation

My aunt denies needing help even though I know she does. I have no idea if my parents will outlive their money because they refuse to discuss financial planning with me. My husband won't get a hearing aid even though he can't hear a thing. Where there's family, there's conflict.

Initiating eldercare conversation is stressful enough, and not having the skills or the know-how to get our point across successfully can drive an even deeper wedge between us and those we love. And when we find ourselves being misunderstood or our motives questioned, conversations lead to nowhere. Historical and unresolved relationship conflicts will impact the success of our interactions. If we haven't already forgiven the other person for past hurts, the possibility of getting our way is a long shot. Resentments, emotional detachment, and personal agendas prevent people from being cooperative.

Let's say it's obvious to you that your mom can no longer live safely at home. While she may know in her heart that moving into an assisted-living community is the right thing to do, she may resist as a way to restore her personal power within the family. Rather than go along with what you are suggesting, she'd rather argue for the sake of arguing. Irrationality, defensiveness, denial, and even outright lying are signals that a personal struggle for power and control is taking over the conversation.

Despite conversation challenges in the eldercare process, there are communication techniques that can work in your behalf. This section of *The Complete Eldercare Planner* offers tips on persuading the other person to do what is best. Making a commitment to put these suggestions to good use will likely result in your being one of the lucky ones who finally hear these words from loved ones: "Thank you for all you've done for me" and "I love you."

TURNING CONFLICT INTO COOPERATION

- The art of negotiation comes into play during *every* eldercare conversation. A little bargaining know-how can bring you big results.

- It is rare that one person is causing all the problems. You must be willing to look at the ways *you* contribute to the conflict.

- You are not dealing with difficult *people*, you are dealing with difficult *behavior*—and all difficult behavior is rooted in fear.

The past doesn't go away, and people don't change overnight. The quality of family relationships is determined by how well the family members cooperate with one another.

OBJECTIVES

After completing "Turning Conflict into Cooperation," you will be able to:

Anticipate and respond to disagreements and differences of opinion.

Manage big issues one small step at a time.

Use techniques that get conversations back on track.

Make your own plans if things don't work out.

PLAN ONE

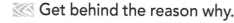 Get behind the reason why.

"Mind your own business." "I'm not moving, and that's final." "Stop telling me what to do." Resistance and defiance are no strangers to eldercare conversations, and conflicts can occur when we least expect them no matter how much love exists between us and our elders. We typically have the best of intentions in mind when we open up the dialogue about their future well-being, and when conversations go south we wonder, "Don't they realize how much I care?"

What triggers an argument is often more than meets the eye. Older people are uncooperative for many reasons, including:

- They are afraid.
- They don't trust you.
- They are restoring their personal power within the relationship and/or the family.
- They're stalling and avoiding making a decision they're not ready to make.
- They're using conflict as an attention-getting device. Arguing is an effective way to keep the focus on *them. Think about it, once the problem is solved, will you continue to give them your love and undivided attention?*

No one likes to be told what to do. When our elders feel as though they are losing their inherent right to be in charge of their decisions, they may override our good intentions and go about their business without seeking cooperation or approval. People respond better when they are *constantly reassured* that they are in control of their own lives.

PLAN TWO

Curb the urge to take over.

Whose life is it, anyway? It doesn't matter if what you have to say is "the truth." It doesn't matter if you are "right." It doesn't matter that you are the voice of reason *if they would only listen to you.* Imposing your will, offering unsolicited advice, doing too much, forcing your values, and coming across as experts on *their* lives will only result in your being perceived as manipulative and overbearing, rather than loving and caring.

If your elders are close-minded about anything you have to say, and you want to get the relationship and conversations back on track, brush up on your communication skills by reviewing the section "Take a Deep Breath and Jump In" in this chapter. (**Note:** Don't disagree or get into an argument via e-mail.) Conduct a quick assessment on your communication style and approach by asking yourself these questions:

Am I trying to do for my elder what he or she can do for himself or herself?

Am I being sensitive to his or her issues of loss?

Am I struggling with my own issues of loss?

Am I keeping his or her autonomy in mind in solving this problem?

Am I making assumptions about what I think he or she needs?

Am I really listening?

Am I being open-minded?

Am I driving the conversation by asking questions and holding back unsolicited advice?

Do I know enough about this subject to offer an opinion?

Am I empowering my elder to solve his or her own problems?

Am I communicating caring?

PLAN THREE

⫸ Not you, not me, but *us*.

If your elder has a problem, *you* have a problem. If whatever is happening is costing you time, energy, money, and sleep, you have every right to remind your elders that they are impacting you and the entire family in one way or another. When they say, *"It's none of your business,"* your immediate response is, *"Oh, but it is."*

Eldercare issues are *family transition* issues. What happens to your elders happens to your family. Reminding them of this fact during conversations keeps them focused on the big picture. Here are some words to say that can help accomplish this goal:

> *This isn't about you alone; it's a family issue.*
>
> *What happens to you happens to me, too.*
>
> *This isn't for me. It's for everyone in the family.*
>
> *Hiring a housekeeper will help me more than you.*

PLAN FOUR

⫸ Appreciate the elder time zone.

Nobody likes deadlines. Conflicts may arise if you use time as a motivator and your elders don't agree with your sense of urgency. Whether you're dealing with a major, life-altering decision or simply planning a special outing, they move to the beat of their own drum. For example, you've asked Mom to be ready at a prearranged hour to go shopping and she's still in her nightgown when you arrive. Expecting her to adhere to *your* timetable sets you up for a day of frustration. Asking her to be ready perhaps an hour before the "real" pickup time may help minimize those agonizing, stressful moments when we're running against the clock.

Visualize for a moment a day in the life of your elders. *Do you really know how long it takes for them to accomplish certain tasks?* Many of us lead busy lives, including juggling work and life responsibilities. Our elders, on the other hand, may exist in a more "meandering" lifestyle. With no bosses to report to or schedules to keep, they may not be the least bit concerned about time: Tuesday could be Friday and April could be September. Forcing them to fit their plans into your busy schedules probably isn't going to work, and may be the impetus they need to dig in their heels and be uncooperative, just because they can. Before bringing deadlines and time frames into a conversation with your elder, be prepared to live with the consequences should things turn out otherwise.

The elder time zone issue will also come into play when you do not allow enough time between one eldercare-related conversation and the next. We are a society of problem solvers. We want quick answers to resolve all of the family's eldercare issues at once so we can get on to something else. Older adults do not respond well to that kind of pressure. Raise one issue at a time, and allow enough time between talks for everyone to adjust and react to the last conversation.

PLAN FIVE

Let's make a deal.

You think Mom should get a dishwasher and she won't spend a dime on herself; Dad thinks traveling alone overseas is doable and you know a ten-hour flight will do him in; Grandma is lip-reading and she refuses to get a hearing aid. The situations are endless, and yet the foundation for conflict is the same: "You want what you want, and I want what I want." We are *equally* determined to get our own needs met and protect our interests.

When we are having trouble seeing eye-to-eye with our elders, perhaps fine-tuning the art of negotiation will win them over. The goal is to create an atmosphere of *inter-dependence.*

Be prepared.

Just as you wouldn't start a cross-country car trip without a road map or GPS, you can't begin to negotiate with another person without knowing your position and defining how conflicts will affect your point of view. Preparing a written response in advance will help maintain your composure and keep you from doing or saying something you may later regret. You can also use this list as a yardstick to measure your progress. Do your homework by taking these steps:

- Put in writing what you want, and what the other person wants.
- Define other factors that impact the outcome, such as costs, time, resources, and location.
- Gather facts and documentation—the more you know, the better.
- Brainstorm all the possible ways you could settle this disagreement.
- Outline all favorable options you are willing to live with.
- Anticipate resistance—write down how the other person may respond that could otherwise catch you off guard.

Put the ball in their court.

Don't assume you know what the other person is thinking and feeling. The more you feel that you have to have the answers, the more forced your efforts become, and the less likely you are to succeed. When your elders aren't sold on what you are saying, find out why. Ask for feedback:

> *Dad, in order for us to come up with some other options, can you explain to me why my suggestion is a bad idea?*
>
> *Mom, can you tell me how staying in your home alone will help you get over feeling depressed?*

Give it a try.

Explore the possibility of a trial run. Employ a time limit, and follow up when you say you will so your elder know you're serious. Sometimes, making the other person happy first, for a short while, opens them up to accepting the alternative plan sooner. When the trial period is over, discuss what worked and what didn't work, and what could be rearranged or added to make the idea work. Here are a few examples:

> *Okay, Mom, I understand you don't want help now. Can we take another look at this situation in two weeks to see how you're doing?*
>
> *Let's move this chair into the other room for a week and see how you like it.*

Offer choices.

Giving people choices puts them in a more agreeable mood. When it's time to present alternatives, be sure that your questions offer options that work for you:

> *Mom, do you want me or Jimmy to drive you to the store?*
>
> *Would you like to talk about this now or wait until I am there in person?*
>
> *Will you take the bus or call a taxi?*
>
> *Is it better for you if Betty cleans the house on Tuesday or Saturday?*

PLAN SIX

Inch them closer to the goal.

Gently ease into action when your elders resist new ideas. Let's say Mom refuses to go to the doctor. Suggest a less-threatening environment, such as a health fair or a pharmacy, where she can be tested for cholesterol and blood pressure. If you want to encourage Uncle Bob to exercise, invite him to a lecture on nutrition at the local community center. Keep your eyes open for shopping-mall events, and suggest you attend them together.

PLAN SEVEN

Validate feelings.

Dad is on a tirade about the cost of prescription drugs, Aunt Betty hates the assisted-living community, and Mom is fed up with being sick all the time—lashing out may be their only emotional outlet. In response, you may be tempted to respond with questions like *"Why are you so angry?"* or *"Why do you talk that way?"* Or you might offer the false comfort of the cliché *"Things will be better tomorrow,"* or the cajoling response of *"Now, now, eat this. It will make you feel better,"* making them angrier still that they have been deprived of righteous anger. Trying to talk anyone out of the way he or she feels and thwarting their inherent right to express any and all feelings almost always creates distance and conflict between people.

Undoubtedly, you can become emotionally drained the more you are subjected to your elders' negative thoughts and criticisms. In addition to leaving the room or changing the subject, you have other options. Everyone feels better when his or her point of view is understood. If you wish to say something during times like these, try validating the other person's feelings.

Validating does not mean you agree with what is being said, it simply means that you understand what the person is experiencing in the moment. Even though this can be a difficult process, try not to take what they are saying personally. Do what you can to distance yourself from what is being said, and use these validation techniques to help defuse and lessen their anxiety:

> *This has been hard for you, hasn't it, Mom?*
>
> *I'm sorry this is happening to you.*
>
> *I know you're disappointed.*
>
> *Yes, Dad, you're alone. And I'm sorry you're so sad.*
>
> *I can imagine how difficult this is for you.*
>
> *You must be very angry at . . . I'd be mad too if that happened.*
>
> *Now I understand what you've been going through.*
>
> *You might be right about that.*
>
> *That's upsetting. Tell me, how did this happen?*
>
> *How terrible this must be.*

Sometimes, words can get in the way during times like this. True caring can also be conveyed through the quality of your listening, an exchange of glances between two people who understand each other, and some small gesture of love, such as holding hands.

PLAN EIGHT

Step back if there's a fight.

The content of eldercare conversations is life altering; it's only natural for tensions to build in the communication process. On a positive note, our elders' resistance reminds us that they are the ultimate master of their own lives. Old family conflicts and "hot buttons" have a way of sneaking into conversations, and it takes a lot of maturity to stick to the present issues.

You don't have to respond to your elder's objection or view it as a personal attack. Issues are rarely settled in one sitting. If an argument erupts, take measures to calm yourself down: Take a deep breath and take a sip of water. This will prevent you from saying anything you'll regret later on. Be aware of your body language—sit back, uncross your arms and legs—and when you're ready to speak, you can say:

I'm sure we can find a solution to this.

I'm on your side.

Where do you think we should go from here?

What's the next step to make this better?

I'm always available to talk with you and am committed to working this out.

I'd like to give this some thought. Let's discuss this later when we've both calmed down.

PLAN NINE

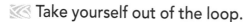 ## Take yourself out of the loop.

Are you the best person for the job? Despite good intentions, your elder may not want to talk with *you* about certain subjects. Here's when the refrain "Mom always liked you best" will work to your advantage. Admit the limitations of your relationship and enlist the help of those who have more influence with that person. Perhaps your sister gets along with Mom better than you.

If situations turn serious, you'll have to override any objections to your getting involved. Leaving the stove on, living alone in a high-crime neighborhood, unsafe driving, and a host of other high-risk situations dictate that it's time to call for a family and/or professional intervention. Power struggles of this magnitude will easily wear you out; trying to reason with irrational people will get you nowhere.

Certain people *outside* the family circle (authority figures) may be helpful, such as the doctor, a member of the clergy, or a geriatric case manager. Tell them of your concerns. When it's time for you to get back in the conversation, you can say, *"Based on what the doctor said about your hearing, Dad, what's your plan about driving?"* In extreme cases, when our elders are hurting themselves and potentially others, and refusing to cooperate with anyone, family members may want to pursue obtaining a court order for guardianship. Review chapter 7, "Legal Matters," starting on page 153. Also, call the local adult protection services office in your city or county, and ask for the assistance of an intervention professional.

PLAN TEN

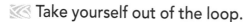 ## The relationship comes first.

Sometimes we get so bogged down in troubleshooting particular situations or solving specific problems that we forget that it's the relationship that brought us together in the first place. If all we do is focus on the problems of eldercare, eventually our elders can be made to feel like worthless and disgraced members of the family. Feeling judged and misunderstood can eat away at relationships, and when our elders feel as though all eyes are on them, they may decide to be unreasonable and uncooperative.

Taking the time to reinforce the personal bond between you can help ease the potential for communication conflicts. There's much to be gained when conversations include other topics; talk about what's going on in *your* world—job, world events, and children. Now is the perfect time to say, *"It's great knowing I have you to talk with."* Smiles and hugs pay big dividends.

PLAN ELEVEN

Give it time.

For months, you've been trying to talk Dad into moving into an assisted-living community. Finally, he's had enough and has cut you out of conversations. For the time being, accept the fact that there is nothing you can do. Give him time and space. Ask other people to speak on your behalf. Write him a letter. Pick up the phone and leave a message telling him how much you love him. Hope for the best.

Low-Cost and Free Resources

Effective communication skills *can* be learned. Consult **communication books** and seek **professional counseling. Assertiveness training programs** can also be helpful. The **Internet** offers a multitude of resources. Do keyword searches on "communication skills," "assertiveness training," "psychology," and "intervention."

Contact your local chapters of **Alcoholics Anonymous** and **Al-Anon** to learn more about how to communicate with elders who have drug and drinking problems.

Locate the local chapter of the **Alzheimer's Association** to find out about support groups, and to learn about recent advances in drug therapy and the communication process.

ORGANIZATIONS AND WEB RESOURCES

Alzheimer Mediation for Dementia Conflict
Karen L. Rice, LNHA Gerontologist
Health & Family Mediator
E-mail: info@alzheimerfamilycaremanage
   ment.com
Website: www.alzheimerfamilycaremanage
   ment.com

American Association for Geriatric Psychiatry
7910 Woodmont Avenue, Suite 1050
Bethesda, MD 20814-3004
(301) 654-7850; fax: (301) 654-4137
Website: www.aagpgpa.org

Anger Clinic
29 S. La Salle
Chicago, IL 60603-1507
(312) 263-0035
Website: www.angerclinic.com

Association for Conflict Resolution
(Find an eldercare mediator)
1015 18th Street, NW, Suite 1150
Washington, DC 20036
(202) 464-9700; fax: (202) 464-9720
Website: www.acrnet.org

Center for Social Gerontology
2307 Shelby Avenue
Ann Arbor, MI 48103
(734) 665-1126; fax: (734) 665-2071
Website: www.tcsg.org

Well Spouse Association
63 W. Main Street, Suite H
Freehold, NJ 07728
Toll-free: (800) 838-0879
Website: www.wellspouse.org

COMMUNICARING ACTION CHECKLIST

(This worksheet is also available online at www.elderindustry.com)

TAKE A DEEP BREATH AND JUMP IN	To Do By	Completed
Understand what's going on behind the scenes		
issues of loss	_____	☐
autonomy	_____	☐
trust	_____	☐
medical issues	_____	☐
mental health	_____	☐
Do your homework before opening up the dialogue		
community services	_____	☐
cost of services	_____	☐
family resources	_____	☐
Review your elder's current abilities	_____	☐
Review conversation dynamics		
conflicting understanding of responsibilities	_____	☐
partnering, not parenting	_____	☐
Try a variety of techniques to open up the dialogue		
seize the moment	_____	☐
plant the seed	_____	☐
ask advice	_____	☐
ask for information	_____	☐
turn the tables	_____	☐
Set the stage for better results		
timing	_____	☐
location	_____	☐

TURNING CONFLICT INTO COOPERATION

Get behind the reason why

    lack of trust   _____ ❑

    restore power   _____ ❑

    stall tactic   _____ ❑

    attention-getting device   _____ ❑

Anticipate disagreements and differences

    curb the urge to take over   _____ ❑

    keep it all in the family   _____ ❑

    limit deadlines   _____ ❑

    make deals   _____ ❑

    put the ball in their court   _____ ❑

    suggest trial runs   _____ ❑

    offer choices   _____ ❑

Inch them closer to the goal   _____ ❑

Use techniques that get conversations back on track

    validate feelings   _____ ❑

    step back if there's a fight   _____ ❑

    take yourself out of the loop   _____ ❑

    relationships comes first   _____ ❑

Review the "Take a Deep Breath and Jump In" section of this chapter   _____ ❑

Make other plans if things don't work out   _____ ❑

5

Emergency Preparedness

Quick and Easy Access

What good is eldercare planning if loved ones can't be accessed if something bad were to happen to them? Imagine your state of mind if you were unable to immediately enter your elders' house because you forgot to exchange house keys. Worse yet, what if a neighbor heard their pleas for help and had no way of entering the residence? And who knows how the scene would unfold if you were unreachable in the event of an eldercare emergency?

Emergency situations also have a way of unveiling the absence of legal and important documents at the least opportune moment. Let's say your dad is temporarily being cared for in a nursing home, and his household bills are stacking up. Do you pay the invoices out of your own pocket or let them go and beg for mercy later on?

Inaccessibility *unnecessarily* complicates the caregiving process. This section of *The Complete Eldercare Planner* will offer simple steps to take *right now* to ensure access to the people who are counting on you to be there when they need you. The process of duplicating keys, creating check-in systems, and preparing legal documents are a few of the many ways you can be prepared to respond to an unforeseen situation.

PLAN ONE

Keep important telephone numbers handy.

Do what you can to complete the "Elder Emergency Information Chart" on page 5. If your time is limited, photocopy your elder's personal address book, and complete the chart when you can.

Obtain a copy of your elders' community telephone directories—the White Pages and the Yellow Pages. If they live outside of *your* 9-1-1 emergency range, make sure you know the telephone numbers of the police and fire departments. Update emergency contact information as needed. Keep this information handy.

QUICK AND EASY ACCESS

- In an emergency, minutes count, and getting help could make the difference between life and death.
- Studies have shown that people are more likely to return to independent living after a fall if help comes *quickly*.

The list of conditions of vulnerability for older adults includes living alone and falling, and no one would know.

OBJECTIVES

*After completing "**Quick and Easy Access,**" you will be able to:*

Provide assistance 24/7.

Create access in an eldercare emergency.

Have greater peace of mind knowing someone is always close at hand.

- If you are computer savvy, download emergency contact information to a flash drive and keep the flash drive on your key chain.
- Post the emergency contact list near the telephone and on the refrigerator at your home and your elder's home.
- Distribute copies of the information to family and trusted friends and neighbors.
- Make hard copies of the list, and keep copies at work.

PLAN TWO

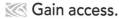 Gain access.

Duplicate plastic access cards. Know the location of electronic door openers. Write down combinations to locks and safes. Learn access codes to computers and telephone answering devices.

In order to draw money from another person's checking and savings account, most banks require power of attorney prearranged on *their* forms. If your elder agrees to these arrangements, accompany him or her to the bank and fill out the appropriate forms. Another strategy is to set up a second signature on designated accounts.

Duplicate and label keys, and selectively distribute them to family, trusted friends, and neighbors. Distribute keys in person if possible. Maintain twenty-four-hour access to keys and to those having access. To locate key duplicating services, see the Yellow Pages under "Locks and Locksmiths."

Know how to access:

alarms	gates
automobiles	luggage
boats	mailboxes
combination locks	recreation vehicles
desks	safes
file cabinets	storage lockers
garage	trunks

PLAN THREE

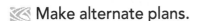 Make alternate plans.

When family members are unwilling (justifiably) to share access to 100 percent of their property and assets, ask them to disclose the names and telephone numbers of those who they have given legal rights to take care of their affairs in the event that something should happen to them. Write down this information so you will remember whom to call in an emergency.

PLAN FOUR

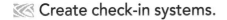 Create check-in systems.

Ideally, your elders will have access to a telephone if an emergency occurs. However, this may not be the case. Make a plan for someone to be in contact with them on a regular basis—by phone and in person. Create a network of people who will agree to stay in touch with your elders on a regular basis. Review chapter 10, "Safe and Secure," in this planner, beginning on page 206, for suggestions on a variety of check-in options.

PLAN FIVE

Consider the protection of a medical-alert system.

Identification of hidden medical conditions and allergies saves lives in an emergency. Simple options such as wallet-sized cards and identification bracelets and necklaces are critical.

Hidden medical conditions may include:

allergies	diabetes
asthma	epilepsy
cancer	heart, liver, and kidney disease

contact lenses	hip, knee, and shoulder
contractible diseases	replacement
such as HIV and AIDS	implants
dementia	pacemaker

PLAN SIX

 Keep vital information accessible.

Store hard copies of information in one safe, accessible place at home or at work. Scan original documents and create backup files on the computer. Important information and documents include:

allergies	power of attorney for health care
blood type	and property (see chapter 7,
driver's license	"Legal Matters")
emergency telephone numbers	proof of insurance
medical history	Social Security number
medications history	financial records

Managing Medications

There is compelling evidence that patients are not taking their medicines as prescribed. One survey reported that nearly three out of every four American consumers report not always taking their prescription medicine as directed.[1] Further, patients may be under the care of several different doctors at the same time, each doctor possibly prescribing different medications. If doctors and pharmacists are not cross-referencing prescription drugs, dangerous interactions can occur. *If your elder is taking any medication, this is one caregiving issue that cannot be ignored.*

This section of *The Complete Eldercare Planner* offers specific guidelines on becoming familiar with your family member's drug usage, and encourages implementing preventative action plans. The use of over-the-counter drugs and herbal remedies also has allowed people to take greater control of their health and well-being. The key is to become an educated consumer. Reading labels, following directions, asking questions, and taking proper amounts of the drug are essential elements of managing medications responsibly.

PLAN ONE

 Investigate which drugs your elder is taking and why.

Get involved. It is imperative that health-care providers are aware that you are monitoring medical treatments and medications. Intervention saves lives. If your elder cannot or does not want to answer questions regarding medications to your satisfaction, it is time to step in.

MANAGING MEDICATIONS

- No single medication-management strategy will *guarantee* that elders will fill their prescriptions and take their medicines as prescribed.
- The risk of falls increases with the number of medications taken.
- If your elders have *not* been told of the side effects of their medications by their doctors, they may be at risk and not know it.

If anyone in the family is taking medications, your involvement in fact-finding and safety precautions could prevent serious mishaps.

OBJECTIVES

*After completing **"Managing Medications,"** you will be able to:*

Know what purpose each prescription serves.

Establish a doctor/pharmacist relationship.

Uncover the possibility of mismanagement of drugs.

Assist family members in managing their medications responsibly.

Ask your elder:

What medicine(s) are you taking?

What is the medicine supposed to do?

Have you been warned of possible side effects?

PLAN TWO

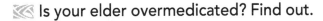 Is your elder overmedicated? Find out.

Older patients who are attended to by several doctors may neglect telling each one about the drugs being prescribed by the others. To lower potentially dangerous levels of drug usage and to prevent deadly drug combinations, remind your elder to inform each prescriber of all routinely used medications, including over-the-counter drugs and vitamins.

BROWN-BAG IT. Gather the prescription drugs, over-the-counter medications, and supplements, including eye drops, cough syrup, pain relievers, cold pills, vitamins, and herbs, and put them in a paper bag. Take them to the next medical appointment or your next trip to the pharmacy and ask for an assessment of the drug usage.

FILL PRESCRIPTIONS AT ONE PHARMACY. The pharmacist can keep track of drug usage by computer and look for the potential of dangerous drug combinations.

DISCUSS ADDITIONAL ALTERNATIVES. Has the doctor recommended alternative methods of treating the medical condition? Is it possible that weight loss, special diet, exercise, massage therapy, and acupuncture, among other treatments, would be effective?

CREATE A DRUG-USAGE CHART. Use the chart below as a guide and bring the chart to *every* appointment. Record current drug and over-the-counter drug usage information. Complete new prescription information in the doctor's office. NOTE: If you think this is too much trouble, be assured that interaction saves lives. Any physician or physician's assistant who avoids answering questions or gives family caregivers little time to ask questions should be reported.

DRUG-USAGE CHART

(This worksheet is also available online at www.elderindustry.com)

PRINT AS MANY COPIES AS THE DRUGS YOUR ELDER IS TAKING.

Today's date _____

Patient name _____

Drug name _____

Drug purpose _____

Drug color and shape _____

Amount to take _____

When to take _____

How to take_____

How long to take _____

Possible side effects _____

PLAN THREE

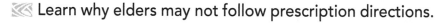 Learn why elders may not follow prescription directions.

Older people sometimes discontinue, resume, or change medications without the physician's consent, which can be quite harmful.

The reasons include:
- The drugs make them feel worse than the symptoms of the illness.
- There appears to be no clear evidence that the drug is working.
- Medications are too expensive.

- They would rather spend their money on something else.
- They feel better and don't believe they need to continue the medication.
- Taking drugs gives them a feeling of loss of independence.
- Drugs are a constant reminder of "being sick."
- Short-term memory loss makes it hard to track drug usage.

PLAN FOUR

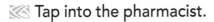 Tap into the pharmacist.

A certified pharmacist, registered with the state pharmaceutical board, is trained to answer questions about medications and over-the-counter remedies.

Ask the pharmacist . . .
- any questions regarding drugs
- about generic substitutions
- for written information about the medicine
- to keep tabs on your elder's drug usage and medical history
- for easy-open containers as long as there are no children present
- about discounts
- for large-print labels
- about emergency prescription services
- about prescription home-delivery services
- about year-end tax and insurance statements

PLAN FIVE

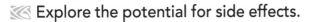 Explore the potential for side effects.

Does your elder know the answer to these questions? Find out.
- What medicines are you currently taking?
- Do each of your doctors know about the other medications you are taking?
- What is the medicine supposed to be doing for you? Is it working?
- How and when do you take this medication?
- Are you experiencing side effects? Is that normal?
- Is it safe to drink alcohol or caffeine beverages? Are certain foods to be avoided?
- Is driving to be avoided?
- Are you allergic to any medications?

PLAN SIX

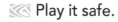 Play it safe.

Mixing two drugs together could make one of the drugs ineffective. The combination also could increase a drug's effect, and be harmful.[2] Researchers say there are several important variables that affect individual differences in how drugs are metabolized, including race, gender, age, and health conditions. For example, very young children and older people have slower drug metabolism than others, and women may metabolize drugs differently than men in some cases.[3]

Discuss the following safety procedures:
- Ask for **large-print prescription labels** and keep a magnifying glass handy. **Braille labeling** is also available.
- When filling prescriptions, check the **name of the drug** on the label *before* leaving the pharmacy.
- **Store drugs as directed.** Refrigerate the drug only if told to do so.
- **Keep pills far from the bed.** This reduces the possibility of taking the wrong dose or the wrong combination when sleepy. The kitchen table or counter may work best.
- Ask the doctor to prescribe a **visiting nurse,** who will come to your elder's home and offer instructions on taking the medications.
- Create a **medications history.** Post the list near the telephone and on the refrigerator. Bring to every doctor appointment and update as needed.
- Do business with just **one reliable pharmacy** and get to know the pharmacist.
- Buy spoons and syringes that are clearly marked with doses for **liquid medications.**
- Use **identification bracelets** for allergies and chronic conditions.

PLAN SEVEN

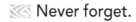 Never forget.

Type the words "medication management" in your Internet browser and you'll be overwhelmed with the number of articles, websites, books, and medication reminder systems offered on the subject. From safety tips to bottles that beep, the methods used to manage medications can be as high-tech or as low-tech as you like.

Discuss the following medication reminder systems and also ask the pharmacist for help finding the right product for your elder.

Medication reminder systems include:
- Reminders that fit on **top of a pill bottle** and special caps that count openings of a prescription vial to tell if the day's doses have been taken.

- A **plastic pillbox** that stores drugs for each day of the week. If you go this route, keep the original prescription containers handy and a sample of each drug in the original vial.
- A **weekly drug usage chart.** List the days of the week, the name of each medication, and the times to take each drug. Cross out the name of the drug each time it is taken.
- **Software** that can handle any drug regimen. Preload your PDA (personal digital assistant) or computer to remind you of when your elders should be taking their medications.
- A medicine container or medicine cabinet that **beeps when it's time for a dose.**
- A **computerized drug organizer-dispenser.**

If Your Elder Is Hospitalized

The hospital environment is a culture all its own. Family caregivers who have little experience dealing with health-care professionals in these highly specialized surroundings may not know what to expect, what to do, and which questions to ask. From the moment you arrive at the hospital, feeling intimidated and confused is not uncommon, especially if your loved one landed there unexpectedly.

This section of *The Complete Eldercare Planner* will help you get your feet planted on more solid ground and quickly focus your attention on what needs to be done. Navigating the hospital setting will require specific action plans to help you gain immediate control over the eldercare emergency situation.

Hospitalization is a traumatic experience for the entire family. Surviving this stressful situation requires asking specific questions and making informed decisions based on facts, not emotions. Veteran caregivers will tell you that a crash course on planning, getting organized, and sharpening communication technique will be the keys to managing this situation. The good news is everything you need right now is within the context of *The Planner*.

PLAN ONE

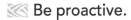 Be proactive.

Being organized is a lifesaving caregiving strategy when a loved one is unexpectedly hospitalized. Keeping track of the many things that are happening all at once will be your goal during these stressful times. Here are a few suggestions.

Create a file or binder. Save all paperwork—reports, lab tests, invoices, and any documents related to the hospitalization. Store all documents in one place. Keep the file or binder with you everywhere you go as long as he or she is hospitalized. You may need it at a moment's notice.

IF YOUR ELDER IS HOSPITALIZED

- The law gives patients the right to refuse care or treatment at any time.
- A modern-day reality of health care is that patients are whisked in and out of the hospital in record time.
- One of the best ways to help ensure a safe and positive hospital experience is to partner with the staff immediately.

Being proactive in the hospital setting will prepare you for hasty hospital discharges.

OBJECTIVES

*After completing **"If Your Elder Is Hospitalized,"** you will be able to:*

Ask meaningful questions during times of confusion.

Gather important health-care information and legal documents.

Make the hospital stay as comfortable as possible.

Research home and health-care-facility options.

Plan ahead for the hospital discharge.

Save receipts on money you spend out of your own funds for possible reimbursement from your elder, the insurance company, other family members, and legal representatives, and for tax deductions.

Keep paper and pen handy at all times. You'll want to document doctors' instructions and anything else that is of importance. Make sure you put the date on your notations.

Obtain legal and important documents—proof of insurance, living will, power of attorney for property, do-not-resuscitate (DNR) order, and power of attorney for health care in this file. Review chapter 7, "Legal Matters," of *The Complete Eldercare Planner* on page 153 for more information on these documents.

Due to Health Insurance Portability and Accountability Act (HIPAA) regulations, you may need to **establish authority** in order to discuss your elder's medical condition with the doctor. Seek advice from the hospital discharge planner and patient advocate.

For the computer savvy, back up any and all computerized files on a **flash drive** and carry the flash drive on your key chain.

PLAN TWO

Take it one step at a time.

With so many questions and so many things to do, you may be overwhelmed to the point of doing nothing, or doing too much with little direction. Follow the action plans in this chapter in the order shown, and go at your own pace.

Get out a sheet of paper, and make a heading titled **Elder Contacts.** List the names, addresses, and phone numbers (day and evening) of the individuals suggested in the lists below. Record this information as soon as you make contact with these people.

IN CASE OF AN ACCIDENT
Police on duty
Victims and witnesses
Insurance agents
Attorney

AT THE HOSPITAL
Hospital name and address
Hospital floor, room, and bed number
Hospital room telephone number
Floor nurses station telephone number
Head nurse and staff
Doctor(s)
Social worker
Discharge planner
Patient representative
Billing director

HOME MANAGEMENT
Housekeeper
House sitter
Pet sitter
Handyman
Home chore services

CAREGIVER SUPPORT
Family/friends
Neighbors
Agency on aging
Family service agency
Home-care agencies
Geriatric case manager
Assisted-living services

POSTHOSPITAL RECOVERY
Rehabilitation center
Assisted-living services
Skilled nursing care
Home hospital equipment rental company
Pharmacy
Adult day services

PERSONAL
Beauty salon or barber
Clubs
Associations
Religious group
Volunteer activities

PLAN THREE

Ask a lot of questions.

If your elder is unable to communicate and in serious condition, and a living will or power of attorney for health care has been prepared in advance, now is the time to review the contents of those documents. If you are the person who is **authorized to make medical decisions on your elder's behalf,** seek the advice of the doctors involved, the hospital social worker, the patient advocate, and the hospital chaplain (this is the generic term used for a nondenominational clergyperson and is the term for people who offer spiritual guidance in the hospital setting). Proactively offer information regarding your elder's medication and medical history. If health-care directives have not been secured in advance, ask to be informed of your rights as a decision-making family member.

As you encounter medical personnel, jot down names, phone numbers, questions, and answers on your legal pad. Remember to put dates on all of your notations.

Medical Emergency Questions Checklist

Ask medical providers . . .

Is there any immediate danger?

What is the medical problem?

What are the short-term effects of this illness?

What are the long-term effects of this illness?

Will my elder require an overnight stay? How long?

Have medications been employed? What are they?

If surgery is recommended, ask . . .

What are the possible complications?

What are the short-term expectations?

What are the long-term expectations?

How often do you perform this procedure?

What is the success or mortality rate?

What is the rate of complications from this surgery?

What are the other choices of treatment?

What are the short-term consequences if surgery is not performed?

What are the long-term consequences if surgery is not performed?

Do I have time to seek a second opinion?

Before your elder is discharged from the hospital, ask . . .

Will my elder need rehabilitation services? For how long?

Will my elder need home-health-care assistance? What kind?

How will the help that is needed be provided?

What is the expected recovery time?

How are these services usually paid for?

If your elder is staying overnight in the hospital, ask him or her . . .

Is there anyone specifically you would like me to contact?

Is there anything you would like me to bring you?

PLAN FOUR

Be prepared for the enormous task of keeping people in the loop.

When a loved one is hospitalized or suddenly becomes ill, the primary caregiver is inclined to let others know what's going on. People who love us and also love our elders will be concerned about what's happening. There will be many phone calls to make and many e-mails to send; follow-up replies to questions people will ask of you will also take a lot of time and energy. You will find yourself telling the story of what is going on over and over again. Friends and family members will ask for details and request that you keep them informed of the course of events as they happen. There also may be rumors and gossip you have to extinguish. People will also share their own experiences whether you ask for them or not. **Keeping people informed can be exhausting**.

To take care of yourself during the course of communicating with others, simplify the process. If you plan to send e-mails, create a new group so sending an update message can go out to many people in your address book at one time. If you are making phone calls, *do not promise to keep everyone informed of your elder's progress (except a select few)*. You will have plenty of other things to do. Instead, ask people to call *you* back.

Also, well-meaning family and friends will ask about telephoning and visiting your elder in the hospital and once they come home. Give them clear instructions if your elder does not want to be disturbed; *don't be surprised if they call and visit anyway*.

The task of making telephone calls and sending e-mail can be overwhelming. Delegate and share this responsibility with other reliable people. Don't underestimate the pressures of this caregiving task. To find important phone numbers, look in your elder's personal address book and appointment book.

Medical Emergency Call List

IF AN ACCIDENT OCCURRED
Police
Lawyer
Insurance agents
Witnesses

CANCEL ELDER'S ACTIVITIES
Place of employment
Appointments
Classes
Religious groups
Travel plans (check if insured
   for cancellation)
Volunteer projects
Social commitments

SUSPEND
Newspapers
Mail delivery

CALL
Family, friends, and neighbors
Banker, accountant, and
   tax adviser
Clergyperson
Landlord (if renting)
Housekeeping services
House sitter
Pet sitter

PLAN FIVE

 ## Take care of business.

Before you leave the hospital, gather your elder's valuables, such as a watch, jewelry, a wallet, or a purse, and take these items home with you for safekeeping until your elder is released. Review the following checklist as a way to take care of your elder's home and other important business while he or she is in the hospital.

Medical Emergency Action Checklist

- Retrieve messages from your elder's telephone answering machine, voice mail, or e-mail. Follow up on high-priority calls.
- Make a list of phone calls to make (review Plan Four).
- Find your elder's personal address and appointment book. Keep them with you or make copies of the contents.
- Find your elder's health insurance policy. Keep a copy of the insurance card with you.
- Go through the mail. Pay time-sensitive bills. If you pay your elder's bills out of your checking account, keep track for reimbursement later on.
- Keep track of all money spent on eldercare-related expenses for possible reimbursement, including travel and lodging expenses.
- Notify creditors and let them know your elder is in the hospital.
- Make duplicate keys to the home, property, auto, and mailbox.
- Make bank deposits on your elder's behalf.
- Pack items to bring back with you to the hospital (see Plan Six).

- Dispose of food that will spoil after too long.
- Check and maintain the security of home and auto.
- Store valuables, jewelry, wallet, purse, credit cards, and driver's license in a safe place.
- Plan for the hospital discharge and make care arrangements (rehab, in-home care, assisted-living services).
- Make temporary living arrangements for your elder's spouse, if necessary.
- If it's near tax time, call the accountant and ask about an extension.
- Gather current medications and bring them to the hospital.
- Arrange to have mail picked up regularly or put on hold at the post office.
- Suspend newspapers that are home delivered.
- Arrange to have the lawn mowed or snow shoveled.

PLAN SIX

Make the hospital stay as comfortable as possible.

Ask your elder what items you can bring back with you to the hospital. Here are a few additional suggestions:

appointment calendar	lipstick and makeup
books/magazines	manicure kit
cell phone and charger	personal address book
chewing gum and mints	portable media player
crossword puzzles	self-standing mirror
deodorant	shaver and shaving lotion
eyeglasses and eyeglass cleaner	slippers
favorite pajamas/robe	snacks and food
hairbrush and comb	stationery and pen
hand and face lotion	stockings and undergarments
handheld game	street clothes and shoes
hearing aid	toothbrush and toothpaste
laptop computer	transistor radio

PLAN SEVEN

Plan ahead as your elder recuperates in the hospital.

You will need to make decisions regarding home or institutionalized health care *before* your elder is released from the hospital. Seek assistance from the **hospital discharge planner** about home and health-care options early on. Hospitals often release patients sooner than you think, so you will want to research care options right away.

The law states that patients are free to leave the hospital upon release from their doctor. The hospital is not allowed to detain patients who have outstanding medical expenses and fees not covered by their health insurance carrier.

Ask the doctor:

Will home nursing care be needed? Full-time? Part-time?

What other kind of care will be needed? Short term? Long term?

What lifestyle changes are expected?

What symptoms could indicate health complications?

Ask the hospital discharge planner:

Whom can I call to get home-health-care assistance?

What are the options for living arrangements during recuperation?

What hospital and home-care costs are covered by insurance?

Get help deciding where your elder will go to recuperate. Also review chapter 2, "Creating a Care Team." Options include:

- their home
- your home
- assisted-living community
- rehab (this is always a temporary option)
- skilled nursing facility

PLAN EIGHT

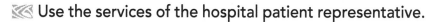 Use the services of the hospital patient representative.

Patient representatives assist family members of patients with health-care problems, concerns, and unmet needs that may have arisen during the hospital stay. Representatives serve as a liaison between patients and the hospital administration.

The patient representative:

- evaluates the level of patient satisfaction
- channels information about care problems to appropriate departments
- directs inquiries and complaints to appropriate hospital staff
- refers patients to services and resources
- investigates patient-care complaints
- assesses responses to incidents

Low-Cost and Free Resources

CPR (cardiopulmonary resuscitation) training has been credited with helping save thousands of lives each year in the United States. Persons interested in learning CPR should contact their local American Heart Association or American Red Cross. Check the Yellow Pages under "First Aid Instruction"; on the Internet, use the keyword search "CPR."

Telecommunications devices for the deaf (TDDs) and **Braille TDDs** are available for telephone customers with hearing and sight disabilities. Contact the special needs center of the telephone company.

Carrier Alert, also known as Postal Alert, is a volunteer program in which letter carriers monitor the possible need of emergency services by examining mail that has not been removed from mailboxes. For more information, contact the local agency on aging or the post office.

Emergency preparedness information of all kinds is available by typing "emergency preparedness" in your Internet keyword search.

ORGANIZATIONS AND WEB RESOURCES

American Heart Association
7272 Greenville Avenue
Dallas, TX 75231
Toll-free: (800) 242-8721
Website: www.americanheart.org

Consumer Health Information Corporation
8300 Greensboro Drive, Suite 1220
McLean, VA 22102-3604
(703) 734-0650; fax: (703) 734-1459
Website: www.consumer-health.com

Medline Plus
(A service of the U.S. National Library of
   Medicine and the National Institutes
   of Health)
Website: http://medlineplus.gov

**National Council on Patient Information
   and Education**
4915 Saint Elmo Avenue, Suite 505
Bethesda, MD 20814-6053
(301) 656-8565; fax: (301) 656-4464
Website: www.talkaboutrx.org

U.S. Food and Drug Administration
5600 Fishers Lane
Rockville, MD 20857-0001
Toll-free: (888) 463-6332
Website: www.fda.gov

EMERGENCY PREPAREDNESS ACTION CHECKLIST

(This worksheet is also available online at www.elderindustry.com)

QUICK AND EASY ACCESS	To Do By	Completed
Set elder access goals		
short-term	_____	☐
long-term	_____	☐
Know the twenty-four-hour emergency phone numbers		
doctor(s)	_____	☐
dentist	_____	☐
neighbors	_____	☐
friends	_____	☐
police	_____	☐
fire department	_____	☐
hospital	_____	☐
hospice	_____	☐
nurse	_____	☐
home aide	_____	☐
pharmacist	_____	☐
electrician	_____	☐
plumber	_____	☐
water company	_____	☐
gas company	_____	☐
electric company	_____	☐
telephone company	_____	☐
alarm company	_____	☐
locksmith	_____	☐
clergyperson	_____	☐
Keep copies of emergency phone numbers		
at home	_____	☐
at work	_____	☐
in car	_____	☐
in wallet or purse	_____	☐

Back up computerized information
on a flash drive _____ ❏

Give copies of emergency phone
numbers to key people _____ ❏

Duplicate keys _____ ❏

Identify and store keys and openers _____ ❏

Distribute keys to necessary people _____ ❏

Have a plan to access finances in an
emergency _____ ❏

Have a backup plan if access to
finances is denied _____ ❏

Consider a medical alert system _____ ❏

Create a check-in system _____ ❏

Elder has access to a telephone _____ ❏

MANAGING MEDICATIONS

Discuss medications with

elder _____ ❏
doctor _____ ❏
pharmacist _____ ❏
family members _____ ❏

Discuss drug

usage _____ ❏
purpose _____ ❏
alternatives _____ ❏
safety _____ ❏

Create strategies for drug safety

**Implement medication reminder
strategies** _____ ❏

Take a CPR class _____ ❏

IF YOUR ELDER IS HOSPITALIZED

Start a file folder _____ ❏

Create a system for recording and filing

    phone numbers _____ ❏

    community resources _____ ❏

    helpers _____ ❏

    receipts _____ ❏

    notes and documentation _____ ❏

    bills _____ ❏

    questions and answers _____ ❏

Create a list of questions for medical
    providers _____ ❏

Back up important information on
    the computer and on a flash drive _____ ❏

Review caregiving options _____ ❏

Make phone calls _____ ❏

Review things to do _____ ❏

Ask what to bring to the hospital _____ ❏

Get additional help from the hospital
    patient representative _____ ❏

6

Money Matters

The Cost of Caring

The financial considerations of caregiving run deep. The possibility of having to shell out tens of thousands of dollars to help cover your elders' care and living expenses is closer to reality than we'd like to admit. The bulk of these expenses are for food, transportation, and medications; assistance with rent/mortgage and home maintenance follow closely behind. Then there are the "hidden" costs to consider, such as your own travel-related expenses and time off work.

Decreasing eligibility and benefits of Medicare and Medicaid are negatively impacting the economic conditions of older people. Medicare does not provide for assisted-living and long-term care, and Medicaid does not kick in until funds are nearly depleted.

Financial problems can go undetected for years. How do you know for sure whether a tight budget is causing your elders to stockpile medications out of necessity, or if they're simply carrying out habitual frugal habits? Lonely and bored people also may be mis-using their credit cards in a variety of ways, including buying overpriced products on tele-vised home-shopping networks. And what are the chances they're sinking deep in debt due to gambling losses from regular excursions to the casino? With people living longer than ever before, the odds are high that they will eventually run out of money.

Naturally, when the money well runs dry, we're motivated by the desire to repay them for all they've done for us over the years, *but mindlessly dipping into our own pockets to help them will cause our financial stability and retirement nest egg to suffer.*

Planning for the economic hit we might have to take addresses our potential role as financial caregiver. This section of *The Complete Eldercare Planner* will help prepare you finan-cially for the cost of caring and also offer personal money-management strategies.

THE COST OF CARING

- Long-distance assistance adds up. Family caregivers can expect to spend their own money on travel, lodging, meals, and much more.
- Parents often want their children to believe that their finances are in better shape than they actually are.
- Eldercare can pose substantial financial challenges for employees who are also family caregivers, due to lost wages from reduced work hours, time out of the workforce, unexpected family leave, and early retirement.

Neither public nor private retirement programs grant credit for caregiving years when calculating retirement benefits; lost work years are factored in as zeros.

OBJECTIVES

*After completing **"The Cost of Caring,"** you will be able to:*

Plan for your long-term financial stability.

Know the limitations of Medicare and Medicaid.

Review dependent-care tax credits and deduction options.

Seek payment for your caregiving services.

PLAN ONE

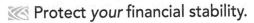 Protect *your* financial stability.

Caregiving will cost you. You might pick up the tab for your elders' groceries or home repairs. You may even end up paying for their expensive assisted-living services. For those who are employed outside the home, there are "hidden" costs to consider, such as unpaid leave from work and lost opportunities for company promotions and transfers. In today's mobile society, we also may find that carrying out caregiving responsibilities from far away is a modern-day necessity, and consequently travel-related expenses and extra days out of the office quickly add up.

Few of us anticipate our elders running out of money, and yet it happens all the time. Compounding the situation, once we dip into our own pockets, we never really know how long the situation will go on. Before saying yes to becoming a financial caregiver, make plans to keep your own finances intact. Consider the following money-management checklist.

Caregiver Financial Strategy Checklist

- Discuss money-management strategies with a financial planner who has attained a financial gerontology certification. With your own longevity in mind, calculate your net worth and outline plans to provide for your retirement needs.
- Put your estate plans in order. Seek the services of an elder-law attorney.
- Purchase long-term care insurance. Employers, businesses, and social organizations often offer group rates to you, spouses, and family members.
- Participate fully in workplace 401(k) plans.
- Purchase disability insurance.
- Keep insurance policies up-to-date and renewed.
- Discuss family-leave options with your employer. Working caregivers may be eligible for unpaid leave under the Family and Medical Leave Act. Some states have also initiated a paid family leave plan.
- Ask employers about tax-advantaged flexible savings accounts (FSAs) for dependent care expenses.

PLAN TWO

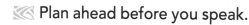 Plan ahead before you speak.

There's nothing like money to break up a family, especially when it comes to eldercare. Family members who are relatively close one day can be torn apart overnight. Disagreements about where to spend the money, who pays for the majority of eldercare services, and deciding who will quit her or his job in order to take on the day-to-day parent care are some of the many financial battles we can expect to both win and lose within the family.

Before you approach the sensitive subject of paying for eldercare-related expenses, and the possibility of comingling family finances is on the horizon, take a moment to fine-tune your communication skills by reviewing chapter 4, "Communicaring," beginning on page 86 of *The Complete Eldercare Planner*.

PLAN THREE

Medicare and Medicaid—find out today what you *can't* count on tomorrow.

Medicare is the government-run health insurance program for those over age sixty-five. This program, in actuality, does not cover most costs that are associated with the kind of extended long-term care older people need. If you are caring for someone with dementia or chronic disease such as Parkinson's, don't look to Medicare to bail you out. The program provides limited assistance for home-health-care and nursing-home expenses.

Medicaid is a federal-state program designed to provide health care to the medically and financially needy; but medical providers know all too well that Medicaid reimbursement continues to lag further and further behind the costs of providing quality care.

Out-of-pocket expenses include prescription drugs, copayments, deductibles, additional services, and non-health-care expenses (such as caregiver respite, housekeeping, and companion services). Most caregivers become acutely aware of how expensive many services can be once they start paying for them out of their own savings.

Even though your elder may be healthy and thriving today, the best-laid plans start with the end in mind; and knowing what Medicare and Medicaid does *not* provide in terms of financial support and care is critical to the health of your personal financial portfolio. Refer to the Medicare and Medicaid topics outlined in this chapter, starting on page 143 in the next section of this chapter.

PLAN FOUR

Who pays for what?

While older adults tap into Social Security, savings accounts, insurance policies, proceeds from the house sale, and other resources to pay for their long-term care and living expenses, there's a likelihood that you and other family members will also have to pitch in to help cover their living expenses. Review the next section of this chapter, "Buying Time," beginning on page 134. Adhere to a family budget, and reevaluate your elders' financial status every six months. Adjust the budget as needed. On the other hand, if you are the only one in the family with cash to spare, ask other family members for their help in terms of time and resources. Here are a few of the many ways they can provide help:

attending doctor appointments
bookkeeping
exterior house repairs
fitness regimens
grocery shopping
home repairs
housekeeping
interior house repairs
laundry
maintaining religious interests
managing mail
meal preparation
personal and beauty care
pet sitting and care
plant care
running errands
social activities
transportation
yard work

PLAN FIVE

Take advantage of dependent-care tax deductions and credits.

As a family caregiver, you may be eligible for savings at tax time if you are providing family caregiving services for relatives. The IRS offers the adult dependent tax exemption to those who qualify. In addition, there are possible deductions and credits that could cut your tax bill a bit more. With the increased expense of caring for a loved one, it is important for caregivers to take full advantage of any and all tax benefits and credits they can.

Take a look at the list below. If you are dipping into your own pocket to pay for these and other care-related expenses, find out how you may qualify for caregiving tax deductions and credits. Talk with your accountant and tax adviser. Also, keep all eldercare-related receipts. You may eventually be reimbursed from your elder's estate, insurance company, and any legal settlements. Here are possible expenses that may be tax deductible:

- cost of diagnosis and treatment of disease
- dental expenses
- adult day services
- cost of home adaptations, such as building ramps and grab bars
- transportation to medical appointments
- long-term care insurance premiums
- prescription drugs
- home medical equipment and wheelchairs
- privately hired in-home assistance and health-care employees
- retrofitting a home or a vehicle to accommodate special needs
- nursing home expenses
- telemedicine and computerized assistive products

PLAN SIX

Consider the consequences *before* you quit your job.

If you are currently working full-time outside the home, and contemplating quitting your job or reducing your workload to part-time status due to caregiving responsibilities, give serious thought before you take any action. While staying closer to home will certainly have its advantages, the decisions you make now regarding your steady income stream will have tremendous impact on your quality of life later on. *If you quit your job, what kind of long-term effect will this decision have on your own family and on your career as a whole? Will you be able to reenter the workforce with ease later on?* This is not a move to make impulsively.

To help in the decision-making process, find out if your employer offers free financial-counseling services to workers and their families. Discuss the following topics with your company financial adviser before you make up your mind to reduce your work hours:

- employee benefits
- health insurance
- family leave policy

- flextime options
- job security
- tenure and sabbaticals
- retirement income and pension plans
- trainings and certifications to sustain licenses
- skills needed to reenter the workplace

PLAN SEVEN

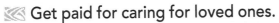 Get paid for caring for loved ones.

The notion that we should care for each other out of love and duty is deeply rooted in our moral code. Yet, because most of us are also employed outside the home in our caregiving years, the financial stakes of eldercare are high. **Family members, partners, and friends deserve to be paid for helping loved ones.** They work long and hard, and the value of their caregiving contributions is priceless. Consider these caregiver payment strategies.

- Hospitals, social-service organizations, and adult education centers offer training programs for caregivers who, upon completion of the program, may qualify to be paid for their services. Call your local agency on aging to see if such a program exists near you.
- If your elder has long-term care insurance, some policies pay for family and friends to provide the care after they have completed a caregiving-training program.
- The Cash and Counseling program for Medicaid enrollees allows participants to pay family members for their services. Contact your local agency on aging or department of social services for more information on government funding.

Sons and daughters provide invaluable parent-care services. Then comes the day of reckoning and both parents are deceased, and the estate gets split equally among all the children. And the caregiver child feels absolutely ripped off. Without an employment contract prepared in advance, the law conveys "no right or entitlement" to family caregivers. Caregiver contracts also may exist between siblings. Hire an attorney to create a written, legal agreement which authorizes the following:

- rate of pay (must be reasonable)
- timing of pay (weekly, monthly, or upon settling of the estate)
- description of services
- travel-related allowance
- reimbursement of expenses and related purchases
- simplified employee pension (SEP)
- prohibition against reassigning the agreement

If the family caregiver contract is drafted correctly, the compensation is not a gift and will not violate any of the transfer rules. Also, there are tax consequences to the caregiver. To make things legal, a caregiver needs to report the income as taxable income since Social Security and other payroll taxes may be withheld.

There are also several programs that allow **low-income caregivers** to care for their elderly relatives, most notably the Personal Care Attendant Program and the Adult Foster Care Program, which pays family members and others to provide care for elders who are Medicaid eligible and need help with the activities of daily living. Call the Medicare office for details or visit the Medicare website at www.medicare.gov.

Buying Time

What does it cost to live a long life? Plenty. Daily headlines continue to drive home the message that because people are living longer than ever before, they also stand the chance of outliving their money. With no long-term financial plans in place, and the fact that older people are spending a fortune on things like senior housing, home repair, prescription drugs, dental expenses, hearing aids, and more, what's not covered by Medicare and supplemental insurance is causing them to dip into their personal savings at an alarming rate.

The unwritten family rule regarding finances is this: It is taboo to bring up the subject of other people's money. In other words, until we learn that our elders are having money problems, we are to assume that they are operating in the black and have planned accordingly to finance a longer life. Another context of *"Don't ask, don't tell."*

So we wonder and worry and wait. *Will Mom be able to afford the house on her own? Does Dad's insurance policy cover prescription drugs? Are Uncle Frank's weekly trips to the casino getting the best of him?* Unless we're willing to open up the dialogue and state our concerns about financing a long life, we won't really know the truth about their ability to remain financially stable in the long run. What we do know is that when the money runs out, the rest of the family typically picks up the tab.

It's never too late to initiate conversations with our elders about their money and their plans for the future. This section of *The Complete Eldercare Planner* is designed to help you review, budget, and understand their current and future financial situation and resources. Before you begin talking to your elders about their money, review the contents of "Communicaring," chapter 4 of this planner, starting on page 86. As you can imagine, talking about this particular hotbed topic will require a kid-glove communication approach.

PLAN ONE

Plan for financial fitness.

Review your elder's current financial state. Use the **"Eldercare Budget Worksheet"** on pages 136–137 to track income and expenses.

BUYING TIME

- Family members may be surprised to find that their parents have far less money than they thought.
- People mistakenly believe that Medicare will pay for their long-term care.
- For many older Americans, retirement will not be a viable option.

If you're a family caregiver and fear that your retirement savings are in jeopardy, start talking today about how to pay for your elders' long-term care.

OBJECTIVES

*After completing **"Buying Time,"** you will be able to:*

Assist in financial planning and saving and spending strategies.

Review resources to pay for long-term care.

Gain access to financial-planning professionals.

Manage elders' money from far away.

PLAN TWO

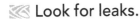 Look for leaks.

Becoming more aware of the vulnerabilities your elders may be encountering on a daily basis will be critical in effectively helping them to make ends meet. **Financial disasters can occur when no one is paying close attention to precarious situations that trigger unplanned expenditures.**

For example, it's no secret that the gaming industry rolls out attractive and elaborate perks and freebies as a way to draw in new consumers and keeping them begging for more. Free meals, complimentary airline tickets, hotel rewards, and instant merchandise are quite appealing when you're on a tight budget and your social life is not what it used to be. Studies that have been conducted on older people and **gambling** reveal interesting and complex psychological issues. Research also indicates that the feelings of independence associated with the gaming process can be intoxicating.

Additionally, older consumers are not immune to **credit-card debt**. People living on a fixed income who also have strong and uncontrollable desires to gift large amounts of money to family members, friends, and charitable causes can replenish their wallets simply by opening up a new charge account. People are also using credit cards to buy basic items, such as groceries and medications, when available dollars don't stretch far enough to cover living expenses.

ELDERCARE BUDGET WORKSHEET

(This worksheet is also available online at www.elderindustry.com)

Today's date_____

Elder's name_____

INCOME AND ASSETS INVENTORY

Wages/commissions _____

Savings _____

Social Security _____

Stocks/bonds _____

IRA/Keogh _____

Pensions/profit sharing _____

Rental income _____

Real estate _____

Investments _____

Other _____

AVERAGE MONTHLY EXPENSES

Housing _____

Home maintenance/repairs _____

Taxes _____

Insurance _____

Cable TV _____

Utilities _____

Food _____

Transportation _____

Auto maintenance _____

License/sticker fees _____

Vehicle insurance _____

Medical _____

Dental _____

Prescriptions _____

Long-term care insurance _____

Assisted-living services _____

Adult day services _____

Eyeglasses, hearing aids _____

Personal care _____

Clothing _____

Laundry/housekeeping _____

Entertainment _____

Memberships _____

Fitness _____

Travel _____

Gifts _____

Donations _____

Children/grandchildren _____

Other _____

TOTAL EXPENSES _____

TOTAL INCOME _____

SUBTRACT TOTAL EXPENSES _____

MONTHLY BALANCE _____

While family members have been known to scam their elders, *outsiders also pose a serious threat*. **Financial exploitation** (the illegal and improper use of another person's funds, property, or assets) by strangers leaves few visible signs of abuse—until the money runs out, and by then it may be too late to recover what has been lost.

PLAN THREE

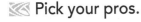 Pick your pros.

Take the time to find the right financial adviser and it will be worth the effort in the long run. Over a half million professionals are now marketing themselves as personal financial advisers to older adults, and some of them are peddling advice that may be inaccurate or downright wrong. Also, a growing number of tax-deferred annuities are now sold inside banks; consequently, trusting bank customers don't realize that they're getting advice from a securities broker, licensed by the bank, who is paid on commission.

Choose financial advisers who understand longevity and bring to discussions an expertise and experience analyzing long-term eldercare financial issues. Start your search for an adviser by soliciting referrals from people you trust. Also look to the professional groups listed in the resource section at the end of this chapter. Before engaging the services of any adviser, conduct a background check and ask for references. Here is a list of potential advisers:

Certified Financial Planner with Financial Gerontology certification
Certified Public Accountant with Personal Financial Specialist certification
elder-law attorney
bank trust officer
insurance agent
investment adviser
Realtor
employer retirement and pension adviser
medical and insurance claims adjuster
health-care professional
Social Security counselor
Medicare counselor
Medicaid caseworker
funeral director

There are a number of questions you should ask before hiring professional advisers.

How long have you been in practice?
What is your work history?
What is your education background?
What license, certification, and special training do you have?
How do you stay current with developments in your field?
What services do you offer? What services do you not offer?
Who will actually do the work? Will it be you or an assistant?
How are your fees determined? What are the terms for payment?
Is there a charge for the initial visit?
What can I expect to pay for the services I need?
Are you compensated by businesses that you refer me to?
Will you provide written reports? How often?
Have you ever been or are you now involved in a lawsuit?
Who are some of your clients? Will you provide three references?

PLAN FOUR

⧉ Look to insurance policies for savings.

Reviewing your elder's insurance policies for discounts and deductions is time well spent.

Mature homeowner and **driver discounts** are available for those over fifty-five years of age.

Multiple policy discounts may be offered to customers who have two or more policies with the same company.

Smoke and **burglar alarm discounts** may apply on homeowner policies. Also ask for discounts for dead-bolt locks and special window locks.

If your elder has **an accident-free driving record, antitheft equipment, automatic seat belts, air bags, antilock brakes, more than one car**, and **low yearly mileage,** he or she may qualify for auto insurance discounts.

Nonsmoker discounts are often offered to home and auto policy holders.

Ask for homeowner discounts for buildings made of **special fireproof materials**.

Long-term policy holders may be eligible for discounts offered to those who keep a policy with the same company for a specified number of years.

PLAN FIVE

⧉ Boost cash flow and dig for discounts.

If your elders' financial resources appear to be dwindling, discuss the possibility of putting some of these strategies in place.

APPLY FOR PROGRAMS

Review the benefits eligibility checklist distributed by the local aging agency.

Ask about the Medicaid application process and Medicaid diversion program.

MANAGE FUNDS

Seek professional financial-planning advice.

Create a realistic budget and stick to it.

Check all incoming bills for errors and overcharges.

Process all medical and insurance claims.

Establish tax and estate-planning strategies.

Ensure adequate insurance coverage.

Get counseling for gambling addictions and credit-card abuse.

REEL IT IN

Collect all money that is owed.

Sell unwanted jewelry, automobiles, and household items.

Consider a part-time or full-time job.

Inquire about life insurance and annuities proceeds.

Investigate the possibility of unclaimed property.

BUY AND SPEND WISELY

Buy at discount stores.

Purchase sale items.

Use money-saving coupons.

Repair house air and water leaks.

Swap skills in terms of time and personal service.

Use public services, such as libraries, transportation, and community centers.

DIG FOR DISCOUNTS

Do your homework and check the Internet for price wars.

Ask for senior-citizen discounts and group rates.

Ask for discounts when paying in full with cash on expensive items.

PLAN SIX

Tap into all potential financial resources.

Be sure that your elders are already receiving money that is rightfully theirs through programs such as Social Security and company pensions. Also investigate programs that are designed for people who are living on limited incomes. Program rebates and reduced rates may also be available for anyone at any income level. You just have to ask. Here are some of your options.

Social Security is a federal income program offered to individuals upon retirement age or upon becoming disabled. Apply for Social Security in person, online, or by calling the local Social Security office.

Veterans benefits and pensions are available for eligible veterans and their dependents. Call the local Veterans Affairs office.

General Relief is allocated to people of low income who are not eligible for federally funded assistance. Contact the local social-services office.

Benefits eligibility lists are available through the local agency on aging and social-services office.

Supplemental security income (SSI) *provides monthly benefits to those with low income, the aged, and persons with disabilities. SSI is available through the Social Security office. If your elder cannot visit the office, ask for a home visit.*

People with disabilities *may qualify for tax postponement, homeowners assistance, and renters assistance. Contact the state tax office.*

Grandparents raising grandchildren *may qualify for a host of government programs. Contact the local social-services office and ask about grandparent-support programs.*

Workers' unions *and* ***fraternal organizations*** *may offer benefits. Call them directly.*

Disease-related organizations *offer a wealth of information and resources on financing care. To locate local chapters on the Internet, type the name of the disease in your search engine.*

Life insurance terms may allow policyholders to pay for long-term care through the use of ***early death benefit withdrawals*** *and* ***viatical settlements*** *(the sale of a life insurance policy by the policy owner before the policy matures). But beware. There are tax questions, commission claims, and other concerns that need to be clarified before signing an agreement. Discuss options with the insurance agent.*

Local ***religious groups*** *may sponsor volunteer programs to help older people with a variety of daily tasks.*

PLAN SEVEN

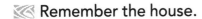 Remember the house.

The house where your elders reside is typically their greatest single asset when faced with paying for day-to-day living expenses and long-term care. Include the expertise of a certified financial adviser in your discussions about using the equity in the family home to defray expenses because taxes and estate plans will come into play.

Older people who want to remain at home may consider a ***house-sharing arrangement*** *with renters. Or they may* ***rent the residence*** *and move to a smaller home, apartment, or other housing option.*

If your house-rich, cash-poor elder is willing to move, ***downsizing*** *to a smaller house or apartment may be an option.*

Government ***deferred-payment loans*** *are available to low-income persons at low-interest rates. The loan permits homeowners to defer payments of all principal and interest until the homeowner dies or when the house is sold.*

If the house appeals to you as an investment, you could buy the home and lease it back to your elder. But be aware, ***sale-leaseback*** *arrangements are legally complex and can impact a person's eligibility for Medicaid and similar benefits.*

Homeowner equity accounts *offer homeowners a line of credit secured by the value of the real estate. Terms vary, as do interest rates. Shop around.*

> A **reverse mortgage** allows people sixty-two or older to convert home equity into cash without having to move or assume extra debt. There are limitations and costs. **Note:** Reverse mortgages do not guarantee homeowners lifelong income or the right to remain in the home. Be fully informed.
>
> Your elder may choose to **gift his or her home** to a person or an institution. The gift recipient then agrees to pay the homeowner a set income.

PLAN EIGHT

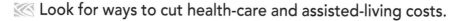 Look for ways to cut health-care and assisted-living costs.

Living a longer life can mean more trips to the doctor. Perhaps some of the following strategies will help lessen the financial load of paying medical-related expenses.

Medical Services

- Avoid hospital emergency rooms for nonemergencies.
- Buy long-term care insurance.
- Ask first if Medicare covers the cost of services.
- Discuss *all* costs with doctors, including telephone consultations.
- Ask if tests in the doctor's office can be performed without the full office visit charge.
- Ask for written estimates and refunds for overcharges, if any.
- Negotiate all medical fees.
- Get routine tests done before checking into the hospital.
- Fill prescriptions at the local drugstore rather than at the hospital pharmacy.
- Check out of the hospital before the checkout hour.
- Make sure the medical equipment supplier is enrolled by Medicare.
- Review invoices and insurance claims for errors.

Assisted-Living Services

- Ask about additional fees and negotiate all costs.
- Ask about less-expensive rooms (views and balconies cost more).
- Find a community in a less-expensive neighborhood.
- Reduce the square footage of the living quarters.
- Consider a shared apartment or bathroom arrangement.
- Look for new communities with special move-in rates.
- Ask your family to help with housekeeping and transportation.
- Purchase medications and supplies outside of the community.

PLAN NINE

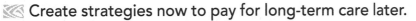 Create strategies now to pay for long-term care later.

Sticker shock has new meaning when it comes to long-term-care expenses. Even the process of death and dying comes at a high price. Take an inventory of the methods your elder will use to pay for long-term care and make good use of professionals who can offer specific insights on medical-related financial strategies. Review the following options.

Private Pay

Expect to pay out of pocket for medications, copayments, insurance deductibles, assisted-living services, skilled nursing care, and non-health-care expenses such as caregiver respite programs, housekeeping services, and companion services. Increasingly, people are purchasing discount cards for prescription drugs, among other expenses. Discounts offer modest savings but, unfortunately, hardly make a dent in long-term-care expenses.

Medicare

Medicare is a federal health-insurance program for people age sixty-five and older, regardless of income, and pays limited hospital and medical expenses. In order to create a more realistic eldercare budget, discuss what Medicare does and does not pay for with a qualified Medicare caseworker:

- Hospital (Medicare Part A) and medical (Medicare Part B)
- HMO (health maintenance organization) and PPO (preferred provider organization) plans (Medicare Part C)
- Medicare prescription drug plan (Medicare Part D)
- veterans benefits
- Medigap insurance policies
- Qualified Medicare Beneficiary program
- medical savings accounts
- preventative and outpatient services
- assisted-living and skilled nursing care
- medical transportation and ambulance services
- dental, vision, and hearing coverage
- coverage for mental health and dementia patients
- chronic care
- oxygen and home medical equipment
- foreign-travel coverage
- caregiver respite programs and adult day services
- hospice and grief counseling

Medicaid

Medicaid is a state program available to low-income individuals who fit into an eligibility group. Each state sets its own guidelines. Be aware that patients may be asked to pay a portion of the medical expenses. For example, if the patient owns a home, the proceeds from the sale of the home help to cover the cost of care services. Ask a geriatric caseworker at the local Medicare office to evaluate your elder's particular financial situation for eligibility for Medicaid benefits. Discuss the following topics:

- eligibility requirements, including the "look-back" period
- the impact of family caregiver employment contracts on qualifying for Medicaid
- bookkeeping and record-keeping guidelines
- copayment plans
- protecting the assets of a spouse

Managed-Care Plans and Long-Term Care Insurance

Medicare managed-care plans, such as HMOs and PPOs, and long-term care insurance help pay medical expenses. Review "Insurance," chapter 8 of this book, starting on page 166. Also consult a certified financial adviser to explore the advantages of combining insurance policies with other financial strategies.

PLAN TEN

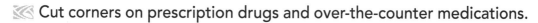 Cut corners on prescription drugs and over-the-counter medications.

Most prescription drugs are expensive, and many older Americans who are feeling the pinch have resorted to drastic measures in order to make ends meet. Some people skip doses of their medications, while others forgo taking their medications altogether. There are also unfortunate reports of people selling valuable items, such as wedding rings, and others robbing the medicine cabinets of friends who have recently died in search of leftover drugs. People are also willing to flout the law and are buying their medications from Canada and Mexico, where they cost much less.

The Medicare drug discount program (Part D) is not the answer for everyone. Consequently, drug companies may provide the cure for higher prices, since the competition among them to serve Medicare beneficiaries is fierce. Here are a few money-saving tactics to review with your elder.

- Ask the doctor to **eliminate drugs from regimens** that are no longer useful.
- Discuss **generic substitutes** with the doctor and pharmacist.
- Ask the doctor for a **prescription of the over-the-counter version.**
- **Compare costs** and ask the pharmacy to meet the price of the competitor.

- Look for **discounts** offered through employers, insurers, senior organizations, memberships, and pharmacies.
- **Compare prices** at deep-discount stores, warehouse clubs, the Internet, and mail-order suppliers.
- Research **consumer websites** for "best buys" for prescriptions and over-the-counter drugs. Computerless? Your local library has one you can use.
- Review eligibility for **veteran** and **union drug plans.**
- Ask the local agency on aging about **state low-income drug assistance programs.**
- Drug costs can be lower in **Canada** and **Mexico** due to trade laws and lower manufacturing costs. But proceed cautiously.

The Medicare Drug Discount Program

Medicare beneficiaries are eligible for prescription drug coverage, regardless of income, health status, or current prescription expenses. Those who currently receive full Medicaid services will automatically get extra help. Know the exact names, dosages, and costs of prescriptions if no insurance coverage applied. Look to the following resources for free advice:

- pharmacist
- the local agency on aging
- social-services agency
- community centers
- Medicare customer service representatives

PLAN ELEVEN

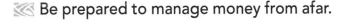 Be prepared to manage money from afar.

There are legal considerations that must be resolved ahead of time when assuming the financial chores of another. Before anything else, review chapter 7, "Legal Matters," in this book, starting on page 153. **Importantly, discuss any potential liability and risks with an attorney** *before you sign papers that put you in the position of joint owner of bank accounts, power of attorney, trustee, or guardian.*

Once the legalities are in place, you can perform a variety of money-related tasks, including paying bills, filing claims, tax preparation, banking, and more. Becoming a financial caregiver is a delicate situation, so continue sharing information with other family members. Consider the following strategies for managing money from afar.

- Establish a **budget.** Make good use of computer software.
- **Organize** financial and insurance records.

- Keep tabs on **deadlines** and **due dates,** especially property, federal, and state taxes.
- **Forward mail** to your address.
- Establish **online bank accounts.**
- Set up **direct deposit** of checks and **automatic payment** of recurring bills.
- Discuss **"representative payee"** alternatives with the Social Security office.

Outside help from money managers, mail organizers, bank trust officers, attorneys, and accountants is also readily available if personally performing the responsibilities of financial caregiver is not an option for you. Compare fees, check references, verify agencies, and ensure that individuals are bonded before hiring. *Importantly, of all the bookkeeping tasks you decide to delegate to others, be sure to retain all check-signing responsibilities.*

PLAN TWELVE

Consider the advantages of a part-time job.

Employment opportunities aren't limited by experience or age. Many businesses welcome older employees. If money is tight, and your elder wants to work to help pay for daily living expenses, chapter 13, "Quality of Life," starting on page 272 in *The Complete Eldercare Planner,* offers numerous employment ideas. **However, be aware that a working status may affect your elder's Social Security benefits.** Review all government benefit regulations before taking on a job that brings in extra income.

Low-Cost and Free Resources

In need of a wheelchair, walker, or cane—but only for a temporary basis? Many communities have loan closets that make **medical supplies and equipment** available for loan—free of charge. Contact the local chapters of the American Cancer Society, the United Way, Easter Seals, and disease-specific organizations, the local aging agency, and religious groups.

Financial support programs may be available by contacting the local social-service agency, religious organizations, charities, and family service agencies. The local disease-specific organizations, including the American Cancer Society, the Alzheimer's Association, and the National Parkinson Foundation offer financial resources.

Contact the local health-care and family services agency for programs that defray costs of medicine. **Free prescription medicines** may be available to those who qualify.

The Internal Revenue Service offers **free tax advice** plus in-home visits to homebound people. Call the local IRS office.

Call the state treasurer's office for a list of **unclaimed money, property,** and **valuables** in safe-deposit boxes.

ORGANIZATIONS AND WEB RESOURCES

Alliance of Claims Assistance Professionals
Website: www.claims.org

American Association of Daily Money Managers
526 Brittany Drive
State College, PA 16803
(814) 238-2401
Website: www.aadmm.com

American Institute of Certified Public Accountants
1211 Avenue of the Americas
New York, NY 10036-8775
(212) 596-6200
Website: www.aicpa.org

American Institute of Financial Gerontology
1525 NW 3rd Street, Suite 8
Deerfield Beach, FL 33442
(954) 421-1403; toll-free: (888) 367-8470
Website: www.aifg.org

Benefits CheckUp
(Explore rebates and discounts)
Website: www.benefitscheckup.org

Low-Income Home Energy Assistance Program
(Help with utility bills)
Website: http://liheap.ncat.org

Financial Planning Association
1600 K Street, NW, Suite 201
Washington, DC 20006
Toll-free: (800) 322-4237
Website: www.fpanet.org/public

Food Stamp Program
(Research local low-cost nutrition programs)
Website: www.fns.usda.gov/fsp

Internal Revenue Service
Toll-free: (800) 829-1040; TDD: (800) 829-4059
Website: www.irs.gov

National Association of Insurance Commissioners
(Search consumer insurance issues)
2301 McGee Street, Suite 800
Kansas City, MO 64108-2662
(816) 842-3600; fax: (816) 783-8175
Website: www.naic.org

National Association of Personal Financial Advisors
Website: www.napfa.org

National Association of Unclaimed Property Administrators
Website: www.missingmoney.com

National Center for Home Equity Conversion
(Consumer information on reverse mortgages)
Website: www.reverse.org

National PACE Association
(Affordable care programs)
801 N. Fairfax Street, Suite 309
Alexandria, VA 22314
(703) 535-1565
Website: www.npaonline.org

Social Security Administration
Toll-free: (800) 772-1213;
    TDD: (800) 325-0778
Website: www.ssa.gov

Society of Financial Service Professionals
17 Campus Boulevard, Suite 201
Newtown Square, PA 19073
(610) 526-2500
Website: www.financialpro.org

University of Minnesota Extension Service
(Family finance planning tools)
Website: www.financinglongtermcare
    .umn.edu

U.S. Department of Veterans Affairs
810 Vermont Avenue, NW
Washington, DC 20420
(202) 273-5771; toll-free: (800) 827-1000;
    fax: (202) 273-5716
Home-care benefits toll-free: (879) 222-8387
Website: www.va.gov

U.S. Securities and Exchange Commission
(File a complaint and conduct background
    checks)
Toll-free: (800) 732-0330
Website: www.sec.gov

Women's Institute for a Secure Retirement
1725 K Street, NW, Suite 201
Washington, DC 20006
(202) 393-5452
Website: www.wiserwomen.org

Debt Relief

Gamblers Anonymous
Website: www.gamblersanonymous.org

National Foundation for Credit Counseling
801 Roeder Road, Suite 900
Silver Spring, MD 20910
(301) 589-5600; toll-free: (800) 388-2227
Website: www.nfcc.org

Health Care

All About Vision
Toll-free: (800) 222-3937
Website: www.allaboutvision.com

American Health Assistance Foundation
(Financial assistance for needy caregivers of
    Alzheimer's patients)
22512 Gateway Center Drive
Clarksburg, MD 20871
(301) 948-3244; toll-free: (800) 437-2423;
    fax: (301) 258-9454
Website: www.ahaf.org

Centers for Medicare and Medicaid Services
(410) 786-3000; toll-free: (877) 267-2323;
    TTY toll-free: (866) 226-1819; TTY: (410)
    786-0727
Website: www.cms.hhs.gov

Medicare Rights Center
Website: www.medicarerights.org

My Medicare
Website: www.mymedicare.gov

Partnership for Prescription Assistance
Toll-free: (888) 477-2669
Website: www.pparx.org

Work/Life

National Partnership for Women and Families
(Information about family leave)
1875 Connecticut Avenue, NW, Suite 650
Washington, DC 20009-5729
(202) 986-2600; fax: (202) 986-2539
Website: www.nationalpartnership.org

Pension Rights Center
1350 Connecticut Avenue, NW, Suite 206
Washington, DC 20036
(202) 296-3776; fax: (202) 833-2472
Website: www.pensionrights.org

MONEY MATTERS ACTION CHECKLIST

(This worksheet is also available online at www.elderindustry.com)

THE COST OF CARING	To Do By	Completed

Become familiar with eldercare-related expenses

	To Do By	Completed
elder's home	_____	☐
household items	_____	☐
basic living	_____	☐
in-home health care	_____	☐

Consider the cost of long-distance assistance

	To Do By	Completed
travel	_____	☐
back home	_____	☐
at destination	_____	☐

Review your own finances

	To Do By	Completed
keep written record	_____	☐
retain advisers	_____	☐
implement important documents	_____	☐

Consider ability to contribute to expenses

	To Do By	Completed
	_____	☐

Budget eldercare expenses

	To Do By	Completed
short-term	_____	☐
long-term	_____	☐

Protect personal financial stability

	To Do By	Completed
	_____	☐

Review elder's financial stability

	To Do By	Completed
	_____	☐

Develop a family plan

	To Do By	Completed
current expenses	_____	☐
future expenses	_____	☐

Create eldercare account

savings _____ ❑
checking account _____ ❑

Record and file eldercare expenses receipts _____ ❑

Evaluate elder's financial needs every six months _____ ❑

Ask family to give time and resources _____ ❑

BUYING TIME

Complete Eldercare Budget Worksheet _____ ❑

Review your elder financial stability

sources of debt _____ ❑
housing and living expenses _____ ❑
medical costs _____ ❑
insurance costs _____ ❑

Consider the services of a financial adviser

get referrals from reliable resources _____ ❑
ask specific questions _____ ❑
do background checks _____ ❑

Set financial goals

short-term _____ ❑
long-term _____ ❑
tax planning _____ ❑
planning for incapacity _____ ❑
estate planning _____ ❑

Increase your elder's income via

Social Security _____ ❑
veterans' benefits _____ ❑

pensions   _____ ❑

relief programs   _____ ❑

life insurance   _____ ❑

homeownership   _____ ❑

gifts and loans   _____ ❑

employment   _____ ❑

Review Medicaid spending policy   _____ ❑

Budget for your elder's

housing expenses   _____ ❑

living expenses   _____ ❑

in-home care   _____ ❑

medical expenses   _____ ❑

insurance   _____ ❑

service providers   _____ ❑

funeral expenses   _____ ❑

**Record the phone numbers of
your elder's**

tax preparer   _____ ❑

accountant   _____ ❑

legal adviser   _____ ❑

bank   _____ ❑

financial adviser   _____ ❑

insurance agents   _____ ❑

Keep phone numbers

at home   _____ ❑

at work   _____ ❑

in wallet or purse   _____ ❑

**Distribute phone numbers to key
family members**   _____ ❑

7

Legal Matters

Estate Planning

There are many advantages to estate planning, yet few people take the time to do it. *Why?* They may not be aware of the necessity, so are unaware as to the many benefits. They hold to a common misconception that estate planning is only a concern of the wealthy. They simply find it hard to make decisions now about what will occur after their death. Failing to engage in estate planning is an example of benign neglect; many people assume their affairs are legally in order because they own everything jointly with their heirs. **This can be a potentially costly mistake.**

As a way to take action, you might ask yourself this important question: What might happen to *your* financial future if the person you are caring for lives longer than expected? In addition to planning for distribution of family assets in the event of death, a key element of estate planning also includes the preservation and distribution of wealth *before* death.

This section of *The Complete Eldercare Planner* simplifies the process of estate planning. You will gain a basic understanding of elder law and legal terms, and insights on how proper planning provides for orderly distribution of assets while minimizing court delays, fees, and taxes. Now more than ever before, people have the potential to live a long life, and it is wise for you and your elders to investigate estate-planning strategies now.

PLAN ONE

Get to know the terms.

Estate planning is less intimidating and easier to grasp once you have an understanding of the legal terms.

A **will** instructs an executor how an individual wants his or her estate to be distributed upon death. The document may include provisions for various trusts, and names an executor.

ESTATE PLANNING

- If someone dies without a will, the state will divide his or her property as per statutory guidelines and potentially leave unnecessarily large "bequests" to the tax collectors.
- Estate planning not only focuses on property distribution after death, but also protects hard-earned assets during a person's lifetime.
- If people don't take steps to plan for incapacity, the state has the authority to set standards as to what the incompetent person would want.

If your elders are avoiding estate planning, perhaps taking the process step-by-step will help ease them into it.

OBJECTIVES

*After completing "**Estate Planning,**" you will be able to:*

Gain a basic understanding of the estate-planning terms and legal documents.

Access affordable elder-law resources.

Make plans for decision making in the event of your elder's incapacity.

Avoid the devastating consequences of inadequate legal documentation.

An **executor** is designated by the creator of the will **(testator)**. His or her job is to carry out the provisions of the will, and pay estate taxes, debts, and expenses of the decedent. The executor need not be a family member, nor even an individual, as is the case when a corporate executor, usually a bank, is designated.

A **trust** is a way for the creator of the trust **(grantor)** to bequeath money or property that takes advantage of tax benefits and accomplishes the desires of the person setting up the trust. A trust can provide greater flexibility and control over the release of money, including attaching conditions of disbursement, before or after death. A **testamentary trust** is one that is created by and does not take effect until the death of the creator of the will. A **trustee** manages the trust. As with executors, a trustee may be an individual or a corporation (bank).

A **living trust** establishes ownership of stocks, property, and other items from individual people to a separate legal entity, avoids probate, and also protects in the event of incapacity. A **revocable living trust** gives the creator of the trust the right to change the terms of the trust, or even to end it.

A **letter of instruction** is prepared for the beneficiaries of a will or trust. The letter is meant to serve as a guide for closing out the affairs of an individual upon his or her death. Although this letter is not a legal document, the composition should be consistent with the individual's will, and can be notarized, though that is not a requirement. A separate letter of instruction should include a list of the people to notify when death occurs and cover the disposition of possessions and specify any particular wishes regarding the funeral.

A **power of attorney over property** is a designation by the principal authorizing an individual **(agent)** to act on behalf of the principal as to the full range of financial and/or property transactions. This document must be executed while the principal is still legally competent, and can be terminated at any time upon the principal's written direction. The agent need not be a family member. The breadth of the responsibilities placed in the hands of the agent mandates that the principal should be highly selective as to whom he or she would entrust with these duties. **Note**: Banks and other financial institutions may not honor power of attorney forms other than their own. Contact each banking institution to obtain proper documents. Also be aware that some states order safe-deposit boxes sealed upon the lessee's death and may not permit them to be opened without following strict procedures. Other states require a court order to open a box that was rented in the decedent's sole name.

PLAN TWO

Seek legal advice.

It is never a good idea for anyone to draft his or her own will. State law sets forth specific requirements as to the execution and witnessing of wills. Documents not prepared in accordance with the law might not accomplish what was intended, and are more likely to be invalidated or contested in court. Heirs might end up paying more estate taxes than they should. A simple will, prepared by an attorney, can cost as little as a few hundred dollars. Keep original copies of legal documents in a safe, twenty-four-hour accessible location. Give copies of the documents to the attorney. A yearly review of the will and other legal documents is advised because financial circumstances and relationships may have changed. Discuss updates and changes with an attorney.

Further, it is especially important for domestic partners and unmarried cohabitants to seek legal advice. At this writing, most states do not give legal standing to such relationships, and therefore no property rights are established or enforceable. In these complex and litigious times, it is better to define the relationship *yourself*—by utilizing the previously mentioned documents—rather than have it defined for you by family members or by the courts.

An estate-planning attorney and an elder-law attorney can be found through personal referrals and attorney referral services, and by calling the local bar association. Check the attorney's qualifications and shop around to compare fees, services, and experience.

PLAN THREE

Implement gift-giving strategies.

Money and property are not the only assets your elder may have. A residence may be filled with furnishings, photographs, books, collectibles, and other items that will need to find a home. Some people prefer to dispose of personal possessions to loved ones while they are alive and enjoy the giving process as they go, while others prefer to distribute personal possessions through a letter of instruction as part of their will.

PLAN FOUR

To gain better control, anticipate incapacity.

Few people plan for disability or incapacity during their lifetime. The result is often a loss of control over *who* will make decisions in a person's behalf, and *how* these decisions will be made. Proper eldercare planning includes legal documentation that allows financial and health-care decisions to be made by a designated person in order to avoid court intervention or guardianship/conservatorship proceedings.

A **power of attorney over property** is a legal document transferring decision-making authority to a designated person and continues that authority in the event of incapacity. Review the description of this document in Plan One of this section.

A **power of attorney for health care** gives another person **(agent)** legal authority to make medical decisions in the event of incapacity. Individuals must be of sound mind and able to give informed consent when composing this document. The power of attorney for health care specifies how life-support decisions are to be made, and under what conditions. It is not necessary to hire an attorney to complete this document; the forms are available free of charge at hospitals, doctors' offices, community centers, and nursing homes. Each state has its own form, so be sure you obtain the correct form where your elder resides. You might ask a geriatric case manager at the local agency on aging to review the form for accuracy. Advice on filling out this form is usually provided free of charge.

A **living will** is a form of communication to health-care providers that death-delaying life support is not wanted. A living will can be prepared by an attorney, though it is not a requirement. On a practical level, the effectiveness of this document is extremely limited, and, in fact it is likely to be ignored if a power of attorney for health care is in effect. Since the medical profession is set up to save lives, doctors may refuse to honor this document.

A **directive to physician** instructs doctors to withhold medical treatment if it would not aid in recovery but only prolong illness or delay death. If the doctor disagrees ahead of time with any key terms, consider switching physicians. **Include these instructions in the power**

of attorney for health care. Instruction also should be left by those who do not want their lives ended by the withdrawal of treatment, no matter how ill or long they are incapacitated.

Legal guardianship (also sometimes called **"conservatorship"**) is a formal appointment by a probate court that authorizes others to assume total control over an incapacitated and/or disabled individual's affairs. This is almost never the choice of the incapacitated person—in fact, it is often *contested* by such person. It grants authority to make decisions on behalf of the disabled person and includes the responsibility to ensure the care and well-being of such person, as well as to protect his or her assets. A court hearing is required. The process of acquiring a legal guardianship can be quite expensive and lengthy. Be aware that state laws and probate courts lean heavily in favor of keeping the disabled person independent to as great a degree and for as long as reasonably possible.

PLAN FIVE

Discuss and distribute estate-planning instructions.

Legal documents and letters of instruction are not useful unless other people are made aware of their existence. Be sure that your elder has distributed and discussed the contents of important and legal documents with designated family members, doctors, friends, nursing-home directors, and other key people.

Keep *original* documents in a safe-deposit box or other twenty-four-hour accessible place. Give the attorney copies, instead of originals. You and your elders may be consulting with different attorneys from time to time. Record the location of all important and legal documents in "The Documents Locator" chapter of *The Complete Eldercare Planner*, starting on page 327.

Power of attorney for health-care agents should be prepared to present proof of this document at a moment's notice. If your elder enters the hospital or a nursing home, insert copies of notarized forms and directives into his or her medical file. Ask nursing-home directors to agree *in writing* that they will comply with your elder's wishes. Update all documentation as needed.

Justice for All

According to U.S. Census Bureau projections, a substantial increase in the number of older people will occur during the period from 2010 to 2030. The older population in 2030 is projected to be twice as large as in 2000, growing from 35 million to 72 million and representing nearly 20 percent of the total U.S. population at the latter date.[1] With this kind of growth in an aging population, government programs that serve the elderly are in serious financial jeopardy. *Every year, policy makers cut the budgets and staffs of social-service organizations, placing increasingly more of the burden of eldercare on the backs of family, friends, and volunteers.*

The current dearth of accessible and affordable eldercare programs makes the family caregiver's task a test of endurance. To make matters worse, many older Americans do not meet the rigid criteria to qualify for the government's free and low-cost services; and Medicare does not cover the costs of the day-to-day care and assistance older adults need.

Elder advocacy also includes taking on a bigger role in the fight against Medicare fraud. Billions of dollars are lost to health-care fraud every year.[2] Double billing, charging for services not provided, and performing unnecessary services are among the Medicare abuses. To combat this loss, Medicare beneficiaries are being asked to report activities that they believe are fraudulent and abusive.

There is mounting evidence that family caregiving and the needs of older Americans are finally on the minds of policy makers. This section of *The Complete Eldercare Planner* is a wake-up call for all of us to become **active advocates** for improvements in government-funded eldercare and family caregiving programs and services. **If we don't get involved, everything's at stake:** family leave, caregiver tax credits, ombudsman services, Social Security, Medicaid, Medicare, respite care, and much more. The time is now to focus our attention on urgent elder-rights concerns.

JUSTICE FOR ALL

- Most older persons with long-term-care needs—65 percent—rely exclusively on family and friends to provide assistance.[3]
- Like other unpaid work, the contribution caregivers make to society is not highly valued.
- National Family Caregivers Month, observed every November, seeks to draw attention to the many challenges facing family caregivers, and raise awareness about community programs that support family caregivers.
- Overt acts of discrimination are a daily occurrence for older people.

Be willing to speak up and keep your eye on the ultimate goal—protecting not only the health and safety of loved ones, but yourself as well.

OBJECTIVES

After completing "Justice for All," you will be able to:

Stay informed of political activities that concern older Americans.

Make contact with politicians who are creating public policy.

Recognize and report incidents of Medicare fraud and abuse.

PLAN ONE

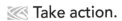 Fight for improved eldercare and caregiver policies and programs.

We must advocate for the passage, authorization, and implementation of local, state, and federal legislation supporting the rights of caregivers and elders. Issues requiring immediate attention include:

affordable housing	LGBT aging and family caregiving
aging in place and in-home care	life-span respite care
caregiver education and training	mental illness and dementia
death and dying	mobility and transportation
elder abuse	nursing-home policies
elder law	paid family caregivers
employment and older workers	prescription drugs
food and nutrition programs	retirement and pension policies
grandparents as parents	Social Security, Medicare, and Medicaid
health care	tax deductions and credits
health insurance	technology and aging
homeless and incarcerated aging	workplace employee benefits

PLAN TWO

Get involved.

Monitor the activities of politicians. Knowing what's happening at local, state, and federal levels can lead to numerous benefits for the savvy researcher. Eldercare programs and family caregiver rights exist as a result of the hard work of individuals who are dedicated to improving the lives of older Americans and the people who care for them.

As a member of an advocacy group, you will be asked to voice your concerns and write letters to legislators. You also may be asked to make telephone calls and send e-mails to a variety of audiences. **Writing letters and taking action works, especially during elections, when politicians need your vote to get or stay in office.** Elder advocacy requires dedication and energy. Join others in making important improvements in eldercare and caregiving policies and services, locally and nationwide. Make good use of the advocacy and legislation resources listed at the end of this chapter.

PLAN THREE

Take action.

On a local level, if you suspect that an older person's rights are being violated, contact the following advocates:

police department

long-term-care ombudsman

family service agency

hospital social-services director

agency on aging

adult protection services

attorney

state's attorney

PLAN FOUR

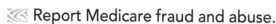 Report Medicare fraud and abuse.

It's only natural that when we hire someone to do a job for us, we discuss how much it will cost, and ask for written estimates of the services to be provided. After the job is complete and the bill comes, we compare the final invoice to the estimate. When the invoice doesn't appear to be in sync or is considerably higher than expected, we have the option of asking service providers for an explanation and an adjustment.

Medicare service providers should not be exempt from these fair expectations. Everyone loses when Medicare beneficiaries are the victims of billing errors, overcharges, and wrongdoings. The system is already fragile; fraud and abuse further threaten the financial soundness of Medicare.

What Is Medicare Fraud?

Medicare fraud is defined as an incident or practice that intentionally deceives or misrepresents claims against the Medicare program. The violator may be a physician or other practitioner, a hospital or other institutional provider, a clinical laboratory, an employee of any provider, a billing service, or any person in a position to file a claim for Medicare benefits.

Fraudulent acts include:
- Billing Medicare for services not furnished
- Overcharging for services and supplies
- Billing Medicare patients at a higher rate than non-Medicare patients
- Offering or accepting kickbacks, bribes, or rebates
- Fraudulent diagnoses on the Medicare claim form
- Waiver of patient deductibles and copayments
- Billing for services not furnished
- Falsifying certificates of medical necessity
- Using another person's Medicare card

Report Medicare Fraud and Abuse

Most health-care providers are honest, and a questionable charge may be the result of a clerical error. That's why many people call their provider first. Otherwise, call the **Medicare Fraud Hotline (1-800-447-8477)** to discuss concerns. Be prepared to offer the following information:

1. Provider's name and identification number
2. Item or service in question
3. Date on which the item or service was provided
4. Amount approved and paid by Medicare
5. Date of the Explanation of Benefits
6. Name and Medicare number of the person who supposedly received the item or service
7. Reason Medicare should not have paid

Low-Cost and Free Resources

The local **AIDS service organization** and **legal-aid agency** will help protect the rights of individuals who have contracted HIV, and also assist with establishing guardianship, if necessary.

Free legal advice may be available for elders with limited incomes. Contact the local agency on aging, the local bar association, or the district attorney's office. Also, call a local law school to find out if community services are offered.

The **secretary of state's office** has a TDD (telecommunications device for the deaf) for voter registration and election information. For persons with visual disabilities, audiotapes of state and county candidates are available in the county clerk-recorder's office.

Free copies of the **power of attorney for health care** forms are available at your local agency on aging, doctor's office, community center, nursing home, and hospital senior services department. Many hospitals provide free assistance in filling out these forms. These documents are governed by individual state laws, so you will want to get the document that is applicable in the state in which your elder resides.

ORGANIZATIONS AND WEB RESOURCES

AARP Legal Hotlines
Website: www.legalhotlines.org

American Bar Association
321 N. Clark Street
Chicago, IL 60610
Toll-free: (800) 285-2221
Website: www.abanet.org

Commission on Law and Aging
Website: www.abanet.org/aging

ElderLawAnswers
Website: www.elderlawanswers.com

National Academy of Elder Law Attorneys
1604 N. Country Club Road
Tucson, AZ 85716
(520) 881-4005; fax: (520) 325-7925
Website: www.naela.org

National Conference of State Legislatures
444 North Capitol Street, NW, Suite 515
Washington, DC 20001
(202) 624-5400; fax: (202) 737-1069
Website: www.ncsl.org

National Guardianship Association
526 Brittany Drive
State College, PA 16803
(814) 238-3126; fax: (814) 238-7051
Website: www.guardianship.org

National Network of Estate Planning Attorneys
10831 Old Mill Road, Suite 400
Omaha, NE 68154

Toll-free: (800) 638-8681
Website: www.netplanning.com

National Senior Citizens Law Center
1101 14th Street, NW, Suite 400
Washington, DC 20005
(202) 289-6976; fax: (202) 289-7224
Website: www.nsclc.org

Advocacy and Legislation

Administration on Aging
(Information about the Older Americans Act)
1 Massachusetts Avenue, Suites 4100 and 5100
Washington, DC 20201
(202) 619-0724; fax: (202) 357-3555
Website: www.aoa.gov

ElderCare Rights Alliance
2626 E. 82nd Street, Suite 230
Bloomington MN 55425
(952) 854-7304; toll-free: (800) 893-4055; fax: (952) 854-8535
Website: www.eldercarerights.org

Federal Government Websites
White House: www.whitehouse.gov
U.S. House of Representatives: http://house.gov
U.S. Senate: http://senate.gov

FedWorld
(Makes it easy to locate government information)
Website: www.fedworld.gov

Gay & Lesbian Association of Retiring Persons
Website: www.gaylesbianretiring.org

Global Action on Aging
Website: www.globalaging.org

Gray Panthers—National Office
1612 K Street, NW, Suite 300
Washington, DC 20006
(202) 737-6637; toll-free: (800) 280-5362;
    fax: (202) 737-1160
Website: www.graypanthers.org

Institute for the Future of Aging Services
2519 Connecticut Avenue, NW
Washington, DC 20008
(202) 508-1208; fax: (202) 783-4266
Website: www.futureofaging.org

Leadership Council of Aging Organizations
Website: www.lcao.org

National Academy on an Aging Society
Website: http://agingsociety.org

National Committee to Preserve Social Security and Medicare
10 G Street, NE, Suite 600
Washington, DC 20004
(202) 216-0420; toll-free: (800) 966-1935;
    fax: (202) 216-0451
Website: www.ncpssm.org

National Governors Association
Website: www.nga.org

National Partnership for Women and Families
1875 Connecticut Avenue, NW, Suite 650
Washington, DC 20009-5729
(202) 986-2600; fax: (202) 986-2539
Website: www.nationalpartnership.org

Older Women's League
3300 N. Fairfax Drive, Suite 218
Arlington, VA 22201
(703) 812-0687
Website: www.owl-national.org

Thomas
(Federal legislation tracking)
Website: http://thomas.loc.gov

U.S. Senate Special Committee on Aging
Website: www.aging.senate.gov

USA.gov for Seniors
Website: www.usa.gov/topics/seniors.shtml

LEGAL MATTERS ACTION CHECKLIST

(This worksheet is also available online at www.elderindustry.com)

ESTATE PLANNING	To Do By	Completed
Set estate-planning goals		☐
Locate elder-law resources		☐
Draw up		
will		☐
trust		☐
letter of instruction		☐
power of attorney for property		☐
power of attorney for health care		☐
Duplicate, distribute, and review documents with key family members		☐
Review assets		☐
Make plans to review and update legal documents		☐
Store documents in a safe, twenty-four-hour-accessible location		☐
Obtain important legal telephone numbers		☐
Distribute legal phone numbers to key people		☐
JUSTICE FOR ALL		
Research advocacy groups		☐
Know how to reach		
city hall		☐
village of		☐
mayor's office		☐

city council members   _____   ☐
senator   _____   ☐
congressman   _____   ☐
governor's office   _____   ☐

**Vote in local and national
    elections**   _____   ☐

Stay informed

community newspapers   _____   ☐
city newspapers   _____   ☐
political flyers   _____   ☐
Internet   _____   ☐

**Recognize Medicare fraud
    and abuse**   _____   ☐

8

Insurance

Insurance Coverage for a Longer Life

In today's world, it seems inconceivable that a person would allow his or her entire personal wealth to be at risk. You certainly know better. You carry many different types of insurance: on your car, on your home and belongings, on your life. *But do you really have any idea whether your elders let a policy or two lapse over the years? Have they upgraded their coverage to match their current assets?*

Making sure your elders have **adequate insurance** can be a matter of economic survival for the entire family, and taking an in-depth look at existing insurance policies may reveal under- and overcoverage. It also may disclose an absence of insurance coverage that should be in place. Insurance needs may have changed since the purchase of the original policy, and now, rather than under emergency conditions, is the time to gather and review their insurance documents.

This section of *The Complete Eldercare Planner* will take you through the action steps that will ensure insurance coverage is adequate and up to date. Establishing a relationship with the insurance agent and asking for explanations on policy coverage and limitations will also help eliminate potential insurance mishaps down the road.

PLAN ONE

✄ Review each insurance policy.

Homeowner, auto, life insurance, disability, personal property, business insurance, and more—do you know for a fact that your elders have **adequate insurance coverage**? Obtain copies of each insurance policy and review the conditions under which they were purchased. Note possible family changes that may affect the beneficiary status.

The most important role of insurance is to protect the policyholder from catastrophe.

INSURANCE COVERAGE FOR A LONGER LIFE

- Insurance needs may have changed since the purchase of the policy.
- The most important protection you can have against accidents is knowing how to avoid them.

If it has been more than one year since insurance policies have been reviewed, now would be a good time to check to see whether your elders have too much or too little protection.

OBJECTIVES

*After completing **"Insurance Coverage for a Longer Life,"** you will be able to:*

Know if an insurance policy is in place.

Bring insurance coverage up-to-date.

Examine an insurance company's financial stability.

Extended personal liability insurance (umbrella coverage) can be coordinated with your elder's home and auto insurance. The cost of insurance depends on numerous variables, including the rate of the deductible. Renewing present insurance policies for adequate coverage may be less expensive than purchasing additional insurance.

Insurance is big business. Television ads and direct-mail offers with celebrity spokespeople can be misleading, since they are paid by the insurance company to endorse the product. Also keep in mind that agents are salespeople, and asking them to offer an opinion on one policy versus another is like asking a car salesman if it's better to buy the blue car or the red car. Do your homework and be informed.

To find a licensed insurance agent, ask for a referral from someone you trust. The local agency on aging also can offer family members the names of insurance advisers who advocate the special insurance needs of older adults. Insurance policies should always be reviewed by a third party before signing.

Insurance Coverage to Consider

HOMEOWNER. If their home and personal possessions were destroyed by fire or water damage, or if the home was burglarized, would your elders have the funds to rebuild and replace their belongings? Could they afford temporary housing during reconstruction? Homeowner policies cover these issues and more.

VALUABLES. Collectibles, paintings, antiques, jewelry, and furs, among other specialty items, should be insured individually because coverage under homeowners and renters insurance policies is limited.

AUTO. The cost of owning a car goes well beyond the sticker price and includes all the expenses of keeping that car running year after year. Insurance premiums, a vital expense element, can account for more than one-fifth of ongoing car costs.

LIFE. Elders may want to carry life insurance for dependents who would suffer financially upon the policyholder's death. People also buy life insurance to cover the cost of funerals and other death-related expenses.

DISABILITY. Experts agree that anyone who has a full-time job outside the home should consider a disability policy. Proper coverage averages 60 percent of a person's salary for as long as the policyholder cannot work. Employed family caregivers would be wise to consider this insurance option.

PLAN TWO

Take inventory.

Prepare inventory lists and photographs of household and business possessions to help establish the proper amount of coverage needed. Videotaped records and digital images work just as well. Itemize all valuables. The insurance company will require sales receipts and appraisals for all valuables. Keep receipts and important documentation in a safe-deposit box.

The insurance company will need **documented proof** in the event that an insurance claim must be filed. Photographs and videos will be of great value in obtaining a fair settlement.

PLAN THREE

Go behind the scenes.

You can examine the financial stability of any insurance company. Insolvencies do happen as a result of bad investments, and some states don't guarantee funds when an insurer goes broke. Investors cannot count on warnings of impending insolvencies from regulators.

Insurance company ratings are conducted by A.M. Best Company, Moody's Investors Service, Standard & Poor's, and Duff & Phelps. If the insurance company is assessed by only one of these companies, that could indicate a problem. You will find these companies' rate books at the public library, or you can obtain rating information on the Internet.

Another method is to contact the insurer's home office and request the most recent quarterly and annual reports. Review the quality of the insurer's investments, which provide the income it needs to meet financial obligations to policyholders.

Beyond Medicare

Medicare, the government health-insurance plan for older Americans, offers minimal coverage for health-care costs. Existing gaps in this basic insurance program mean that your elders may be unprotected from today's soaring health-care expenses. A chronic illness such as arthritis or diabetes can put the financial resources of the entire family at serious risk, since Medicare won't pay for the kind of day-to-day care these illnesses demand.

To help customers make informed health-care-insurance decisions, Congress imposed tougher standards on supplemental insurers (also known as Medigap insurers). Companies are required to sell standardized policies so that customers can easily compare competitive products. To ease comparison procedures, insurers must also provide potential buyers with detailed outlines of policy coverage.

This section of *The Complete Eldercare Planner* explains the interplay between Medicare and private supplementary insurance and suggests specific questions to ask when purchasing health and long-term care insurance. Additionally, states across the country have expanded counseling programs on Medicare and other health-care issues. Encourage

---

BEYOND MEDICARE

- If medical bills aren't at least partially covered by an employer's insurance plan and your elders have opted out of a Medigap policy, what's the plan to pay for their health care?
- An assisted-living residence offers personalized supportive services for older adults who need help with activities of daily living and assistance managing medications. Residents generally pay the cost of assisted living from their own financial resources and/or a long-term care insurance policy. *Government-subsidized programs for assisted-living services are extremely limited.*
- The key to buying supplemental health insurance is to review and compare policy differences. If what the insurance company offers sounds too good to be true, it probably is.

Since Medicare doesn't cover all of a patient's medical expenses, buying some form of health insurance supplement is essential.

OBJECTIVES

After completing "Beyond Medicare," you will be able to:
Distinguish Medicare from supplemental health insurance policies.
Locate insurance advisers.
Review Medicare, HMO, and long-term care insurance options.
Protect against insurance denial coverage and policy cancellation.

Medicare-qualified family members to take advantage of this free advice to ensure a wise choice when purchasing a health insurance supplement.

PLAN ONE

🗲 Become familiar with Medicare and Medicaid options.

Medicare beneficiaries are offered a range of choices in how they receive health-care services. The range of coverage will depend on the plan package. Knowing what Medicare does *not* provide is critical when deciding how much and what kind of additional health insurance to buy. Refer to the Medicare topics starting on page 130 in chapter 6, "Money Matters." Apply for Medicare at the local Social Security office.

What Does the Medicare and Medicaid Menu Include?

The Original Medicare Plan is a federal insurance program that covers a portion of medical and hospital bills for those age sixty-five and older, regardless of income, and those already receiving Social Security benefits.

Medicare Part A is hospital coverage and **Part B** is medical. Part B is optional and requires a monthly premium payment. **Part C** is additional coverage offered by private insurance companies that have been approved by Medicare. These health-care plans offer some coverage of prescription drugs. **Part D** is prescription drug coverage.

PLAN TWO

🗲 Explore the need for additional health insurance coverage.

While enrollees in the Original Medicare Plan are allowed to use any doctor or hospital that accepts Medicare, the plan doesn't cover all outpatient prescription drugs or long-term care. Consequently, backing up Medicare with additional health insurance is a smart idea.

Start the process by reviewing health-care policies that are already in place. People who retire before age sixty-five may be covered by a previous employer or insured if a spouse is still working. Others may be receiving benefits from a trade union, the Railroad Retirement Board, the Department of Defense, and the Department of Veterans Affairs. However, many retirees have no such coverage. In that case, the options for Medicare supplemental insurance coverage are **Medigap** policies and **Medicare Advantage Plans**.

Medigap

A Medigap policy is health insurance that fills the "gaps" in the original Medicare plan. These policies are sold through private insurance companies and help pay some of the health-care costs that Medicare doesn't cover. Medicare and a Medigap policy will pay both their shares of covered health-care costs.

Insurance companies have "standardized" Medigap policies and are clearly identified as "Medicare Supplement Insurance." Each plan offers basic and extra benefits and costs vary. With the Medigap option, in addition to paying the monthly Medicare Part B premium, participants also pay a premium to the Medigap insurance company. A Medigap policy does not cover the health-care costs of a spouse. Each person must buy a separate policy.

Medicare Advantage Plans

Medicare Advantage Plans are part of the Medicare program and are run by private companies. When individuals join a Medicare Advantage Plan, they are still in Medicare and continue to have Medicare rights and protections.

Medicare Advantage Plans provide Part A (hospital) and Part B (medical) coverage and cover medically necessary services. They offer extra benefits, and many include Part D (drug coverage). Generally, individuals must see doctors who belong to the plan and go to certain hospitals to get covered services. Options for coverage include:

Medicare Health Maintenance Organizations (HMOs)
Preferred Provider Organizations (PPOs)
Private Fee-for-Service Plans
Medicare Special Needs Plans

Medicare Special Needs Plans are specially designed for people with certain chronic diseases or disabling conditions, and use a care coordinator to develop personal-care services and health-care efforts between Medicare and Medicaid.

PLAN THREE

Implement health insurance safeguards.

Keep your elder's health insurance coverage in check with these basic tips.

- Arrange for automated payment of premiums and ask the insurance company to send *you* duplicates of invoices.
- Buy only *one* Medicare supplemental policy. *(It's the law.)*
- Medicare cannot deny enrollment because of preexisting health conditions.
- Know the rules for coverage *before* leaving one plan for another.
- Medicaid beneficiaries do not need additional health insurance policies.

If your elders are considering the Medicare HMO option, here are the questions they need to ask.

QUESTIONS REGARDING PHYSICIANS

If I'm unsatisfied, may I switch primary care physicians?

What happens if the plan doesn't include a specialist that I need?

Do doctors get a bonus if they make fewer referrals to specialists?

How many doctors leave the plan each year?

QUESTIONS REGARDING PRESCRIPTIONS

Do you carry my current prescription?

Do you ever remove drugs from your list?

What recourse do I have if you remove my prescription from your preferred list?

QUESTIONS REGARDING CARE

When I need to see the doctor, how long must I wait for an appointment?

Will I get prompt care in a medical emergency?

Who decides what is "medically necessary" in my case?

How do I appeal a medical decision?

Is dental care available?

Are there any extra services covered with the plan?

How are chronic ailments covered with this plan?

Which hospitals, nursing homes, and home-health-care agencies do you use?

What are the procedures for filing complaints or leaving this plan?

How do members get emergency care while traveling outside the HMO service area?

QUESTIONS REGARDING COSTS

What are the monthly premiums? What about copayments? Deductibles?

What is your policy on rate increases?

How long is the open-enrollment period before I am locked into this plan?

PLAN FOUR

Know the Medicaid spending policies.

State Medicaid spending policies protect the assets of one spouse should the other require care in a nursing home. Without professional advice sought ahead of time, overspending can leave the remaining spouse virtually penniless, and family members may be penalized for implementing certain spending strategies. Seek advice from an elder law attorney or certified financial planner.

PLAN FIVE

Long-term care insurance—yes or no?

There is good reason why the government is giving us the hard sell on buying long-term care insurance for ourselves and for our older dependents, and handing out tax incentives to do so: Long-term care is costly, and long-term care insurance policies help with the escalating costs of skilled nursing care. Persons of moderate income and limited savings can exhaust their money if they pay out of pocket for nursing-home care.

Assisted living is a special combination of care. From housing and supportive services such as bathing to getting dressed in the morning, when a person needs help with these simple yet knotty problems, the costs involved are typically prohibitively expensive, and must be paid for privately—either out of pocket or through insurance policies that cover the services.

Medicare does not pick up the tab for long-term care, and looking to Medicaid as a health-care plan will seriously restrict a person's ability to access quality care.

Long-term care insurance—under the right circumstances—can be a pretty good deal, but it's not for everybody. If the need is already just around the corner, most likely the premiums are going to be prohibitively high. Customers may not qualify if they are in poor health or have an alcohol or drug addiction. At the very least, it's worth investigating whether long-term care insurance is the right choice for your elder, and for you.

What Does Long-Term Care Insurance Buy?

Long-term care insurance can provide an aide who carries out the basic support tasks of daily living when a person is incapacitated due to an illness, injury, or cognitive impairment. More than nursing-home care, policies cover help with activities such as eating, dressing, mobility, bathing, and homemaker chores, besides providing supervision for the elder and respite (time off) for the family caregiver. Long-term care can be administered in the person's home, in adult day centers, an assisted-living facility, or a nursing home.

Where Can You Find Long-Term Care Insurance?

employers
membership associations
private insurance companies
senior organizations
fraternal societies
continuing-care retirement community (CCRC)

PLAN SIX

Shop around for a quality long-term care insurance policy.

In order to capture their share of the market, insurance companies offer policies that cover long-term care such as domestic help and personal-care services so that older adults can remain in their own homes, if that's what they desire. However, there may be a substantial gap between what consumers think they have bought and the level of help they actually receive.

Many policies do not provide *immediate* at-home assistance, and don't go into effect until sixty or ninety days have elapsed. Also, strict criteria must be met before a policy covers assistance to someone who is not completely disabled but simply needs help with eating, dressing, bathing, or domestic chores. The situation has to be far more serious than most people expect. **Caveat:** Insurance coverage or benefits may be denied completely if the company can prove that untrue statements were made on the application.

Here are some tips and guidelines to follow when shopping for a long-term care insurance policy.

THE APPLICATION PROCESS

- The applicant—not the insurance agent—should fill out the medical history questions on the application.
- Make sure questions are answered truthfully and completely. If an agent tells the applicant not to list a health condition, find another agent.
- During the free-look period (thirty days after the policy is delivered), check the application to make sure that the agent answered the questions correctly and has not changed any answers. If you spot an error, notify the company immediately and insist that the company respond in writing.
- Submit a currently dated physician's statement along with the application. Request written confirmation from the insurance company that they are in receipt of this information and have filed it with the insurance policy. Keep a copy of the physician's statement in your files.

THE INSURANCE CARRIER

- Beware of agents who say they can get coverage in a very short period of time (twenty-four to forty-eight hours).
- Check with your state insurance department to see if they have information on how the company in question pays claims or engages in "post-claims underwriting"—the practice of health insurance companies who check policyholder's medical history only after a claim is filed, instead of at the time of application.
- Look for an "A" or better rating in the A.M. Best Company insurance reference guide found at the public library.
- Know that insurance coverage is governed by laws of the state in which it's issued.

- If switching insurance companies, be sure the coverage under the old policy stays in effect until the new coverage kicks in.
- Make sure the policy defines complaint-filing procedures.

THE CONDITIONS OF CARE

- No prior hospital stay should be required.
- Medicare approval should not be required.
- Be wary of the limits on both the maximum daily benefits and the number of days (or visits) per year for which benefits are paid.
- Identify the waiting period before benefits begin.

THE LEVELS OF CARE

- Benefits can be used at home or in an assisted-living community or nursing home.
- The choice of the doctor who will certify the care must be retained by you (rather than someone hired by the insurance company).
- The benefits should include personal grooming and homemaker services.
- The policy should include the use of in-home medical equipment and personal safety devices.
- The plan should cover caregiver programs for family members.
- There must be full coverage for Alzheimer's disease and other dementia.
- The plan should provide coverage for respite care (time off for the family caregiver), adult day services, home health care, and hospice.
- The policy should cover all levels of care—skilled, intermediate, and custodial.
- Payments should be made for any type of care in *any* licensed facility.
- Payments should reflect the same daily rate no matter where the care is given, although there may be reduced payments for some services and programs.
- The policy should provide automatic increases in benefits, or the ability for the insurer to upgrade to higher benefits or less-restrictive coverage.
- There can be no reduction in policy benefits.

FINANCING THE POLICY

- Age and current health status are the key determinants of cost.
- You can save money on the policy by buying only three or four years of coverage.
- If you agree to pay for the first ninety or one hundred days of care, you can cut premium costs (much like raising the deductible on a car insurance policy).
- You can request a spousal and dependent discount when purchasing coverage for two lives or more.
- The policy should be guaranteed renewable.

- Premium levels are locked; they cannot be raised due to health or age.
- The policy should explain "class basis" as a condition of raising premiums.
- The policy should have inflation protection.
- The death of the insured immediately terminates premiums.
- The policy should waive the premium payments once you start using the benefits.
- The benefits received from the policy must be income-tax free and cannot affect seniors' Social Security benefits.
- The premiums may be tax deductible on itemized returns, since they are considered a medical expense, although there are some restrictions.
- Ask how benefits are paid. Some companies demand that the insured submit nursing-care receipts for reimbursement, others will pay providers directly, and others simply send a check for the agreed upon monthly benefit.

PLAN SEVEN

Take action to file a complaint or appeal a health insurance decision.

Health insurance is a complex business, and being assured of quality care can be challenging. When things don't go right and when insurance decisions are not in the patient's favor, you and your elder have the right to file a complaint and appeal an insurance decision. Even if the patient has since died, the estate of that person can appeal a decision when the delivery of items and services did not meet your expectations.

The reasons for filing a grievance may include:

You think a service or item should be covered and it isn't.

Payment for a service or item is denied.

The amount paid for a service or item is questionable.

The drug plan won't cover a prescription.

A prescription drug costs more than you think it should.

Unexpected bills show up in the mail.

There is evidence of discrimination against the patient (on the basis of race, age, religion).

Health information privacy has been breached.

The hospital is making a patient leave too soon.

There is no response to a complaint or an appeal.

ADDED MEDICARE PROTECTION. If your elders have Medicare coverage and are admitted to a Medicare-participating hospital or skilled nursing facility, or they are receiving services from a comprehensive rehabilitation facility or home health agency, they should automatically be given a document titled **"An Important Message from Medicare,"** which explains their rights as a patient. Any complaints regarding Medicare-related services should be directed to the local Medicare office immediately. The Quality Improvement Organization will review the case.

ACT QUICKLY. Most health insurance claims, including Medicare, have a time limit on appeals. If you miss a deadline, file a complaint anyway.

FILE A FORMAL COMPLAINT. Every insurance carrier, including Medicare, offers instructions and documents to assist in the process of filing complaints and appeals. Keep logs of all conversations, including names and dates. Also, refer to the resources listed at the end of this chapter.

CONSIDER THE SERVICES OF A PROFESSIONAL. Social workers and geriatric case managers help with insurance issues and the coordination of nursing-care plans. Claims assistance professionals can help you track health insurance payments, file insurance claims, and work with you to challenge any claims that are denied by the insurance company. To find a local claims assistant, review the resources listed at the end of this chapter.

Low-Cost and Free Resources

The Senior Health Insurance Program (SHIP) has volunteer counselors available free of charge to assist Medicare beneficiaries and their caregivers with Medicare, prescription drugs, long-term care, and related issues. Look in the Blue Pages of the telephone directory under "State Government." Conduct a keyword search on your Internet browser using "senior health insurance program" and include the state where your elder resides in the search box.

To obtain information on **Medicare health insurance coverage**, visit or call the local Social Security office. Home visits from agency representatives are also available.

The local **agency on aging** assists individuals with Medicare billing problems and insurance policy selections, and offers lists of Medicare health-care providers.

State medical services are available through the local **county bureau of health services.** People can make use of these care facilities if they have insurance, are on Medicare or Medicaid, or have no health insurance. For more information, contact the county office where your elder resides.

ORGANIZATIONS AND WEB RESOURCES

Alliance of Claims Assistance Professionals
(For help with filing insurance claims and
  complaints)
Website: www.claims.org

**American Association for Long-Term Care
Insurance**
3835 E. Thousand Oaks Boulevard, Suite 336
Westlake Village, CA 91362
(818) 597-3227
Website: www.aaltci.org

American Health Quality Association
(Professionals working to improve health-care
  quality and patient safety)
1155 21st Street, NW
Washington, DC 20036
(202) 331-5790; fax: (202) 331-9334
Website: www.ahqa.org

America's Health Insurance Plans
601 Pennsylvania Avenue, NW, South
  Building, Suite 500
Washington, DC 20004
(202) 778-3200
Website: www.ahip.org

Center for Medicare Advocacy
PO Box 350
Willimantic, CT 06226
(860) 456-7790
Website: www.medicareadvocacy.org

Centers for Medicare and Medicaid Services
Medicare Service Center: (800) 633-4227
Medicare Service Center TTY: (877)
  486-2048
Report Medicare Fraud and Abuse: (800)
  447-8477
Website: www.cms.hhs.gov

Consumer Coalition for Quality Health Care
1101 Vermont Avenue, NW, Suite 1001
Washington, DC 20005
(202) 789-3606; fax: (202) 898-2389
Website: www.consumers.org

Insurance Information Institute
111 William Street
New York, NY 10038
(212) 346-5500
Website: www.iii.org

Medicare Beneficiary Ombudsman
(To report problems, submit complaints, and
  obtain appeals forms)
Toll-free: (800) 633-4227

Medicare HMO
Website: www.medicarehmo.com

Medicare Rights Center
Toll-free: (888) 466-9050
Website: www.medicarerights.org

National Association of Insurance Commissioners
(To locate your local state insurance commission)
2301 McGee Street, Suite 800
Kansas City, MO 64108-2662
(816) 842-3600; fax: (816) 783-8175
Website: www.naic.org

National Committee for Quality Assurance
(Health-care-plan assessment for quality care)
2000 L Street, NW, Suite 500
Washington, DC 20036
(202) 955-3500; toll-free: (888) 275-7585; fax: (202) 955-3599
Website: www.ncqa.org

National Committee to Preserve Social Security and Medicare
10 G Street, NE, Suite 600
Washington, DC 20004
(202) 216-0420; toll-free: (800) 966-1935; fax: (202) 216-0451
Website: www.ncpssm.org

National Insurance Consumer Helpline
(Ask to be directed to the kind of information you are seeking)
Toll-free: (800) 942-4242

Social Security Online
(To find a local office)
Website: www.ssa.gov

U.S. Department of Health and Human Services
200 Independence Avenue, SW
Washington, DC 20201
(202) 619-0257; toll-free: (877) 696-6775
Website: www.hhs.gov

U.S. Department of Veterans Affairs
810 Vermont Avenue, NW
Washington, DC 20420
(202) 273-5771; toll-free: (800) 827-1000; fax: (202) 273-5716
Health-care benefits toll-free: (877) 222-8387
Website: www.va.gov

INSURANCE ACTION CHECKLIST

(This worksheet is also available online at www.elderindustry.com)

INSURANCE COVERAGE FOR A LONGER LIFE	To Do By	Completed
Review insurance policies for proper coverage		
homeowner	_____	☐
auto	_____	☐
life	_____	☐
disability	_____	☐
business	_____	☐
valuables	_____	☐
Set insurance coverage goals		
short-term	_____	☐
long-term	_____	☐
Review life insurance company for stability	_____	☐
Review policies with insurance adviser	_____	☐
Take inventory		
photographs	_____	☐
inventory lists	_____	☐
video	_____	☐
Keep inventory documents in a safe, twenty-four-hour accessible place	_____	☐
Know phone numbers of your elder's insurance agents	_____	☐
Keep proof of insurance accessible	_____	☐

BEYOND MEDICARE

Become familiar with Medicare

Part A   _____ ☐

Part B   _____ ☐

Part C   _____ ☐

Part D   _____ ☐

Explore Medicare supplementary insurance options

Medigap policies   _____ ☐

Medicare Advantage Plans   _____ ☐

Medicare HMOs   _____ ☐

PPOs   _____ ☐

Fee-for-Service Plans   _____ ☐

Medicare Special Needs Plans   _____ ☐

Ask specific questions of HMO providers
   _____ ☐

Review Medicaid qualifications and plan

State Medicaid programs   _____ ☐

QMB plans   _____ ☐

SLMB plans   _____ ☐

Research Medicaid spending policy
   _____ ☐

Review health insurance safeguards
   _____ ☐

Review the need for long-term care insurance
   _____ ☐

Shop around for long-term care insurance
   _____ ☐

File formal complaints
   _____ ☐

Know the phone numbers of

Social Security office _____ ❏

Supplementary insurance company _____ ❏

Medicare _____ ❏

Medicaid _____ ❏

**Keep health insurance phone
numbers accessible** _____ ❏

Make copies of insurance cards _____ ❏

9

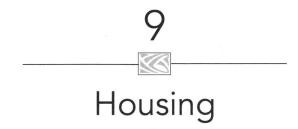

Housing

Move or Stay Put?

Few experiences can be more devastating for older people than having to move out of their home. Independence and home ownership are the cornerstones of the American dream. An overwhelming majority of elders say they want to remain in their homes for as long as possible; physical limitations, memory problems, and the inability to drive can cut that dream short.

Whether our elders move or stay put will depend on many things, but one thing is certain: *The subject of housing and all its implications has the potential to cause a tremendous amount of anxiety for family caregivers.* We are witness to elders who refuse to move out of their house in spite of obstacles such as having to climb stairs; we contend with elders who are lonely and isolated by choice; we worry and wonder how they get by when they are sick; and we wait in the unrealistic hope that if a move is inevitable, the process will be quick and stress free.

If there's one topic that does not necessarily obey the natural laws of being reasonable and using common sense, it is the issue of housing. When it comes to where and how we live, we all tend to do as we please. Much of who we are is tied up in our choice of residence and the stuff that surrounds us. Moving means saying good-bye to something—memories, routines, and neighbors—and staying put means not having to go through all that.

This chapter of *The Complete Eldercare Planner* offers an array of housing options, including tips on when and how to bring up the delicate subject of moving out of the family home. The more *you* know, the better your chances of a positive outcome. You may be able to minimize the normal negative reactions to changes in your elder's living environment by proceeding thoroughly and slowly. Bringing up the subject of moving is unquestionably a traumatic experience for everyone.

MOVE OR STAY PUT?

- As health declines, being near family can be of greater importance, as elders want the security of knowing a loved one is nearby.
- A study of American women age forty-five and older suggested that women in general are having conversations with their parents about their ability to live independently; however, less than half of their parents have begun to plan for the possibility of needing assistance with independent living.[1]
- The need to limit driving or giving up the car keys altogether may spark a conversation about moving out of the family home.

With adequate planning, people can control their housing destinies and prevent last-minute, regrettable decisions down the road.

OBJECTIVES

*After completing **"Move or Stay Put?"** you will be able to:*

Create a "friendlier" home environment.

Assess the need to make housing changes.

Review housing and long-term-care options.

Tap into resident-centered housing initiatives.

Manage the moving process.

PLAN ONE

Determine specific needs when choosing senior-housing options.

The "ideal" place for older adults to live may change over time. While remaining in one's own home is often the most desirable housing option, it may not be the final residence in the long run. The decision to move or stay put is assessed on current and future needs and also on a combination of other factors, including income, location, health, safety, availability of help, transportation, and personal preferences.

Typically, the onset of a physical or mental impairment begins the conversation about moving. Elders may develop limitations that affect where they live, how they live, and with whom they live. Reviewing chapter 2, "How to Tell When Your Elder Needs Help," on page 33 in *The Complete Eldercare Planner* is a good way to assess housing needs.

Specialized housing for older adults falls into three ownership groups: not-for-profit, for-profit, and government-owned. There are also several different housing categories by type, including conventional and shared housing; supported housing; unassisted age-restrictive communities; and assisted and skilled care facilities. Here are the housing options to consider.

CURRENT HOME. People who are physically and mentally fit and can manage their own well being often choose to stay put. Even if more frequent care is needed due to illness, elders who want to "age in place" can arrange for services such as meals, nursing, housekeeping, personal care, transportation, and more. Bringing in additional help will require often expensive private-pay arrangements.

SHARED HOUSING. This is a new name for an old custom: two or more unrelated people sharing living quarters. This option stretches available dollars while providing added security and companionship for older homeowners. Occupants share expenses and in return have private bedrooms and access to common areas, such as the kitchen and living room.

NATURALLY OCCURRING RETIREMENT COMMUNITIES WITH SUPPORTIVE SERVICE PROGRAM (NORC-SSP). People who live in neighborhoods with an above-average concentration of older adults may have the option of remaining at home. Members pay annual fees, and services such as personal care, social activities, and limited nursing services are included in a membership or offered at a discount on an "à la carte" basis.

SENIOR VILLAGE. A variation of the NORC-SSP idea, the village is not a place but rather a membership program that helps people stay in their own homes by providing support— everything from cooking and fixing the air conditioner to making doctor appointments and getting dressed. Members pay the providers, but the village staff and volunteers select and screen them, and can help coordinate these appointments. Villages may also provide social outlets, linking residents with similar interests.

SUBSIDIZED HOUSING. Such housing offers affordable rents to qualified low-income seniors or individuals with disabilities as established by the U.S. Department of Housing and Urban Development (HUD). Financial assistance is available through a number of federal programs. The demand for affordable housing is on the rise. Finding a vacancy takes time and effort because there's a limited supply of affordable buildings. Waiting lists are long; but being on several waiting lists at the same time is not prohibited.

THE MOBILE HOME. These days, the term *mobile home* has new meaning. From small motor homes to large recreational vehicles, elderly nomads are traveling all over without a permanent home. Some people are seeking work or volunteer opportunities, while others are looking for sunshine and relaxation. Living on a cruise ship is another mobile option. While on "the endless cruise," as it's sometimes called, people enjoy restaurants, movies, casinos, driving ranges, spas, room service, and more. Many cruise ships have doctors and nurses on call 24/7.

AGE-RESTRICTED RENTAL APARTMENTS. Independent, healthy residents who want to socialize with other adults are attracted by the lifestyle offered at age-restricted rental apartments. Fitness centers, gardens, cafés, housekeeping, and handyman services are attractive features. Apartments are specifically designed for comfort and include important modifications such as wide doorways, emergency buttons, and bathroom grab bars. Some apartments may charge a "community fee" in addition to monthly rent. These housing complexes generally don't include on-site medical care.

GROUP HOMES. These homes offer three or more residents separate rooms or apartments with common areas for dining, socializing, and activities. While this option usually provides housekeeping services, group homes are designed for people who are relatively mobile and self-sufficient. The cost of rent, housekeeping, utilities, and meals is shared.

COHOUSING. Opting to age with friends in housing developments or communal homes offers togetherness and opportunities to share the care. Would-be neighbors spend time working out community rules and responsibilities, and share in the management of the community, as well as chores, expenses, social activities, and meals (which may be served in a common building). Although cohousing can accommodate different generations, it has emerged as a way for like-minded people to tackle growing old together. On-site health care is most likely not available. Some communities set aside space for live-in caregivers.

ACTIVE-ADULT COMMUNITY. Single-family homes, town homes, cluster homes, and condos provide maintenance-free living and social activities. In addition to the cost of the home, homeowner association fees are extra. Homes are senior-friendly, with features such as wide doorways and bathroom grab bars. Developments typically offer common areas for meetings and special events, and also may include a library, a fitness center, and a dining room with meal service. This option does not necessarily provide health-care services.

CONTINUING-CARE AND LIFE-CARE RETIREMENT COMMUNITIES. These communities promote healthy living and active lifestyles, and provide priority access to a full continuum of health care in one setting. A full range of amenities can include choices in dining rooms, fitness centers, spas, art studios, and more. Traditionally, this living arrangement requires a sizable entry fee, plus monthly maintenance fees. More recently, communities have begun to make this option available on a rental basis. A guide to understanding the financial arrangements of a continuing-care retirement community is available. For additional information, review the "Low-Cost and Free Resources" section of this chapter on page 201.

ASSISTED-LIVING RESIDENCE. This offers a combination of housing, supportive services, and personalized assistance, and appeals to people who can no longer live safely alone at home. Meals, housekeeping, medication supervision, social events, wellness programs, and transportation are among the amenities offered. Large residential communities can accommodate as many as one-hundred-plus people, who live in individual apartments. Board-and-care homes may be smaller (four to six residents), and are typically private homes that have been converted into a care community. Sliding-scale eligibility is available in most states.

ADULT FOSTER CARE. This is a living arrangement in a single-family residence where non-related adults live with a foster family that provides meals, housekeeping, and personal care.

ALZHEIMER'S AND DEMENTIA CARE. People who have been diagnosed with Alzheimer's disease require a highly specialized home environment because the disease may lead to a loss of abilities to carry out daily life activities; moreover, residents may exhibit wandering behaviors. Housing modifications and precautions that are appropriate in the earlier stages of the disease may not work for middle and later stages. Care is available in smaller homes (four to six residents) and in communities as large as a hundred people or more. In all cases, this type of housing is specifically designed to meet the needs of loved ones who have been affected by dementia issues.

SKILLED NURSING CARE. Nursing homes provide specialized services for people needing twenty-four-hour medical attention. Nursing homes also provide rehabilitation services after a hospital stay and also may serve as temporary housing for families seeking short-term respite from caregiving responsibilities. Facilities are licensed by the state department of health services.

PLAN TWO

Don't move. Improve.

Simple home modifications can convert your elder's house into a safer, more senior-friendly space, and lessen day-to-day caregiving demands on you. Lifting, transferring, and bathing are the top three physical burdens faced by family caregivers. The bathroom is perceived to be the most problematic room in the house. Installing adequate lighting, confining living quarters to one floor, and adding grab bars and shower benches are common alterations.

If your plan is to modify the home's environment, start the process by taking a walking tour of the house—inside and out—accompanied by your elder. If he or she uses a wheelchair or walker, use the device as a way for you to experience the living space from that perspective. For additional tips on creating a safe environment, review chapter 10, "Safe and Secure," starting on page 206.

Retrofitting the home to meet current and future needs may also require a major redo. Observe the requirements for obtaining building permits and meeting zoning laws and building codes.

Home improvement plans require making observations and asking questions. Follow these suggestions as you begin to formulate your plans.

OUTSIDE THE HOUSE. Is there parking close to the house? Is there space to safely get in and out of the car? Are the sidewalks and entrance leading to the front door in good shape? Are handrails available and in safe condition? Are ramps an option? Is lighting adequate?

LIVING SPACES. Are doorways wide enough to accommodate a wheelchair? Are living, sleeping, and cooking areas on one level? Is there adequate space to move around? Are floor surfaces nonskid? Are closets and drawers easy to negotiate? Are lighting and ventilation systems adequate? Are electrical outlets within reach?

KITCHEN. Are appliances and electric cords up to safety standards? Are controls easy to reach and grasp? Can appliances be opened safely and easily? Are counter heights reasonable? Is the sink within reach and the water controls easy to operate? Is the kitchen table sturdy? Are cabinets within reach and easy to open? Are supplies within reach?

BATHROOM. Is the sink a comfortable height? Are the water controls easy to operate? Is the mirror accessible? Is the medicine cabinet within reach and easy to open? Are supplies within reach? Is the toilet a safe height? Is the bathing area easy to access? Does the shower-head include a handheld spray? Are grab bars available and sturdy? Are towel racks being used as grab bars?

BEDROOM. Is a full bath available on the same floor as the bedroom? Is there space for a portable toilet? Could a first-floor room accommodate a bed if the need arises?

DOORS. Are peepholes at an accessible height? Is it easy to open and close doors? Are thresholds low and easy to negotiate? Are door knobs and locks easy to operate?

Creating a more senior-friendly home environment may include buying items that make negotiating the living space and performing day-to-day tasks easier and safer. Plus, they make great gifts. Here are a few ideas:

automatic jar openers	mobile and cordless telephones
automatic-turnoff appliances	night-lights
bath mats	nonbreakable glasses and dishes
clip-on battery-operated fans	nonskid slippers and socks
easy-grip kitchen utensils	programmable thermostats
easy-on/easy-off Velcro clothing	"reaching" devices
electric hand mixers	shower/bath stool
elevated toilet seats	talking clocks
glow-in-the-dark, large-dial clocks	universal remote control
illuminated light switches	whistling tea kettles

PLAN THREE

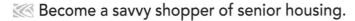 Become a savvy shopper of senior housing.

People shop for senior-housing options when they are healthy and also when a chronic illness makes the independent-living environment obsolete. Finding suitable housing *and* care takes time and effort. There's homework to do and questions to ask before signing on the dotted line. The "Senior-Housing Checklist" will help in your research process. Include your elder's long-term-care needs when considering housing options.

SENIOR-HOUSING CHECKLIST

(This worksheet is also available online at www.elderindustry.com)

Today's Date: _____

Name of Establishment: _____

Address/City/State/Zip: _____

Name of Contact Person: _____

Telephone/E-mail of Contact Person: _____

GETTING STARTED

- During the initial phone call, inquire about levels of care offered. If the housing option does not offer any levels of on-site health care or in-home assisted-living services, weigh that fact against the possibility of having to move your elder again down the road.
- Find out if a wait list exists. It may be worth putting down a small deposit now, especially if this housing option is one of the best around.
- Check with local consumer organizations, the Better Business Bureau, and state regulatory agencies to see if complaints or lawsuits have been filed.
- Visit as many different choices as possible. Stop by the community unannounced and at different times of day and night. Typically, you'll find different staff members on duty on certain days and on weekends.

The On-site Visit

- You'll want to be sure that the facility in question has been properly accredited and licensed. Ask for written documentation.
- Ask for copies of current state inspection reports.
- Find out who is behind the scenes. Ask questions about the owners and the sponsors, as well as consulting firms they have employed in the past.
- You'll want to ask for proof of long-term financial stability.
- All legal agreements as well as billing procedures should be offered to you in writing.
- Ask for written policies on how all levels of care are provided, especially in cases of increased frailty and the diagnosis of dementia and health assessments.

- Ask specific questions about the staff, including their qualifications and licenses regarding administering medications.
- Ask for proof of state and federal criminal checks for *all* workers.
- Be advised on how the staff handles advance medical directives, including do-not-resuscitate (DNR) orders.
- Ask about medication-management procedures. How does the facility guard against mistakes and mishaps?
- Get copies of menus, activity calendars, and resident newsletters.
- Obtain resident-satisfaction rating reports and ask permission to attend a resident/family/staff council meeting.
- Ask for written copies of the resident rules and regulations.
- Find out resident termination conditions and procedures.
- Ask to meet the on-site resident advocate representative.
- Ask how family members of residents are kept informed.
- Discuss complaint-filing procedures.

Health-Care Questions

- How are medications managed?
- What is the availability of the doctor and the nursing staff?
- How are medical emergencies handled?
- Do you have a standard policy for residents to "age-in-place" even upon the onset of an illness?
- Who decides when a resident is transferred to the health-care unit?
- What is your policy if an ill resident refuses to move to the care center?
- How is a resident transported to the hospital or care center?
- What is the health-evaluation procedure?
- Will the staff work with my elder's current physician?
- What are the physical and chemical restraint and bedrail policies?
- How long will an apartment be held if a resident has to be hospitalized?
- Are on-site physical therapy and rehab services offered?

Financial Questions

- What are the total costs? What is not included in the costs? Ask about "hidden fees," such as catheters, rubber gloves, bandages, lotions, and wheelchair rental.
- What costs are covered by Medicare and Medicaid insurance policies?
- How does one qualify for Medicaid?

- What veterans benefits are available?
- Are fees refundable? Under what circumstances?
- Is there a reduction in fees for part-time residents?
- What fees are residents obligated to pay for while being cared for in the nursing units?
- Are there cost adjustments for a couple when one is relocated for health-care reasons?
- What are the resident's costs upon remarriage?
- How will future expansion and refurbishing building plans affect costs?
- How are residents kept informed of the community's financial status?
- Are residents required to have long-term care insurance in place?
- What happens if the resident's money and insurance coverage runs out?
- Does each resident have an individual savings account for incidentals?

Quality-of-Life Considerations

- Review the location of this housing option in terms of proximity to your elder's family and friends.
- Ask about visitation and overnight guest policies.
- Find out about flexible dining and menu options, including food preparation preferences.
- Obtain information on food services options, especially when a resident is too ill to cook or dine in the community dining area.
- Ask questions about the staff, including the ratio of staff to residents, staff trainings and certifications, and staff turnover rate.
- Find out what services are included, especially housekeeping, laundry, linen services, and transportation.
- Review the activities calendar to explore the extent of the wellness program. Look for the implementation of all of the dimensions of successful aging: physical, social, emotional, and spiritual.
- Ask about educational programs, computer classes, and resident in-room computer hookup.
- Get written policies on safety procedures and security measures.
- Find out if the resident is allowed to control his or her own heat and air-conditioning system.
- Ask about the right of residents to bring their own furniture and personal belongings.
- Ask about the availability of on-site and easily accessible storage space.
- Ask about the extent of resident-driven activities.
- Find out if there is an active family-member council.
- Review the outdoor area and ask about resident outdoor activities.
- Find out about intergenerational activities.

- Obtain a list of on-site personal grooming services, such as a hair salon and pedicures.
- Ask about on-site banking and financial-planning services.
- Find out if personal-assistance services are offered, such as help with dressing and running errands. Ask about the additional costs of these services.
- If more care is needed, ask about in-home care and caregiver options.
- Review the mail-management system and outgoing mail services.
- Ask for copies of the resident and family newsletter.
- Explore the extent of religious and spiritual programs, as well as ethnic and cultural activities.
- Get policies regarding smoking and alcohol consumption in writing.
- Review the pet policy.
- Ask about resident and family support groups.

Assisted-Living and Skilled Nursing Care Considerations

- Background checks on the staff have been conducted and completed.
- I have researched any and all formal complaints and lawsuits filed against this facility.
- I felt at ease and was warmly greeted the moment I entered the building.
- Staff and management have been accessible to me.
- Staff and management have treated me respectfully, and I like and trust them.
- I feel that this is a safe and caring environment.
- Residents appear to be happy and well cared for.
- This is a resident-centered environment; residents are given choices and offered a customized living environment.
- So far the staff has responded to my requests in a timely manner.
- My elder's cultural, spiritual, and emotional needs will be met here.

GO THE EXTRA MILE

- Give several housing options a test drive. Make reservations to eat several meals at the community. Arrange for your elder to stay the weekend.
- Get opinions on several housing options from trusted sources, such as a geriatric care manager, friends in similar situations, or your elder's doctor.
- Conduct background checks on the financial stability of the community, rate-increase history, the owner/developer's track record, and any past complaints and lawsuits.
- Negotiate all costs and fees.
- Seek the advice of a financial planner to help create long-term financial and tax strategies and plans to pay future health-care expenses.
- Review housing and care contracts with an attorney and financial planner before signing.

PLAN FOUR

Insist on resident-centered living.

Everything in this country is being affected by the growth of the older adult population. Simultaneously, professionals in senior-related industries are revolutionizing the process of aging. Today, resident-centered living certification and training programs are lessening the plagues of loneliness, helplessness, ageism, and boredom that adult-housing residents can experience. Resident-centered living begins with the idea that each resident is unique and deserves to be treated as such. Programs help to maintain the independence and dignity of each resident and, consequently, provide the best possible lifestyle and service options.

As you explore the adult-living-community option, ask about resident-centered programs. **Masterpiece Living** and **Eden Alternative**, for example, ensure quality living not only for the residents, but also for their families, the employees, and the community at-large.

Special staff certifications provide evidence of the quality of life a resident experiences when living at a particular adult housing community. On your visit, ask how many staff members have completed a national professional certification program called **CASP,** which stands for **certified aging services professional.** The program is designed to educate and train professionals involved in the management of assisted-living facilities, continuing-care retirement communities, senior housing, and other types of aging services.

PLAN FIVE

Review the nursing-home residents' bill of rights.

Under federal law, all nursing homes must have a written description of the rights of the residents. A copy of the bill of rights must be made available to any resident and family member who requests it. Highlights of the bill of rights include the following.

- The resident must be informed of his or her rights.
- The resident is to be informed, in writing, of the nursing home's policies.
- The resident is to be informed of the nursing home's services and charges.
- The resident is to be informed of charges not covered by Medicare or Medicaid.
- The resident is to be informed of his or her medical condition, unless restricted by the doctor's written orders.
- The resident is allowed to participate in the planning of his or her own care.
- The resident can refuse medical treatment.
- The resident has the right to choose his or her own physician.
- The resident has the right to manage his or her personal finances and has the authority to authorize someone else to manage their finances for them.
- The resident can expect privacy and to be treated at all times with dignity and respect.
- The resident has the right to wear his or her own clothing.

- The resident is allowed to use his or her own possessions as long as the items do not infringe upon the rights and safety of others.
- The resident must be free of mental and physical abuse.
- The resident has the right to be free from chemical and physical restraints unless authorized in writing by a physician.
- The resident has the right to voice opinions and grievances without fear of coercion and retaliation from others.
- The resident has the right to be discharged or transferred only for medical reasons.
- The resident can appeal any and all discharges and transfers.
- The resident has the right to be accessible to visitors or to refuse visitors.
- The resident must be allowed immediate access by family members.
- The resident has the right to receive visitors during at least eight hours of a given day.
- The resident is allowed privacy and confidentiality for meetings or conversations with visitors.
- The resident has the right to receive assistance from an advocate in asserting their rights and benefits at the nursing home.

PLAN SIX

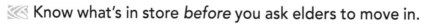 Know what's in store *before* you ask elders to move in.

We mean well when we ask our loved ones to move in with us; but we may not realize the potential negative consequences—emotionally, financially, and otherwise. For example, if parents move in and contribute to the cost of remodeling the house to accommodate their needs, do they gift their portion of the house to the caregiving child? How do siblings feel about this financial arrangement? Should parents have a contract in which they pay their children for caring for them? How does this living arrangement affect a person's eligibility for Medicaid?

Sharing one's home with their elders is not for the faint at heart. Seeking the advice of an elder-law attorney will offer solutions and help avert resentment and guilt among family members. Consider the following discussion points.

QUESTIONS TO ASK YOUR ELDER

Do you want to move in and share a household with my family?

Are there relationship conflicts that need to be resolved before you move in?

Do you feel that you can talk openly with me about your feelings?

Are you prepared to help with any costs?

Are you comfortable switching doctors if you have to?

How long are you prepared to live here?

QUESTIONS TO ASK OTHER FAMILY HOUSEHOLD RESIDENTS

Would anyone resent this living arrangement?

What adjustments would you have to make to your lifestyle?

Will you pitch in and help?

Are you willing to treat this person as a family member, not to be ignored or isolated?

QUESTIONS TO DISCUSS WITH NONRESIDENT SIBLINGS

Will you help care for our parents in the event they get sick and need extra care?

How will you pitch in when it's time for me to take a break or a vacation or if I get sick?

Are you prepared to contribute financially to this arrangement?

QUESTIONS TO ASK YOURSELF

Will my spouse and children get the attention they need?

How will this decision affect my personal and professional goals?

Is there another family member who already requires time and attention?

Am I good at delegating responsibilities?

Will my elder have access to a full range of activities outside the home?

Will we create ways for my elder to contribute to the family and feel needed?

Is there a plan to preserve privacy and autonomy for everyone?

Is my family financially and emotionally stable enough to take this on?

PLAN SEVEN

 Keep elders close yet independent.

An **accessory dwelling** is one possible alternative to making room for loved ones under the same roof. Converting space over the garage into living quarters or adding a separate wing or stand-alone house in the backyard may make better sense for older family members who want privacy and also want to be close enough if help is needed. Building codes and zoning laws dictate whether this option is allowed in your area.

PLAN EIGHT

 Gear up for the task of downsizing and moving a lifetime.

The day your elders decide to move out of the family home is the day downsizing takes on a whole new meaning. The process of sorting and getting rid of decades' worth of accumulations, not to mention the potential for explosive family squabbles, is exhausting.

Helping your elders sort through a lifetime of possessions, reminiscing about the good old days, and saying good-bye to the family home is nothing less than traumatic for everyone, and may be more than you can handle emotionally. Considering the possibility that a **professional senior-move manager** may be better equipped to handle the job may be the best move of all. Our elders need to make their own decisions about what to keep and what to toss. They also need to feel in control of the move, and we may not have the patience for this kind of work or the knack for coordinating. Enlisting a professional service that specializes in moving older adults helps create a smooth transition for everyone. Sources for relocation professionals are listed at the end of this chapter.

Every move begins with the process of creating a **floor plan** of the new location. Knowing the exact amount of living and storage space and accurate furniture measurements will determine what comes with and what stays behind.

If the responsibility of downsizing your elder's home has landed on your lap, the guidelines below will help in the process. Make moving a team event and **ask siblings to pitch in** and do their fair share. If they refuse, ask if they'll contribute financially to your hiring a professional senior-move manager to help you complete this enormous task.

Start the downsizing process by **purchasing supplies**—boxes, paper to wrap items, bubble wrap, tape, markers to label boxes, colored dots to label furniture, box cutters, and industrial-strength garbage bags. As you approach each room, categorize the household goods accordingly:

- Take it along.
- Give it away.
- Sell it.
- Donate it.
- Store it.
- Toss it.

TAKE IT ALONG
- Measure and label furniture and large items that are going to the new location.
- Set up several open boxes of varying sizes in each room within easy reach for items that are going to the new location.

GIVE IT AWAY
- Getting rid of unwanted items may be easier when we picture someone else benefiting from them. One way to part with possessions is for **elders to ask family and friends** if what they have may be of value to them or someone they know. Artwork, keepsakes, jewelry, and photos memorialize family history and can be cherished for years to come.
- Ask anyone who has stored items in the house to **make arrangements to come get them.** Set a deadline, and let them know of your plans to dispose of those items at

your discretion if they are not removed by that date. Also, **return all borrowed and rented items.**

SELL IT
- Ask the **people who bought the house** if they have any interest in purchasing items.
- **Retail outlets** for selling valuables include antique and consignment shops and fine jewelers. Consider the services of an estate-sale professional and auctioneer.
- Sell items **online** through auction and "garage sale" websites.
- **Used bookstores** may purchase interesting book collections.
- Participate in a neighborhood **yard sale** or host a garage sale of your own.
- Place a **classified ad** in the local newspaper and church bulletin.
- Post a "For Sale" advertisement on **bulletin boards** around town.

DONATE IT
- **Clean, usable items.** Kitchen dishes, glassware, rugs and furniture, and other household items are accepted by local charity outlets. Drop off or arrange for a pick up. Items may be tax-deductible. Look in the Yellow Pages under "Thrift Shops" and "Social Services Organizations."
- **Used clothing.** Community theaters, church missions, thrift stores, and women's shelters may accept items if they are in good condition.
- **Books, magazines, and videos.** Contact community centers, assisted-living communities, nursing homes, libraries, rehab centers, and women's shelters.
- **Clean blankets, linens, and towels.** Contact shelters, community centers, church missions, and animal shelters.
- **Fitness equipment.** Ask a fitness trainer for recommendations.
- **Unused toiletry items (toilet paper, unwrapped soap, unopened shampoo, toothpaste, and new toothbrushes).** Contact shelters and church missions.
- **Games, toys, holiday decorations, arts and crafts supplies.** Contact child and adult day-services centers, assisted-living communities, schools, church groups, rehab centers, and community centers.
- **Record collections, musical instruments, sheet music.** Ask music teachers and music store owners for recommendations. Contact child and adult day-services centers, assisted-living communities, schools, record shops, music schools, church groups, and community centers.
- **Computers.** Call a local school, community center, or church groups.
- **Televisions, cameras, slide projector, and screen.** Call shelters, community centers, child and adult day-services centers, assisted-living communities, schools, and church groups.
- **Tools, workbenches, wood scraps, and yard equipment.** Contact community centers, church groups, high schools, and community colleges.

- **Unwanted hearing aids and eyeglasses.** Service organizations such as the Rotary Club and the Lions Club run hearing aid and eyeglasses recycling programs. Call the local chapters for drop-off locations. Some community centers also have programs to recycle used hearing aids and eyeglasses.

STORE IT

- You may be tempted to rent storage space when elders can't or won't let go of particular items and when space in the new location is an issue. However, think twice before going this route. **Storing items** simply postpones sorting and dispersing later on. Also, the monthly tab can add up fast.

TOSS IT

- **Large appliances (refrigerators, stoves, etc.).** Call the local sanitation department for proper disposal procedures. Ask village officials if leaving items on the curb or in alleyways is permissible.
- **Bulky items or large loads.** Call professional haulers when tossing large items or if a houseful of unwanted items is too big to handle.
- **Computers and electronic waste.** Contact the local department of the environment. Also, look online for programs that allow users to send used computers and components back to the computer manufacturer to be recycled for free or a small fee.
- **Hazardous waste.** Dispose of items responsibly. Swimming pool chemicals, household cleaners, aerosol cans, batteries, bug sprays, pet flea collars, mothballs, medicines, gasoline, antifreeze, motor oils, paint, and charcoal can be dropped off at the local recycling center. Look in the Yellow Pages under "waste removal, recycling center." Contact the city's department of public health or department of the environment.

Manage Mountains of Papers

When scaling down in preparation of a move, it's not unusual to encounter piles of paper accumulated over the years—bills, junk mail, newspapers, legal documents, insurance policies, catalogs, magazines, receipts, newsletters . . . you name it. The task of **downsizing paperwork** appears to be overwhelming at first. However, to start somewhere (anywhere) is the best approach of all. Here are a few suggestions.

- While some documents require **immediate action** (bills and unfilled prescriptions), others can be put aside **until further notice** (appointment and information requests).
- Some paperwork requires long-term storage (legal and tax papers) while other items need attention from time to time (warranties and instruction manuals). **Grouping papers** eases the stress of knowing what to keep and what to toss.
- Outdated documents are best shredded before they are disposed of. Unfortunately, identity theft is here to stay, and **destroying confidential information** is a must. Before

making any decision on what to keep or discard, check with an accountant and attorney. Buy a shredder or call in a professional service. Look up "Paper Shredding" in the Yellow Pages.

- Finally, papers that need to be saved should be compiled, boxed, and clearly labeled for **storage**.
- **Sort, follow up, file, and toss**—do a little each day and you'll be amazed at how quickly the paperwork will be organized for the move ahead.

PLAN NINE

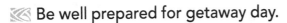 Be well prepared for getaway day.

There are certain items that should be **packed separately** and easy to access on move day. Items include:

alarm clock	move-related phone numbers
book elder is currently reading	moving-related paperwork
cash and checkbook	overnight bag of clothing
cell phone and cell-phone charger	paper and pen
computer files backup disks	personal address book
cosmetics and toiletries	prescription drugs
eyeglasses and extra eyeglasses	snacks and special foods
keys to old house and new house	TV remote control

Household items that are irreplaceable and of greater value should be transported by family members. Items include:

computer backup CD-ROMs	jewelry
deeds, wills, and other important and legal documents	paintings and artwork
	photo albums
high-priced clothing, such as fur coats	stamp and coin collections

PLAN TEN

Plan for an easy move.

Eight Weeks Before

- Shop for a moving company.
- Have a general idea of what is being moved before obtaining move estimates.
- Get three estimates and compare services.

- Ask about price breaks and low-season discounts.
- Ask how payments are made.
- Ask about insurance claim procedures for damages.

One Month Before

- Request a moving checklist from the moving company.
- Review the moving agreement details.
- Start packing.
- Finalize downsizing process—discard, distribute, and donate unwanted possessions.
- Photograph valuable possessions before having them moved.
- Fill out change of address cards (available at the post office).
- Transfer prescriptions to the new pharmacy.
- Arrange for disconnection and connection of utilities and telephone.
- Arrange for the transportation of pets and plants.
- Reserve the elevator in high-rise buildings.

Final Week

- Make arrangements for payment of movers.
- Pack final items.

Moving Day

- Be home when movers arrive.
- Watch as belongings are inventoried, packed, and loaded on truck.
- Check the bill of lading.
- Review new location address and contact information with movers.
- Give movers your telephone number.

Delivery Day

- Be home when movers arrive.
- Be prepared to pay with cash or money order upon delivery.
- Keep moving-related receipts for tax purposes.

Low-Cost and Free Resources

Assisted-living products that help elders to remain safe and more independent are available online: type "independent-living products" in your Internet browser. Helpful products are also listed in the Yellow Pages under the following headings: "Home Health Care," "Home Health Care Equipment & Supplies," "Hospital Equipment & Supplies" and "Medical Supplies."

Universities with gerontology centers can provide information about housing options, home safety, and chore services.

The **local agency on aging** can provide information on community programs that assist individuals who want to age in place and have services brought into the home. Also ask for home modification financial assistance available for eligible older people in both urban and rural settings.

If your elder was recently hospitalized, the **hospital discharge planner** can help assess the appropriate levels of care and housing.

Retrofitting one's home for older residents is a popular topic in magazines and interior-decorating books. Also visit the **public library** and search for books that offer information on making the home more "senior-friendly."

The decision to move to a continuing-care retirement community (CCRC) requires a significant personal financial commitment for the consumer. In return, the CCRC has an obligation to the consumer to have the resources necessary to provide services as outlined in the contractual agreement. You may want to download a report titled **"Consumer Guide to Understanding Financial Performance and Reporting in Continuing Care Retirement Communities"** (www.carf.org/pdf/ccrc.pdf).

Affordable Housing

U.S. Department of Housing and Urban Development
(Find a housing counselor)
Toll-free: (800) 569-4287
Website: www.hud.gov

Aging in Place

Alzheimer's Association
(Home modification suggestions)
Website: www.alz.org

Elder Cohousing Network
1460 Quince Avenue, Suite 102
Boulder, CO 80304
(303) 413-8066; fax: (303) 413-8067
Website: www.eldercohousing.org

National Aging in Place Council
1400 16th Street, NW, Suite 420
Washington, DC 20036
(202) 939-1784; fax: (202) 265-4435
Website: www.naipc.org

National Association of Home Builders
Website: www.nahb.org

National PACE Association
(In-home programs for the elderly)
Website: www.npaonline.org

National Resource Center on Supportive Housing and Home Modification
Andrus Gerontology Center
University of Southern California
3715 McClintock Avenue
Los Angeles, CA 90089
(213) 740-1364
Website: www.homemods.org

Naturally Occurring Retirement Communities
Website: www.norcs.org

Rebuilding Together
(Repairing the homes of those in need)
Website: www.rebuildingtogether.org

The Wright Stuff
(To buy independent-living products)
Website: www.thewright-stuff.com

Housing Options

Administration on Aging Housing Programs
Website: www.aoa.gov

American Association of Homes and Services for the Aging
2519 Connecticut Avenue, NW
Washington, DC 20008-1520
(202) 783-2242; fax: (202) 783-2255
Website: www.aahsa.org

American Seniors Housing Association
5100 Wisconsin Avenue, NW, Suite 307
Washington, DC 20016
(202) 237-0900; fax: (202) 237-1616
Website: www.seniorshousing.org

Assisted Living Federation of America
1650 King Street, Suite 602
Alexandria, VA 22314-2747
(703) 894-1805; fax: (703) 894-1831
Website: www.alfa.org

Commission on Accreditation of Rehabilitation Facilities (CARF)
(Look for CARF accredited programs as assurance for the highest possible standards)
CARF International website: www.carf.org
CARF Canada website: www.carfcanada.ca

Consumer Consortium on Assisted Living
(Focuses on the needs, the rights, and the protection of assisted-living residents)
Website: www.ccal.org

International Association of Homes and Services for the Ageing
2519 Connecticut Avenue, NW
Washington, DC 20008
(202) 508-9468; fax: (202) 220-0041
Website: www.iahsa.net

National Accessible Apartment Clearinghouse
(Connects individuals with disabilities with apartments adapted to meet their needs)
Website: www.accessibleapartments.org

National Center for Assisted Living
Website: www.ncal.org

National Citizens' Coalition for Nursing Home Reform
1828 L Street, NW, Suite 801
Washington, DC 20036
(202) 332-2276; fax: (202) 332-2949
Website: www.nccnhr.org

SeniorHousingNet
Website: www.seniorhousingnet.com

U.S. Department of Agriculture Rural Housing Service
(202) 690-1533; toll-free TTY: (800) 877-8339
Website: http://www.rurdev.usda.gov

Later-Life Move

Moving Station
(Total relocation management)
Website: www.movingstation.com

National Association of Professional Organizers
Website: www.napo.net

National Association of Senior Move Managers
Website: www.nasmm.org

Seniors Real Estate Specialists
Toll-free: (800) 500-4564
Website: www.seniorsrealestate.com

Resident-Centered Housing Initiatives

Eden Alternative
Website: www.edenalt.com

Masterpiece Living
Website: www.mymasterpieceliving.com

HOUSING ACTION CHECKLIST

(This worksheet is also available online at www.elderindustry.com)

MOVE OR STAY PUT?	To Do By	Completed
List circumstances for possible change in housing	_____	❑
Set housing goals		
short-term	_____	❑
long-term	_____	❑
Determine modifications		
short-term	_____	❑
long-term	_____	❑
Check laws and codes for home modifications	_____	❑
Research loans and funds for home modification plans	_____	❑
Determine in-home assistance needed		
homemaker	_____	❑
personal grooming	_____	❑
home health care	_____	❑
quality of life	_____	❑
Research Realtors to help sell the family home	_____	❑
Review housing options		
ECHO housing	_____	❑
Retirement residence	_____	❑
Life-Care or CCRC	_____	❑
Group home	_____	❑
Public housing	_____	❑
Intermediate care	_____	❑
Skilled nursing facility	_____	❑
Family member's home	_____	❑
Shared housing	_____	❑

Create senior-housing questions
   and checklists   _____   ❏

Secure contracts and
   documents   _____   ❏

Review contracts and documents
   with attorney   _____   ❏

Obtain family consensus before
   asking your elder to move in   _____   ❏

Develop moving strategy   _____   ❏

10

⟨⟨⟨

Safe and Secure

Minimize Distress over Distance

We are a society on the move. Family members are going their separate ways in pursuit of professional and personal interests and looking to improve the quality of their lives. The impact of a mobile family undoubtedly affects our family eldercare issues. *How do we care for and watch over each other from far away?*

Being separated from each other can create a disturbing mixture of anxiety and fear on both sides. Family members don't really know what's going on in their elders' lives on a day-to-day basis and are increasingly concerned that they won't be able to respond immediately to an eldercare emergency. Older family members fear that something bad may happen to them and no one would know. How, then, do we help them balance a desire to remain at home—measurably independent—while ensuring their safety and security?

The answer requires family caregivers to take necessary precautions: making the home a safer place to live; staying alert to con artists and scams; and creating a stronger family and community network of support. The action plans listed in this section of *The Complete Eldercare Planner* will specifically guide you in ensuring your elders' well-being.

However, no matter how much you plan for safety, feelings of anxiety may remain. When these emotions surface, you can sometimes find reassurance simply by picking up the telephone and calling faraway relatives just to hear their voices.

PLAN ONE

⟨⟨⟨ Home safety is no accident.

Impaired vision and hearing, arthritis, dementia, and side effects from medications are all factors that bring potentially dangerous consequences to living at home. To lessen the possibility of a visit to the emergency room, here are some suggestions on creating a safer home environment.

MINIMIZE DISTRESS OVER DISTANCE

- It is very difficult when loved ones live far away. You worry because they may need care and there's no one looking out for them.
- The notion that older people cannot or will not adopt technologies has changed. Many adults have embraced technology to help keep them safe and in touch with others.
- A study prepared for the National Center on Elder Abuse found that self-neglect (an adult's inability to perform essential self-care tasks) was the most common category of investigated elder-abuse reports, followed by caregiver neglect and financial exploitation. Fifteen states reported that 65 percent of elder-abuse victims were female.[1]
- Scam artists play on people's fears about maintaining a comfortable lifestyle on a fixed income. The telephone is the most popular vehicle for committing fraud.

Putting common sense into play helps avert the possibility of becoming a victim of a scam. When family members feel as though "something's not right," it probably isn't.

OBJECTIVES

*After completing **"Minimize Distress over Distance,"** you will be able to:*

Address existing and potential home hazards.

Implement home safety precautions.

Create check-in systems.

Use technology to supplement caregiving tasks.

Report incidents of elder abuse, neglect, and exploitation.

Basic Emergency Items

Dedicate one place to store the following items. The location should be one that is found easily in the dark, and these items should also be ready to go at any time.

- first-aid kit
- two flashlights with working batteries
- cell phone and cell-phone charger
- battery-powered radio tuned to the emergency station
- extra batteries for radios
- extra batteries for medical equipment
- current medications
- extra pair of eyeglasses

Communications Center

Family members and friends as well as emergency workers such as firefighters should find it easy to locate vital and emergency contact information. Many people use the kitchen as a convenient location, and often use the front of the refrigerator as a makeshift message board for important information.

Post the following information on the refrigerator:

- photo of the elder would be helpful
- photostat of last EKG
- list of current medications
- living will/power of attorney for health care (see chapter 7, "Legal Matters")
- do not resusciate (DNR) (see chapter 12, "Managing Medical Care")
- Elder Emergency Information Chart (see page 5 of *The Complete Eldercare Planner*)

Home-Safety Inspection Services

Typically offered as a collaborative effort between police officers, firefighters, and health-care professionals, an **in-home safety inspection** will ensure that an older person's home is free from safety hazards.

For example, inspectors will see to it that smoke detectors are installed and in proper working order. They will also check for loose rugs that can cause a fall and perhaps suggest getting rid of area rugs altogether. They will also examine doors and window locks to keep intruders from easy entry. Air ventilation, water temperature, and adequate lighting throughout the house will also be included on their safety checklist. Contact the local agency on aging to inquire about the availability of this service where your elder resides.

PLAN TWO

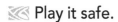 Play it safe.

Considering that home injuries send millions of people for medical attention each year, conducting a basic home safety survey with your elder will help minimize mishaps. Here are a few suggestions.

FALL PREVENTION
- Remove clutter on floors and objects on stairways.
- Clear all exits and passageways.
- Make sure that carpets are free of snags and securely in place.
- Remove area rugs and runners that slide.

- Ensure that stairways are not slippery.
- Provide stable step stools with a top handrail and store in handy locations.
- Make sure that long-handled grippers are available for easy reach of lightweight items.
- Verify that handrails, grab bars, and nonskid decals are sturdy and in use.
- Make sure that elevated toilet seats and shower seating are in use.
- Ensure that nonskid slippers and socks and low-heeled shoes are being used.
- Make sure that robes and pajamas are not too long.
- Safely tuck away hanging fabrics, such as bedspreads and curtains.
- Ensure that room traffic patterns provide clear and easy access to doors and windows.
- Make sure that the kitchen table is sturdy.
- Take only current medications prescribed by the doctor and in the prescribed dosages.
- Provide cane, wheelchair, walker, or scooter and use at the first sign of need.

LIGHTING
- Install motion sensors to turn on lights for nighttime bathroom and kitchen visits.
- Make sure that night-lights are installed in hallways, bedrooms, bathroom, and kitchen.
- Light switches should be available at the top and bottom of stairs and room entrances.
- Show how to change fuses and operate circuit breakers.
- Stairwells should be well lit.
- Working flashlights should be handy.

FIRE PREVENTION
- Smoke detectors must be working properly.
- Space heaters should be placed one yard away from objects and wall.
- Electrical outlets should not be warm to the touch or overloaded.
- Electrical cords must be in good condition, not frayed or cracked.
- Outlets and switches must have cover plates and no wiring should be exposed.
- Arc fault circuit interrupters (AFCI) must be installed.
- Small appliances should have an auto-off feature.
- Long-sleeved clothing should not be worn while cooking.
- Electric appliances must be a safe distance from water.
- Lightbulbs must be the appropriate wattage for light fixtures.
- Containers of volatile liquids should be tightly capped.
- There should be a policy of no smoking in bed.

SAFE AIR AND WATER

- The heating system should be checked annually for carbon monoxide leaks.
- Smoke and carbon monoxide detectors must be present and working.
- The water temperature should be adjusted to prevent scalding.

INTRUDERS

- Make sure that any outgoing message on a telephone answering device does not indicate that no one is home.
- Use discretion as to who knows your elder lives alone.
- The door should never be opened to unannounced visitors.
- Don't let service people in the house unless the work was ordered.
- Peepholes and deadbolts should be installed at the appropriate height.
- Make sure your elder has befriended helpful and watchful neighbors.
- Blinds and drapes must be drawn at night.
- Lock systems should be in working order on windows and entranceways.
- Notes should not be left on the door when going out.
- Lights, the radio, or the television should be left on when going out.
- Don't put second set of keys in the mailbox or under doormat.
- Report suspicious neighborhood activities.

PLAN THREE

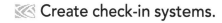 Create check-in systems.

There's a consistent message from older people everywhere: They cherish their independence, yet they want the peace of mind knowing that someone is near should something bad happen. With the likelihood of family members living miles apart, we are increasingly turning to a variety of **safety check-in systems** and **technology** to relieve long-distance concerns. Technology already has transformed our lives—from cell phones to e-mail—and while it is meant to complement human resources, it doesn't obviate the need for human contact.

Whatever method we choose to ensure our elders safety and security, we need to be flexible about adjusting it. What works today may not work well next year or next week. Here are a few suggestions that may help ease the physical and emotional issues that typically surface when caring for loved ones from a distance.

Neighborhood Network

People who interact with our elders on a consistent basis can be lifesavers. For example, a neighbor may notice that Dad hasn't retrieved his morning newspaper, or the hairstylist is alarmed when Mom doesn't show up for her weekly appointment. To create a network of support, first ask your elders whom they recommend and feel comfortable with you contacting. An informal circle of community-minded people is one of the most effective ways to get help fast should an emergency occur.

Telephone

The **cell phone** is an invaluable communication tool, allowing users to stay in contact with others anytime, anywhere. Cell phones equipped with personal digital assistant (PDA) features offer extra benefits, including text messages, photos, global positioning system (GPS), e-mail, Internet access, videoconferencing, reminder systems, and medical data collection.

Now that the cell phone has shrunk to the size of a credit card, older people often complain that keypads are hard to use and handling the phone is a nightmare. Look for phone units that are specifically designed for people with physical impairments. Today, you can purchase **cell phones that offer special features,** including larger buttons, a comfortable ergonomic shape for easy gripping, easy-on-the-eyes text, volume control, and hardware for visual- and hearing-impaired users.

In addition to cell phones, also consider buying **cordless phones, picture phones, walkie-talkies,** and **intercom systems** for home usage.

Emergency Response Device

A **personal emergency response system (PERS)** links individuals with a monitoring station that can immediately notify an ambulance service, a family member, or a medical care-giving team. A PERS can be activated with a button click or voice activation link or detect the physical action of a person falling and make the call automatically.

A PERS offers **special features for people with hearing and visual impairments**, including flashing keypad for incoming calls and oversized numbers; other systems include reminders for medications and appointments. Depending on the level of services, prices vary. Devices can be purchased, rented, or leased. Typically a PERS is not covered by Medicare, Medicaid, or insurance companies.

Programs for Homebound Elders

Telephone reassurance programs and postal alerts provide daily contact with homebound elderly people. Here's how telephone reassurance programs work: Failure to answer the call brings a second call within minutes; no answer to the second call results in a visit from a designated person who physically goes to the home. Other programs may require elders to phone in at a specified time of day. If the person doesn't call within a certain time frame, someone is sent to the residence. This service is typically offered through the local agency on aging.

Homebound people may want to register to participate in a **postal check-in program**. A sticker is placed inside the mailbox to alert the mail delivery person in the event of accumulating mail. The post office then calls the phone number on the sticker or the emergency number listed at the post office.

Computer

The use of a computer as a caregiving tool is a reality of our mobile society and offers a variety of ways for families and elders to stay connected.

E-MAIL. This is best used as a method of information sharing. If older family members shy away from using the computer or find the process of e-mailing too difficult and confusing, keep them in the loop by purchasing a computerless e-mail mailbox, such as Presto (www.presto.com). (The Presto looks like a fax machine and sits on a desk or counter. No keyboard is necessary since the Presto is a one-way communication device. E-mails are printed instantly on regular copy paper.) The use of e-mail as a sole check-in system is not recommended because it's far too easy for people to hide a multitude of problems.

INSTANT MESSENGER. This is real-time communication between two individuals. A text message is displayed on the computer monitor immediately after it is sent, permitting the receiver of the message to respond. Free software comes with most computers.

VOICE. Microphones (or headsets) and speakers allow individuals to communicate verbally on the computer. Conversations happen in real time, with each individual hearing the voice of the person who is speaking with surprising clarity.

VIDEO CHAT. Computers equipped with a sound card, a microphone, speakers, and a video cam transmit simultaneously the voice and picture of the sender and receiver. Family members can see and speak with each other in real time, giving everyone a better sense of how things are going on a day-to-day basis. Online video chat services are also available by typing "online video chat service" in the Internet browser search window.

Geriatric Care Manager

When regular on-site visits are not possible or practical, **geriatric care managers** can be hired to check in and offer valuable feedback on how well (or not) your elders are doing. Care managers typically have backgrounds in nursing or social work and offer a wide range of services. If complex medical problems are present, you'll probably want a nurse. If your elder is lonely and has social issues, a social worker might be a better fit. If health issues escalate, care managers can also help coordinate assisted-living services.

This kind of assistance is expensive, though in many cases well worth what it costs. Geriatric care managers usually charge $80 to $200 an hour, depending on the services provided, and Medicare does not pick up the tab. For referrals, references, and proof of certifications, contact the National Association of Professional Geriatric Care Managers.

PLAN FOUR

Home monitor system—yes or no?

An increasingly transient and technology-friendly world means supportive family members are making greater use of coordinated, centralized computer networks to observe, respond to, and communicate with elders, professional caregivers, and medical staff. By installing **in-home video cameras** and **sensor monitor systems,** family caregivers are receiving images and data by way of computers, cell phones, and pagers.

If the concept of using technology and home monitor systems to help supplement your caregiving responsibilities appeals to you, be aware that your elders may not initially welcome the idea. Privacy is a big issue. Most people don't want anyone looking over their shoulder, and the fear of others knowing that help is needed is reason enough for them to be close-minded.

Do what you can to convince them that at some point it's not about privacy but about being connected and maintaining a safe and secure living environment. Review chapter 4, "Communicaring," of *The Complete Eldercare Planner,* starting on page 86, before opening up the dialogue on this potentially sensitive subject.

Monitor Systems

Home monitor systems provide families an opportunity to observe loved ones at home and be alerted to eldercare situations that require attention. The goal is to respond to the person in a timely manner and avert problematic situations.

VIDEO CAMERA
- Observes movements and activities
- Relays visual information of dangerous situations
- Records completion of necessary activities (like taking medications or eating)
- Monitors caregivers to ensure that the care is appropriate

SENSOR *(less intrusive alternative than cameras)*
- Sends alarm when person or environment needs immediate attention
- Relays alerts via e-mail, beeper, phone, and computer
- Monitors abnormal activities (e.g., if someone with Alzheimer's wanders from the home)
- Signals emergencies (such as falls)
- Extends home security systems

PLAN FIVE

≋ Raise the home IQ.

Home-assistive devices have evolved to **home-assistive environments**. Technology that supplements caregiving responsibilities can be an invaluable resource when it comes to caregiving from a distance. In addition to enhancing the safety and security of those who want to remain at home, technology assists family members with a variety of caregiving-related tasks, including:

> *fall prevention*
>
> *wandering prevention*
>
> *eating assistance*
>
> *personal grooming*
>
> *medication management*
>
> *medical condition indicators*
>
> *reminders and instructions*
>
> *housekeeping chores*
>
> *mobility aids*
>
> *isolation and entertainment*

To learn more about products and services that are available in the marketplace, type the following keywords into your Internet browser search window: "fall prevention," "independent-living products," "alarm systems," "wandering management systems," "paging systems," "home security," "telephone monitor service," "home monitoring," "home safety," "home fire protection," "home control systems," "medical alarms," "eldercare robotics," "appointment reminder," and "Web-based home control." Additional resources are listed at the end of this chapter.

Fall Prevention

The risk of injury due to a fall increases dramatically with age due to weakness, unsteady gait, confusion, and certain medications. While some falls do little harm, others can have serious consequences: fractures, head injuries, and even death. Falls can be prevented, and costly risks reduced through exercise and strength training. Making environmental modifications, such as removing clutter and installing grab bars, will also be helpful.

In-home products that reduce the risk of a fall include antislip footwear, antislip tub and bathroom floor mats, and wheelchair antirollback devices. Products aimed at reducing the risk of injury when falls occur include hip protectors, bedrails, low beds, and bedside cushions. Fall-detection devices, such as a personal emergency response system (PERS), sense a change in the person's body position and immediately notify caregivers if he or she has taken a fall.

Smart House

Wireless, Web-enabled technology allows us to control and monitor the home environment. Regardless of where we are in the world, we can instruct our laptop or cell phone to perform a variety of tasks, including turning up the heat in Dad's bedroom, double-checking that Mom has turned off the stove, and closing the blinds and switching off the lights so Aunt Bernice can nap. From touch-screen computer monitors to remote-control command stations and voice commands, computers and cell phones play a dominant role in ensuring our loved one's safety and security.

A "smart" house is also a safe house. Most devices have battery backup in the event of a power outage. Systems are also available to send warning messages, such as a lightbulb is about to blow, the kitchen is filled with smoke, or a door has been left open.

Automated Assistants

Home technology and "intelligent" products can assist with a multitude of caregiving functions and offer people even greater control over their own home environment. In addition to monitoring medical conditions and anticipating special needs, in-home systems help residents control dozens of household products. While some are activated with the touch of a screen, others are completely hands-free by either moving a body part or speaking a command. Televisions, stereos, fans, lights and lamps, telephones, blinds and shades, doors, wheelchairs, clock radios, bed controls, and nurse calls can respond on demand.

Robotics has entered the caregiving scene. Personal-assistant robots can watch over Mom, follow her around, assist her with eating, and verbally remind her of time-sensitive events, such as taking medication, watching her favorite TV show, and scheduling medical appointments. Family members must have access to a computer and the Internet to set up robot commands, assign chores automatically, and survey and collect data from the robotic unit.

Accessible Telecommunications

Special devices that help people who have difficulty using a standard telephone are available by contacting the local aging agency. Ask for information about telephone relay services and amplified handsets, among other products and services.

Cognitive Devices

Smart technology is keeping dementia sufferers happy at home, and helping to reduce anxieties for the rest of the family. Sensors that "talk" to household devices, such as the stove and light switches, and products with voice-prompt instructions and reminder systems boost the dignity, independence, and autonomy of individuals who have memory issues.

While some technologies function in a manner similar to alarm clocks, issuing fixed reminders at prespecified times, others employ artificial intelligence to monitor the execution of activities. For example, if Dad is detected opening the front door at inappropriate times, he would be given a prompt to let him know the time and be encouraged to go back to bed. Similarly, if he gets out of bed at night and moves around the house when it is dark, appropriate room lights gently fade up to reduce the risk of him falling.

Other memory-aid products include telephones with monitors that display the photo of the person who is calling; handheld devices that help forgetful people navigate their way home; and talking medication reminders. Also, family websites showing old photos and playing music and relaxing sounds can be used as a therapy to relax Alzheimer's patients.

Wandering Management

Alzheimer's disease and other dementia-related issues cause a high level of concern, even for the at-home caregiver. Consider the use of monitoring devices that can be used to notify family members as soon as the person has wandered past a specific point or enters an unsafe area.

Lightweight, tamper-resistant, and waterproof transmitters come in several styles, including pendants, wrist and ankle bands, fanny packs, and watches. Devices are worn comfortably, and the wanderer's precise geographic location can be viewed by logging on to a secure website or by contacting a call center. Other wandering-tracking devices include bed alarms and wireless door monitors. Contact the local agency on aging and ask for information about community wandering-management programs.

PLAN SIX

Put a stop to elder abuse, neglect, and financial extortion.

The aging of our society presents many challenges. While people are living longer than ever before, many are not living a *better quality of life*. Becoming frail makes older people even more vulnerable. Unfortunately, there are people who take advantage of other people's weaknesses and frailties.

Elder abuse, neglect, and extortion can happen anywhere—at the front door, over the phone, on the street, on the Internet, inside senior-housing and assisted-living communities, and in health-care institutions such as nursing homes and hospitals. Abusers can include family members, neighbors, professional caregivers, health-care providers, service providers, volunteers, and, of course, strangers.

Elder abuse, neglect, and extortion can take on many forms and is best described as action by a person in a position of trust causing harm to an older person. Examples of abuse include:

- exploiting, misusing, or concealment of funds, property, or assets
- physical abuse, including striking, shaking, and rough handling

- emotional abuse, including insults, humiliation, and threats
- isolation and abandonment
- sexual assault
- denying access to food, water, clothing, medication, and health care
- violation of rights (such as opening mail and wire tapping)
- denial of freedom of speech and religious worship

Abuse Prevention Strategies

- Plan for the day your elder may find it difficult to manage his or her own financial affairs. Establish who will have power of attorney for property and who will oversee the accounting of the finances. For additional protection, assign a third party, such as an attorney or a financial planner, to review financial statements on a monthly basis.
- Insist that elders do not commingle their own funds with those of the person granted power of attorney or family members. Commingling funds complicates the financial monitoring process.
- Befriend bank trust officers. Ask them to contact you when something is amiss in a financial situation. Most bankers are trained to recognize potential frauds and report suspicious activity.
- Elders who live with relatives or other people who have a background of violent behavior or drug and alcohol abuse may be subject to constant abuse and neglect.
- When loved ones reside in a nursing home, visit them at all hours. Make certain the nursing home is aware of your visits and whom you're visiting. The most vulnerable residents are those who have no visitors.
- Check references and conduct criminal-background checks on all hired help.

Help for Family Caregivers

The stresses and strains of caregiving can easily wear a person down to the point where the quality of care is compromised. Many cases of abuse arise from a lack of coping skills and not knowing that help is readily available. **If you're a caregiver on the brink of burnout,** here are a few suggestions.

- Consider adult day-services programs.
- Attend support groups that also teach coping skills.
- Arrange for regular breaks. Even three hours a day will make a difference.
- Call the local agency on aging and ask about community caregiving resources.
- Check on the availability and cost of home-health aides.
- Ask if funding is available through local aging agencies for respite care.
- As discussed in chapter 3, attend education classes on anger management.

PLAN SEVEN

Tip-offs to rip-offs.

No one likes to think that a stranger would steal money from an older person; yet it happens all the time. People are scammed at the front door, over the phone, in mailboxes, and in cyberspace. It's never been easier to win their trust—then steal their hearts and their money.

Scammers target older adults who are alone and isolated. When elderly people live far from family, it makes it even easier for con artists to sweet-talk them out of money and valuables. The best prevention is to stay involved; make routine visits and spend time together.

Has a Con Artist Already Struck?

Experts say most people don't realize right away they've been scammed. It's only later they feel something "wasn't right." Intelligent, well-read, and accomplished people have succumbed to slick sales pitches, fearing exposure of the incident might bring their competence into question. Some victims choose to forget about the loss and "keep it a secret."

Have your elders already been victimized? Observe their behavior when you bring up the subject. Do they clam up? Become standoffish? Watch and listen for other clues such as:

- overdue bill notices and bounced checks
- unusual activity in bank accounts and cash withdrawal machines
- withdrawals of large amounts of cash
- unrecognizable signatures on financial documents
- conflicting accounts of incidents
- forgetfulness regarding the whereabouts of checkbooks and bank and credit-card statements
- frequent trips to gambling casinos
- recent changes in wills or the creation of a new will
- increased frequency of incoming and outgoing telephone calls
- large volume of mail that promotes prizes or free trips
- missing valuables, such as artwork, silverware, and jewelry

Cut Off Con Artists at the Pass

- Discuss with elders the importance of setting up a "screening plan." For example, urge them to automatically reply to anyone asking for large sums of money that it's their policy to check with *you* first. Explain to your elder that scammers will most likely go away when they hear that someone is overseeing their spending patterns.
- Encourage them to share official-looking mail and contracts before taking any action and signing on the dotted line.

- Protect private information, such as Social Security numbers, passwords, and phone numbers. Remove Social Security cards from wallets and purses.
- Help prevent identity theft by shredding mail, receipts, membership notices, and financial statements. Keep important documents in locked files. Scrutinize bank and credit-card statements.
- Tell your elders to hang up immediately on all unsolicited sales calls. Better yet, get them a phone with caller ID.
- Stay alert for people with cell phones in hand standing near the checkout counter. Camera phones make it easy to snap a picture of a credit card.
- Do not let them endorse "gift" checks, coupons, sweepstakes entries, or rebates sent by mail. They may be signing an agreement or appointing some unknown person or company to provide unwanted services.
- Discuss the importance of never opening the door to strangers. Install dead bolts and peepholes.
- Befriend helpful, watchful neighbors.
- Before hired helpers arrive, put away valuables, cash, jewelry, watches, and credit cards.

Avert Cybercrime

The Internet is the con artist's playground. Discuss the following important tips regarding Internet security with your elders.

- Immediately delete unsolicited e-mail.
- Do not open e-mail attachments unless they originate from a trusted source.
- Ask someone to oversee purchasing transactions when shopping online, making travel arrangements, and bidding on auction items.
- Never give bank account numbers and Social Security numbers online.
- Do not visit chat rooms or use online dating services.
- Install antivirus and antiphishing (identity theft via computers) software.

PLAN EIGHT

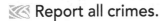 Report all crimes.

Victims of elder abuse, neglect, and financial extortion can contact any one of these crime-reporting and victim-protection resources:

- 911 (to be dialed in the event of an emergency)
- state adult protective services

- local and state agency on aging
- local police department and sheriff's office
- county public guardian's office
- county department of social services
- district attorney's office
- physician
- hospitals and medical clinics
- state long-term-care ombudsman's office
- public health agency
- mental health agency
- facility licensing/certification agency
- state attorney general's office
- State Medicaid Fraud Control Unit
- Better Business Bureau
- Federal Trade Commission

Low-Cost and Free Resources

Telecommunications devices for the deaf (TDDs) and **Braille TDDs** are available for telephone customers with hearing and sight impairments. Contact the Special Needs Center of the local telephone company.

Some communities have **neighborhood watch** programs. Call the local police department to find out how to sign up.

To learn **CPR** (cardiopulmonary resuscitation) contact the American Heart Association, the American Red Cross, or the fire station to find out where courses are given. Check the Yellow Pages under "First Aid Instruction."

To participate in a **self-defense class** geared for the older adult, contact the local agency on aging.

If elder abuse and neglect is suspected, call the department of social services' **adult protection services.** Contact the **state long-term-care ombudsman** for abuse and neglect in senior living communities and nursing homes.

Conduct an **Internet keyword search** for resources and information on these topics: elder abuse, fraud, scams, computer crime, and identity theft.

ORGANIZATIONS AND WEB RESOURCES

Elder Abuse, Neglect, and Financial Exploitation

Better Business Bureau—Canada
2 St. Clair Avenue E., Suite 800
Toronto, ON M4T 2T5
Canada
(416) 644-4936
Website: www.bbb.org

Better Business Bureau—United States
4200 Wilson Boulevard, Suite 800
Arlington, VA 22203-1838
(703) 276-0100
Website: www.bbb.org

Call for Action
(Empowering consumers)
Website: www.callforaction.org

Direct Marketing Association
(To stop unsolicited mailings and
    telemarketers)
Do Not Call Registry: (888) 382-1222
Website: www.the-dma.org
Website: www.donotcall.gov

Elder Abuse Foundation
Website: www.elder-abuse-foundation.com

Federal Trade Commission
Toll-free: (877) 382-4357
Website: www.ftc.gov

Identity Theft Resource Center
Website: www.idtheftcenter.org

National Center on Elder Abuse
1201 15th Street, NW, Suite 350
Washington, DC 20005
(202) 898-2586
Website: www.elderabusecenter.org

**National Committee for the Prevention of
    Elder Abuse**
1612 K Street, NW
Washington, DC 20006
(202) 682-4140
Website: www.preventelderabuse.org

National Consumers League
1701 K Street, NW, Suite 1200
Washington, DC 20006
(202) 835-3323
Website: www.nclnet.org

National Crime Prevention Council
1000 Connecticut Avenue, NW, 13th Floor
Washington, DC 20036
(202) 466-6272
Website: www.ncpc.org

National Domestic Violence Hotline
Toll-free: (800) 799-7233

National Fraud Information Center
Toll-free: (800) 876-7060
Website: www.fraud.org

Nursing Home Abuse Resource
Website: www.nursing-home-abuse-
    resource.com

Privacy Rights Clearinghouse
Website: www.privacyrights.org

Safe Shopping Online
Website: www.safeshopping.org

Smart House Resources

Alzheimer's Association
(Home products and safety tips for people
with Alzheimer's)
Website: www.alz.org

Center for Aging Services Technologies
Website: www.agingtech.org

Lighthouse International
(Home safety tips for the blind and visually
impaired)
Website: www.lighthouse.org

**National Association of Home Builders
Research Center**
(Type "seniors" in search box)
Website: www.nahbrc.org

**National Resource Center on Supportive
Housing and Home Modification**
Andrus Gerontology Center
University of Southern California
3715 McClintock Avenue
Los Angeles, CA 90089
(213) 740-1364
Website: www.homemods.org

National Safety Council
1121 Spring Lake Drive
Itasca, IL 60143-3201
(630) 285-1121
Website: www.nsc.org

**Partnership for Advancing Technology in
Housing**
Website: www.pathnet.org

Project Lifesaver International
(Helps to locate lost and wandering patients)
815 Battlefield Boulevard S
Chesapeake, VA 23322
(757) 546-5502; toll-free: (877) 580-LIFE
(5433); fax: (757) 546-5503
Website: www.projectlifesaver.org

SAFE AND SECURE ACTION CHECKLIST

(This worksheet is also available online at www.elderindustry.com)

MINIMIZE DISTRESS OVER DISTANCE	To Do By	Completed
Set safe and secure goals		
short-term	_____	☐
long-term	_____	☐
Review home hazards		
throughout home	_____	☐
kitchen	_____	☐
bedroom	_____	☐
bathroom	_____	☐
exterior	_____	☐
garage	_____	☐
Have elder's home surveyed by		
police department	_____	☐
fire official	_____	☐
electric company	_____	☐
gas company	_____	☐
Implement safety precautions		
at home	_____	☐
on an extended trip	_____	☐
walking	_____	☐
driving	_____	☐
banking	_____	☐
shopping	_____	☐
Create check-in systems		
visitors	_____	☐
geriatric case manager	_____	☐
telephone	_____	☐
emergency response device	_____	☐
telephone reassurance program	_____	☐
postal carrier alert	_____	☐

computer _____ ❑

computer audio/video _____ ❑

e-mail _____ ❑

home-monitor system _____ ❑

ombudsman _____ ❑

Check for abuse and neglect _____ ❑

Plan to ward off con artists _____ ❑

Make sure an elder with hearing/ sight impairments has access to a telephone _____ ❑

Know the telephone numbers of

police department _____ ❑

fire department _____ ❑

electric company _____ ❑

water company _____ ❑

gas company _____ ❑

plumber _____ ❑

electrician _____ ❑

11

Transportation and Mobility

Meeting Transportation Needs

Few of us plan for a time when we won't be driving, but many of us could eventually outlive our ability to safely operate a vehicle. At the same time, Americans are growing older, and the existing transportation network is not keeping up with the fundamental needs of an aging population.

Alternatives to driving are sparse, particularly in suburban and rural communities, causing significant problems for people who attempt to maintain a desirable mobility level as they age—the kind of mobility required to live life with dignity and independence. The question then becomes, if transportation alternatives were more readily available, might impaired drivers make better choices about how to get from one place to the next?

Better transportation is what is needed. Unless we start thinking both personally and publicly about our dependence on the car for transportation and identity, we could be sentencing our loved ones (and eventually ourselves) to a life of confinement and isolation. Sadly, isolation issues of nondrivers have been known to lead to depression and alcoholism. The transportation problem is not solely about the deterioration of driving skills, it's also about a gross failure of a national transportation policy. *The need for new public and private transportation programs is urgent.* Until then, millions of people may be driving long past when they should.

Today, there are no national standards or systems to identify older drivers who have critical impairments. Ideally, people come to their senses and hand over the car keys and let other drivers pitch in when driving skills become compromised. This section of *The Complete Eldercare Planner* offers specific action steps for older drivers and their family members to make plans for retiring from driving when it is no longer safe, and offers suggestions on how older drivers can get accustomed to the idea of alternate transportation resources.

MEETING TRANSPORTATION NEEDS

- Some medications or combination of medications can cause a variety of reactions and make it difficult to operate an automobile safely. Reactions include sleepiness, blurred vision, and slowed reaction and movement.

- The safety of older drivers can be measured several ways. On a licensed-driver basis, older adults are among the safest. The picture changes somewhat when crash rates are calculated on the basis of miles traveled. Using this measure of exposure, older adults *are* at increased crash risk.[1]

- People suffer an emotional void when driving comes to an end. Long-established patterns of social interaction immediately begin to break down.

Revoking a driver's license over a certain age is not an acceptable solution. Driving skills vary widely at all ages.

OBJECTIVES

*After completing **"Meeting Transportation Needs,"** you will be able to:*

Prepare for confrontational driving-related conversations.

Encourage older drivers to monitor their driving abilities.

Suggest transportation options and resources.

Minimize the potential for former drivers to become isolated and inactive.

PLAN ONE

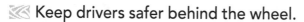 Keep drivers safer behind the wheel.

Everyone's personal dignity is important; a heightened dependency on others when elders can no longer drive has distinctly negative consequences in terms of their perception of self-worth. Helping your elders to maintain the status of "safe driver" is the first approach to extending their driving capabilities. Discuss the following possibilities.

- Arrange a physical exam, including a vision and hearing checkup.
- Review medications with the doctor or pharmacist and discuss side effects.
- Purchase a wide rearview mirror and add a seat cushion, if needed.
- Keep a charged cell phone handy to use in an emergency.
- Plan trip routes ahead of time.
- Avoid left turns as much as possible.
- Encourage daytime driving in good weather and shorter trips.
- Suggest an exercise program to improve overall fitness.

- Consider a driver assessment (see resources at the end of this chapter).
- Keep the car in excellent working condition.
- Make sure auto insurance payments are up to date.

PLAN TWO

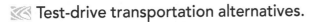 Test-drive transportation alternatives.

Americans have developed a lifelong reliance on automobiles. Not driving is hard to get used to and requires a great deal of planning. One way for people to learn how to get around without driving is to ask other adults who have never driven how *they* do it. Start talking about transportation options early on.

- Ride with family, friends, and neighbors.
- Take taxis or hire professional drivers.
- Rideshare and carpool when night driving becomes difficult.
- Inquire at church groups, clubs, and community centers about volunteers who will offer to drive.
- Ask the hospital, the doctor's office, and the shopping mall about vans and paratransit services.
- Walk and bicycle to nearby places.
- Consider public transportation.
- Move to a retirement housing community, where transportation is provided.
- Move closer to children, shops, services, and public transportation.

PLAN THREE

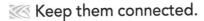 Keep them connected.

Your elders may not balk as loudly at the idea of giving up the car keys if they remain actively engaged with others. Being mobile offers access to other people, and opportunities that lead to self-fulfillment and a life of purpose. On the other side of the coin lies the possibility of isolation and depression. Keep elders connected and active by reviewing these suggestions.

- Invite elders for weekend visits and to family activities, birthday parties, and holiday celebrations, and arrange for family members or friends to provide transportation.
- Arrange for regular home visitors, such as other family members, friends, children, pets, clergy, and volunteers.
- Suggest that elders get involved in clubs and activities where participants carpool.
- Tap into local community centers that provide transportation for social activities.

PLAN FOUR

⚏ Be aware of at-risk driving.

Although many drivers know when they should stop driving, family members typically take it upon themselves to assess the situation and then do something about getting impaired drivers off the road. None of the warning signs listed in the "At-Risk Driving Checklist" automatically means that your elder should immediately give up the car keys. Regular evaluations of driving skills determine the need to alter driving habits or stop driving altogether.

At-Risk Driving Checklist

- Failing to yield to cars or pedestrians who have the right-of-way
- Failing to follow the rules of the road
- Receiving a traffic citation
- Driving too slow or too fast
- Stopping for green lights and in the middle of an intersection
- Ignoring red lights
- Drifting into the wrong lane
- Not using turn signals or using signals incorrectly
- Confusing brake and gas pedals or not finding them
- Consistently asking passengers if the coast is clear
- Forgetting how to get to familiar places or getting lost
- Experiencing near misses
- Hitting curbs and sideswiping parked cars
- Neck muscles are weak, making head turning in both directions difficult
- Not using side-view or rearview mirrors
- Difficulty with seeing and hearing
- Drowsiness while driving
- Reacting to medications or abusing drugs and alcohol
- Increasing aggressiveness while driving
- Noticing new dents and dings on the car
- Hearing others complain about the older person's driving

PLAN FIVE

⚏ Negotiate impaired drivers off the road.

Driving is not necessarily an all-or-nothing activity, and yet *any* conversation with older drivers about lessening the need to drive is going to be a challenge. Much of the misery is about status and flexibility—the freedom to go where they want when they want. A driver's license also symbolizes personal identity and self-reliance.

The goal is to help them plan for "retiring from driving" while preserving independence. Driving issues will not be resolved quickly. Allow enough time between conversations for them to adjust to the idea of a car-free lifestyle. Try different approaches at different times. And don't give up.

Change the "Feel" of the Message

Resist the urge to command them to stop driving and, instead, negotiate them off the road by asking questions. Try to introduce the topic of driving into everyday conversations. Older drivers who are given opportunities to think more about the subject (even if they don't let on) may draw their own conclusions about not driving. Conversation starters include:

Sometimes when I drive at night it's hard to see. Does this happen to you, too?

Do other drivers make you nervous? I know I get jumpy when everybody goes too fast.

I'm surprised at how often vehicles come out of nowhere when I'm driving. How about you?

Other drivers seem to be honking at me a lot. Why do they do that?

Did you hear about the terrible carjacking incident in the shopping mall parking lot?

Appeal to their Pocketbook

Break down the cost of owning, maintaining, insuring, licensing, and parking a car. Even a taxi service can be less expensive than maintaining a car. Transportation costs can also be minimized by making better use of meal-delivery services, arranging medicine delivery by mail, and shopping by catalog. Conversation starters may include:

Owning a car is expensive. And the price of gas! How do you do it?

I'm finding I use my car less and less. I'm even thinking about getting rid of it.

The cost of my auto insurance is out of this world. How much are you paying?

Have you heard about the online grocery shopping service? I use it all the time.

Take It Up a Notch

If conversations seem to be going well, ask more specific questions. Additionally, older drivers who are interested in information on the subject may not know where to turn for practical and unbiased assistance. Come prepared with transportation options and resources. Questions might include:

I just read about AARP's driver safety program. Do you know anything about it?

What does the doctor say about medications and possible side effects when driving?

Do you think your neighbor could take you to the grocery store sometimes?
Have you found anyone who drives at night to the places you want to go?

PLAN SIX

If all else fails . . .

If you feel strongly that your elders cannot drive safely and you have evidence to prove it, you have little choice but to get them to stop driving. If they agree without an argument, hooray for you—and them. If not, you have several options. Importantly, be certain that you have the support or at least approval of other family members, and that you're prepared to handle any feelings of guilt in the process.

- Report bad drivers anonymously. Contact the local department of motor vehicles and explain your concerns. Authorities may insist on a driving test or do nothing more than send a warning letter. This alone might convince impaired drivers to hand over the car keys.
- If your elder insists on driving while heavily medicated, ask the prescribing physician to write a "no-driving" prescription.
- Organize an intervention. Include other family members as well as social workers, a clergyperson, and anyone else who is viewed as an authority figure. During the meeting, people who are willing to volunteer their driving services should speak up.
- "Lose" the car keys; make the car impossible to start; or remove the car altogether. While this may seem extreme, this approach saves lives—your elder's and innocent bystanders.

Putting Ability Before Disability

Everyone has the right to remain mobile and to lead a productive life. Like everyone else, older people want the freedom to do more, when they want, and on their own terms. The Americans with Disabilities Act has dramatically changed the lives of people who live with disability and chronic illness, facilitating everything from employment opportunities to telecommunications relay systems. Advancements in medicine and technology also have played a major role in helping people accept and manage their physical impairments and participate in personal and professional pursuits on their own terms.

Helping, without taking away our elder's dignity, is a balancing act; gaining a better understanding of their special needs will improve *our* ability to cope from day to day. Caring for a person who has a disability and chronic condition is a difficult job—one that requires an iron will, emotional and physical strength, and the patience of a saint. At the same time, the idea of "being a burden" is often the source of great emotional turmoil for care receivers.

The action plans offered in this section of *The Complete Eldercare Planner* will help you manage the caregiving process under these highly demanding circumstances, minimizing psychological and physical risks by helping people become masters of their own domain. In spite of the daily stresses and strains of chronic care, you may gain a new appreciation for your *own* capabilities and strengths.

PLAN ONE

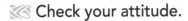 Check your attitude.

When the doctor says, "Your mom has arthritis in her hips" or "Looks like your husband has diabetes," receiving a diagnosis of a chronic illness is only the beginning. From interacting with numerous specialists and undergoing endless tests to rearranging a lifetime of habits and rituals, the entire family goes through a transition of experiencing losses of one kind or another. *Everyone* is afraid of the costs involved. *Everyone* becomes weary of the process. *Everyone* grieves the loss of a former lifestyle. *Everyone* worries about the future.

If you are caring for someone with a chronic illness, you're not alone. Common chronic illnesses such as arthritis, heart disease, diabetes, cancer, multiple sclerosis (MS), and Parkinson's affect nearly every American family.

PUTTING ABILITY BEFORE DISABILITY

- Arthritis is the most common chronic condition older people manage on a daily basis.
- The Americans with Disabilities Act gives every person the right to a productive, independent, and purposeful life.
- Approximately 80 percent of older adults have at least one chronic health condition and 50 percent have at least two. Arthritis, hypertension, heart disease, diabetes, and respiratory disorders are some of the leading causes of activity limitations among older people.[2]

Making life easier for people who are dealing with disabilities and chronic illness starts with the right attitude.

OBJECTIVES

After completing "Putting Ability Before Disability," you will be able to:

Gain a healthier perspective on living with a chronic illness.

Lessen the negative impact of a chronic illness.

Tap into independent-living products and services.

Consider the special needs of the older traveler.

Older adults who have a chronic illness should be considered people *first* and people with disabilities *second*. Living with a chronic illness doesn't necessarily mean living with sickness. Attitudes will greatly influence choices of treatment and quality of life. As caregivers, we must do our best to avoid mischaracterizing our elders as sick or unmotivated people.

For example, we may believe that people in wheelchairs are weak or feeble. To the contrary, it takes enormous energy to sit in one position for several hours, let alone all day. Also, it takes great physical strength to move a wheelchair. Individuals in manual chairs sometimes reject electronically driven chairs, seeing them as a sign of failure or weakness, or one of giving in.

There will be days when caring for the chronically ill will be overwhelming and extremely frustrating. Make sure you ask for and accept plenty of help from others. In the meantime, take a moment to look at life from the perspective of a person who lives with a chronic condition.

People who are living with a disability:

- have psychological hurdles on top of physical disabilities
- feel as though they are perceived as social misfits
- must find ways to feel productive while accepting assistance from other people
- live with the physical reminders of a disability (canes, wheelchairs, walkers)
- may be living in constant pain
- use more energy and take more time to do the same basic tasks as you
- often experience feelings of loss and isolation
- fear abandonment
- worry increasingly about paying for medical bills
- live in fear of losing even more control

PLAN TWO

Regain control.

The best plan is to become your elder's advocate, and together learn as much as you can about the chronic condition. Here are a few suggestions.

- Maintain access to experienced and knowledgeable health-care professionals.
- Seek health-care providers who are willing to entertain new ideas.
- Never stop researching what's new in medical advances. Find out what is correctable, treatable, and curable.
- Separate medical problems from psychological problems. Seek professional counseling. Stifling negative emotions can wear away at immune systems.

- Find role models who are successfully engaged in an active lifestyle in spite of their pain or disability.
- Caregivers and care receivers benefit greatly from support groups. Join one now.
- Review chapter 6, "Money Matters," starting on page 128. Create a realistic plan for how to pay for long-term care and future housing needs.

PLAN THREE

 Make life easier.

The onset of a chronic illness can make it difficult to use everyday products; hobbyists sometimes quit what they enjoy because they have physical limitations with activities. The good news is there are specialty products on the market that keep people functioning at high levels. Fun projects and daily activities of living can be resumed with the right tools.

The **websites** and **resources** listed at the end of this chapter offer a variety of innovative independent-living products. Helping your elder to overcome self-imposed limitations and finding the balance between dependence and independence is a worthy goal.

PLAN FOUR

 Get outta town!

What's stopping older people from being mobile and traveling the world over? These days the answer is . . . not much. Disability and chronic illness don't have to keep people away from the places and people they love.

Senior travel is big business; travel outfitters and experts have figured out that catering to older travelers is smart marketing. If a trip is in your elder's future, you'll want to make sure his or her special needs are addressed along the way. For senior-travel resources, look in the Yellow Pages and on the Internet under the following headings:

alumni travel	national parks
auto club	religious groups
colleges and universities	retreat centers
cruise ships	senior travel
elderhostel	tour guides
museums	travel agency

With a little forethought, travel does not have to come to a complete stop. Besides the typical arrangements that go into planning for an excursion, discuss the following options with your elder.

Extra Precautions

- Keep a **cell phone** and cell-phone charger handy at all times.
- Consider **trip cancellation insurance** and ask about refund policies.
- Make copies of the trip itinerary and trip-related **contact information** and passports, and distribute copies of the information to family members.

Air Travel

- **Wear glasses** and insert **hearing aids.**
- Say yes to airport **wheelchair** and **escort assistance.**
- Wear **slip-on shoes** and **ask for help** when putting shoes on after the security check.
- Review the **airline website** for limitations regarding packing, carry-on luggage, luggage lock restrictions, and oxygen canisters.
- Make every effort to book nonstop flights.
- Keep lots of $1 bills handy to **tip anyone who may help.**
- Inquire about **immunizations** and **passports.**
- Consider an **aisle seat** for quick trips to the restroom.
- Carry a pacemaker and hip-replacement **identification card** or a note from the doctor.

Undoubtedly, air travel has changed dramatically since 9/11. If the revised restrictions and regulations are keeping people from flying, then hiring a **flying companion** might be the way to go. Experienced air travelers and former airline professionals who know the tricks of the trade are making air travel as smooth as possible for older travelers. Companions are fully insured (ask for proof of insurance) and have passed an extensive background check (ask for references before hiring).

Flying companion services include escort from departure airport to destination; wheelchair assistance; airport check-in and security assistance; assistance with connecting flights; luggage handling; and destination companion, among others. Type "flying companions" in your Internet search engine to locate providers of this service.

If special assistance with oxygen and medications is required, ask for flying companions who can address health-care needs and attend to a medical emergency, if necessary. Contact the local agency on aging and local home-care agency and ask for referrals from geriatric case managers.

Medical Needs

- **Consult the doctor** before committing to the trip. Discuss recommendations about dealing with changes in altitude, time zones, and diet.
- Pack all medications in the carry-on luggage. Be sure labels clearly spell out dosages and instructions on how to take medications.

- Pack extra medication in case the trip is delayed. Find out how to arrange for **medication refills.**
- **Carry on a change of clothes and an extra toothbrush in case of lost luggage.**
- **Obtain information in advance** on local hospitals, pharmacies, and suppliers of medical equipment, such as walkers and wheelchairs. Most heavy and bulky items, such as wheelchairs, lifts, and backup oxygen tanks, can be rented at local suppliers.
- **Carry a notebook** listing physicians, phone numbers and medications.
- **Wear a reliable watch** for taking medications on time.
- Arrange for a **private caregiver or geriatric case manager** with a local home-care company as an additional traveling companion.
- Inquire about adequate **health insurance coverage** if traveling out of the country.

Accommodations

- If accommodations require handicap access, **book reservations well in advance**. Special rooms and services sell out fast because they are often in great demand.
- **Be precise**. Simply asking if a room (or bus or train) is "accessible" does not mean it is. Ask about elevators, transport lifts, widened doorways, large bathrooms with grab bars, wheelchair access, and the acceptance of service dogs, among other considerations.

Low-Cost and Free Resources

Telecommunications devices for the deaf (TDDs) and **Braille TDDs** are available for telephone customers with hearing and sight disabilities. Contact the Special Needs Center of the telephone company.

Look to the "City Government" section of the **local phone book** for Dial-a-Ride services and specialized transportation (paratransit) for people who are unable to use city buses.

Conduct an **Internet keyword search** on "senior transportation," "safe driving," "driving instructions," "paratransit," "dial-a-ride," "volunteer drivers," and "department of motor vehicles."

The **American Red Cross** and the **American Cancer Society** may provide transportation for medical-related appointments. Contact the local **Easter Seals** office and inquire about the **Project ACTION** program.

The **Alzheimer's Association** offers information about the effects of early Alzheimer's dementia on driving capabilities.

Call the **local agency on aging** and ask about neighborhood transportation services and voucher programs. Seek advice from a staff member at the local **community center.** **Church groups** and other **service-minded organizations** may have volunteers who provide transportation.

The **local hospital** may maintain vans for patient transportation to outpatient and rehabilitation and radiation services. Call the hospital or the local agency on aging for information.

The local library and bookstore can provide **books and videos** on a chronic illness or disability. The library can also provide lists of organizations that deal with specific diseases (such as the American Cancer Society) and provide toll-free numbers, educational materials, fitness programs, and local chapters with support groups.

There's no need for the physically challenged to stay home. For a wealth of information on **accessible travel**, type the following keywords in the Internet browser: "disability," "disability travel," "independent living," "senior travel," "disabled elderly," and "assistive technology."

ORGANIZATIONS AND WEB RESOURCES

AAA Exchange
(Features for Mature Drivers)
Website: www.aaaexchange.com

AAA Foundation for Traffic Safety
607 14th Street, NW, Suite 201
Washington, DC 20005
(202) 638-5944
Website: www.seniordrivers.org

American Association of Motor Vehicle Administrators
(To find the department of motor vehicles office in another state)
Website: www.aamva.org

American Public Transportation Association
Website: www.apta.com

Canadian Automobile Association
Website: www.caa.ca/agingdrivers

Eldercare Locator
(To locate specialized supplemental transportation)
Website: www.eldercare.gov

GrandDriver
Website: www.granddriver.info

Hartford Financial Services Group
(Family Conversations with Older Drivers)
Website: www.thehartford.com/ talkwitholderdrivers

National Center on Senior Transportation
1425 K Street, NW, Suite 200
Washington, DC 20005
Toll-free: (866) 528-6278; TDD: (202) 347-7385
Website: www.seniortransportation.net

Disability

ABLEDATA
(Access to assistive technology)
8630 Fenton Street, Suite 930
Silver Spring, MD 20910
Toll-free: (800) 227-0216; TTY: (301) 608-8912
Website: www.abledata.com

Americans with Disabilities Act
Website: www.ada.gov

Disability Info Online
(Disability-related government resources)
Website: www.disabilityinfo.gov

Family Caregiver Alliance
(Support for those caring for adults with chronic, disabling health conditions)
Website: www.caregiver.org

Making Life Easier
Website: www.makinglifeeasier.com

Mobility International USA
132 E. Broadway, Suite 343
Eugene, OR 97401
(541) 343-1284 (Tel. and TTY)
Website: www.miusa.org

National Rehabilitation Information Center
8201 Corporate Drive, Suite 600
Landover, MD 20785
(301) 459-5900; toll-free: (800) 346-2742;
    TTY: (301) 459-5984
Website: www.naric.com

Office of Disability, Aging, and Long-Term Care Policy
U.S. Department of Health and Human
    Services
200 Independence Avenue, SW
Washington, DC 20201
(202) 690-6443
Website: http://aspe.hhs.gov/daltcp

Driver Assessment / Driver Training

AAA Roadwise Review
(Senior driver tools and resources)
Website: www.aaa.org

AARP Driver Safety
(To find a class)
Toll-free: (888) 227-7669
Website: www.aarp.org/families/driver_safety

Association for Driver Rehabilitation Specialists
(To find specialists who can assess and provide
    refresher courses for older drivers)
Website: www.driver-ed.org

Independent-Living Products

Silvert's
(Affordable clothing that slips on quick and
    easy)
Website: www.silverts.com

The Wright Stuff
(Full range of products for activities of daily
    living and leisure)
Website: www.thewright-stuff.com

Senior-Friendly Travel

Access to Recreation
(Exercise equipment and much more for the
    disabled)
Toll-free: (800) 634-4351
Website: www.accesstr.com

Elderhostel
Website: www.elderhostel.org

Society for Accessible Travel & Hospitality
Website: www.sath.org

TRANSPORTATION AND MOBILITY ACTION CHECKLIST

(This worksheet is also available online at www.elderindustry.com)

MEETING TRANSPORTATION NEEDS	To Do By	Completed
Implement driver safety precautions		
arrange physical exams	_____	☐
review medications	_____	☐
purchase driving enhancement items	_____	☐
discuss safe-driving habits	_____	☐
suggest driver assessment	_____	☐
maintain auto working condition	_____	☐
proper insurance in place	_____	☐
Monitor elder's ability to drive	_____	☐
Prepare for driving-related conversations	_____	☐
Suggest transportation options		
family and friends	_____	☐
professional drivers	_____	☐
rideshare	_____	☐
car pool	_____	☐
volunteers	_____	☐
health-care transport services	_____	☐
walk	_____	☐
bicycle	_____	☐
public transportation	_____	☐
senior housing with transportation services	_____	☐
Lessen the need for elders to drive	_____	☐
Minimize isolation and inactivity	_____	☐
Know the signs of at-risk driving	_____	☐
Implement intervention support if all else fails	_____	☐

Know phone numbers of

    auto insurance   _____ ☐

    auto club   _____ ☐

    motor vehicle department   _____ ☐

Obtain copy of your elder's

    auto insurance card   _____ ☐

    auto club card   _____ ☐

PUTTING ABILITY BEFORE DISABILITY

Gain a healthier perspective

    review insights list   _____ ☐

Lessen the negative impact of a chronic illness

    access health-care professionals   _____ ☐

    research medical advances   _____ ☐

    separate medical problems from psychological problems   _____ ☐

    seek professional counseling   _____ ☐

    join a support group   _____ ☐

    review the "Money Matters" chapter   _____ ☐

Help your elder maintain an independent lifestyle

    medical goals   _____ ☐

    psychological goals   _____ ☐

    access to professionals   _____ ☐

    environmental barriers removed   _____ ☐

    mobility issues   _____ ☐

    transportation issues   _____ ☐

    elder role models   _____ ☐

Make use of independent-living products   _____ ☐

Investigate senior-travel outfitters   _____ ☐

Exercise travel precautions

keep cell phone and charger handy _____ ❏

consider trip cancellation insurance _____ ❏

make copies of the trip itinerary _____ ❏

distribute trip details to family members _____ ❏

Make special travel provisions

air travel _____ ❏

medical needs _____ ❏

accommodations _____ ❏

12

Managing Medical Care

Partnership for Quality Health Care

When our elders get sick, it's a whole new ball game. Older people are commonly plagued with several chronic illnesses simultaneously—memory deficits, movement disorders, diabetes, heart conditions, vision and hearing loss, and more—and managing their medical care is a job unto itself.

Expect to become extremely frustrated as you encounter long wait times and medical mishaps. Expect to step in if your elders fail to follow—knowingly or otherwise—doctors' orders. Expect to engage in stressful conversations that will impact medical decisions. Expect to use your communication and decision-making skills to the maximum. And expect to get very little sleep.

Managing medical care works best if you approach tasks as you would any other complicated mission: gain basic knowledge of the medical issues at hand; encourage your elders to be accountable for their words and actions; ask a lot of questions; and stay connected to qualified advisers at all times.

This section of *The Complete Eldercare Planner* understands how truly challenging the process of managing medical care can be. No medical or care decision will be perfect, and health-care issues will evolve in time from one situation to the next. Focusing on your elder's quality of life *in the moment*, rather than reacting to the shortcomings of the health-care system, is a more realistic goal.

PLAN ONE

Become familiar with health-care professions.

Gerontology is the study of healthy aging. **Geriatrics** is the study of illness and disease related to aging. Look to physicians and other professionals who have undergone a

---

PARTNERSHIP FOR QUALITY HEALTH CARE

- Ignoring health-care problems can mean the difference between residing at home and being forced to live in a nursing home.
- Older people may have been conditioned to *never* question the doctor's authority.
- Based on two years of fieldwork, the MIT Workplace Center reports that "family care-givers—untrained, undersupported, and unseen—constitute a 'shadow workforce.'"[1] Keeping medical records, coordinating and managing medical care, and advocating quality care on their elders' behalf fills gaps in a system that is uncoordinated, bureaucratic, and impersonal.

Older adults require specially trained doctors. Finding a geriatric physician will become even more difficult over the next twenty years, as the nation's 77 million baby boomers age.

OBJECTIVES

After completing "Partnership for Quality Health Care," you will be able to:

Become familiar with the health-care professions.

Encourage elders to be more in charge of their own health care.

Address spiritual issues in the health-care setting.

Organize the process of medical record keeping.

Advocate patients' rights and quality of care.

---

formal board certification program and have experience diagnosing and treating older adults. The differences between and similarities among various health-care fields are defined in the following pages.

A **general practitioner** (GP) and a **medical doctor** (MD) are physicians who treat diseases and injuries, do checkups, prescribe medicine, and perform minor surgery. They make referrals to specialists.

A **board-certified specialist** is an MD whose practice concentrates on a specific medical field. For example, an FACS (Fellow of the American College of Surgeons) specializes in surgery. If an operation is recommended, check the doctor's credentials. A board-certified MD has to pass rigorous exams to qualify as a specialist in her or his particular field.

An **internist** is an MD specializing in the diagnosis and treatment of diseases.

A **doctor of osteopathy** (DO) uses his or her hands as a primary tool to diagnose and treat illness and injury.

A medical doctor (MD) may refer a patient to any of a number of medical specialists.

Cardiologist—*heart and coronary artery specialist*

Dermatologist—*skin specialist*

Endocrinologist—*specializes in gland and hormone disorders*

Gastroenterologist—*stomach and digestive tract specialist*

Gynecologist—*specializes in the female reproductive system*

Hematologist—*blood specialist*

Nephrologist—*specializes in the function and diseases of the kidney*

Neurologist—*brain and nervous system specialist*

Oncologist—*cancer and tumor specialist*

Opthalmologist—*eye specialist who also performs eye surgery*

Orthopedist—*specialist in bone, muscle, and joint disorders*

Otolaryngologist—*an ear, nose, and throat specialist*

Proctologist—*specialist in disorders of the anus, rectum, and colon*

Pulmonary specialist—*specialist in disorders of the lung and chest*

Radiologist—*X-ray specialist*

Rehabilitation specialist—*specialist in correcting stroke and injury disabilities*

Rheumatologist—*specialist in rheumatism and arthritis*

Surgeon—*specialist in treating diseases, injuries, and deformities by performing surgery on the body*

Urologist—*specialist in the male reproductive system and urinary systems in both sexes*

Mental Health

Clinical psychologist—*not an MD; may have obtained an academic PhD; specializes in the family and one-on-one patient counseling*

MFCC/LCSW (marriage, family, and child counselor and licensed clinical social worker)—*trained to diagnose and treat emotional disorders*

Psychiatrist—*MD trained in the diagnosis and treatment of patients for physical and emotional behavior disorders*

Psychoanalyst—*may or may not be an MD; specializes in the treatment of patients with emotional disorders*

Eye and Ear

Optometrist—*not an MD; prescribes and adjusts eyeglasses and contact lenses*

Optician—*not an MD; fills prescriptions for eyeglasses and contact lenses*

Audiologist—*not an MD; tests patients for hearing loss and impairments*

Dental

Dentist—DDS (doctor of dental surgery); treats tooth decay and gum diseases, provides dentures, can detect mouth cancer, diabetes, and eating disorders

Dental hygienist—not a DDS; cleans and polishes teeth and takes X-rays

Endodontist—dentist who specializes in root canal procedures

Oral surgeon—dentist who performs difficult tooth extractions and jaw surgery

Orthodontist—dentist who specializes in straightening teeth

Periodontist—dentist who specializes in the treatment of gum diseases

Feet

Podiatrist—DPM (doctor of podiatric medicine); diagnoses and treats injuries and diseases of the foot

Additional Health-Care Resources

Many of the following practitioners provide services that are covered by insurance.

Acupuncturist—administers treatment by way of insertion and manipulation of needles into the skin; may be a doctor of acupuncture and Oriental medicine (DAOM)

Chiropractor—not an MD; physically manipulates and adjusts the spinal column, joints, and soft tissues

Hypnotist—guides patients into a hypnotic state to help eliminate and control unwanted habits

Licensed practical nurse—(LPN); assists physicians and registered nurses

Massage therapist—applies pressure and friction upon the muscles and joints of the body for therapeutic or physical responses

Naturopath—practices treatment of disease through manipulation of diet

Nurse-practitioner—(NP); registered nurse also trained to conduct physical exams, counsel, and treat patients

Occupational therapist—(OT); works to rehabilitate patients by helping them regain abilities to perform daily activities of living

Pharmacist—dispenses prescription medicines; knowledgeable about the chemical composition and correct use of medicines

Physician's assistant—(PA); takes medical histories, conducts physical exams, performs routine diagnostic procedures, and offers treatment plans

Physical therapist—(PT); works to restore mobility and strength to body parts affected by illness, disease, or injury

Registered dietitian—(RD); specializes in dietary counseling

Registered nurse—*(RN); can be a staff member at a health-care institution or offers nursing services for private patient care*

Speech or language therapist—*evaluates and treats speech impairments*

PLAN TWO

Be aware of privacy laws.

The Health Insurance Portability and Accountability Act (HIPAA) protects a person's privacy, and limits access to information about another person's medical history. Doctors, dentists, nurses, pharmacies, hospitals, clinics, nursing homes, health-care providers, health insurance companies, and HMOs must have written authorization from the patient to share medical information with others.

HIPAA regulations dictate that medical treatment centers must build walls and partitions around admission desks, block patient charts from view, and prevent the overhearing of private conversations. You may have noticed that the traditional patient charts at the foot of the hospital bed and on the wall upon entering a patient's room have disappeared.

This rule applies to you if you want to be briefed about your elder's medical condition. Unfortunately, some health-care providers are now charging for this service, which can run into hundreds of dollars for a prolonged illness—so ask about costs ahead of time.

To obtain HIPAA authorization:

- Have your elder sign and date the HIPAA authorization form, which will be provided by the health-care establishment, naming the individual(s) whom he or she is authorizing to be briefed and/or to receive medical reports and updates.
- Print copies of the signed and dated HIPAA consent form and distribute to all health-care providers involved with your elder's care.
- Keep the original document with you. In an emergency, you may need proof of authorization with new medical providers.

PLAN THREE

Advocate quality care.

People who are ill are particularly vulnerable. *Who can speak for them when they cannot? Who will be a second set of eyes and ears when the doctor is talking and offering treatment plans? Who will make sure medical errors are kept at bay?*

When caregiving responsibilities include managing medical care, our role as advocates will be *the key* to quality medical care. As advocates in the health-care setting, we guard our elders' interests, protect their rights, and stand up for them when they can't stand up for themselves. No one in the health-care setting will care more than you about the needs, fears, and hopes of your loved ones. Refer to the following guidelines to ensure your elder is getting first-rate medical care.

Medical Consumer Guidelines

Patients are entitled to:

- privacy in treatment
- be treated with dignity and respect
- free initial consultation interviews
- informed, certified, properly trained practitioners
- practitioners who keep scheduled appointments
- be fully informed of medical conditions
- ask questions and participate in planning medical treatment
- refuse treatment and understand consequences of such refusal
- second and third opinions
- prompt and understandable explanations of test results
- twenty-four-hour-accessible medical services
- refuse to participate in experimental research

The health-care team should:

- be board certified and have obtained geriatric certification
- have doctor privileges at the hospital of the elder's choice
- address both the medical and psychosocial needs of the patient
- return phone calls and e-mails in a timely manner
- help patients communicate with the doctor
- make referrals to community resources
- be open to the importance of the family's role
- make time to meet and address concerns

Look for clues that older patients are in good hands:

- Is the elder acknowledged respectfully and attended to?
- Is he or she allowed enough time for explanations and questions?
- Is he or she listened to no matter how busy the staff is?
- Is the elder offered an individualized plan of care?
- Does the elder feel empowered to make choices and decisions?

Create an environment of quality care:

- Check staff credentials, licenses, certifications, and discipline reports.
- Review resident/patient admission policies and agreements.
- Remember that kindness and a positive attitude will result in better service.
- Get educated—read up on medical issues.
- Hire a private nurse to act as an advocate when you are unavailable.

When your expectations aren't met or serious problems are not being resolved, take action. Seek assistance from the staff supervisor, the director of nursing, the staff social worker, and an ombudsman. Enlist the help of the resources listed at the end of this chapter.

PLAN FOUR

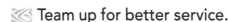 Team up for better service.

While many of us think nothing of proactively discussing our personal medical issues and treatment plans with our doctors, our elders may abide by a different set of attitudes and roles. They may have been conditioned to never question their doctor's authority and consequently believe that their health lies solely in someone else's hands. Seeking second opinions is also something they may resist. Having more of a say in their own well-being and treatment options may mean learning new behaviors. The deep-rooted habits of not challenging authority and not asking questions aren't easy to change, and the idea of taking charge of one's own health may seem foreign at first.

Today, we know that decisions regarding personal-health matters are **cooperative efforts between informed patients and their doctors.** We also know that obtaining a second (and even a third) opinion from another doctor does not necessarily mean we mistrust the physician's judgment; this course of action simply confirms an initial diagnosis.

Do what you can to encourage elders to take a more active role regarding the services they receive in the health-care setting. If you need additional tips on talking about sensitive subjects, review "Communicaring," chapter 4 of *The Complete Eldercare Planner.*

Before the Doctor Appointment

- **Track the pain.** Ask your elder to describe his or her pain and write down the answers to these questions: What hurts? On a scale of 1 to 10 (10 being most intense), what number is your pain? What does the pain feel like—piercing, aching, burning, throbbing? Does your pain change when lying down or standing up?
- **Put *everything* in writing.** Make lists of questions, concerns, pain history. Create a medical history, as outlined on pages 254–256. Include new and changed symptoms

since the last visit. Record major life stresses, such as changes in living arrangements, difficulties getting medications, and recent deaths of loved ones. Use the **"Medications" chart on pages 255–256.**

- **Prioritize health issues.** There's only so much time allowed at every medical appointment. Number the items on the list in order of importance.
- **Dig even deeper.** Some people like to research illnesses and treatment options by asking others how they've fared with the same disease or by conducting research on the Internet or in a medical library. Keep elders involved in the research process to encourage awareness in their own health-care issues.
- **Bring the goods.** Gather notes, proof of insurance, advance directives, medical and medications history, test results, medications, X-rays, photographs, and any other other that will help tell the health-care story during the medical appointment.
- **Accompany elders to *every* appointment.** Advocates help get patients to appointments, translate information, ask questions, take notes, provide comfort and moral support, and help patients recall what the doctor said. Make plans for someone else to be there when you are unavailable.
- **Prevent wasted appointments.** Call the day before to confirm the appointment time, date, and location, and verify that lab results and medical charts have been received and reviewed. Be sure to give the doctor's office advance notice if your elder's medical appointments must be missed or rescheduled.

During the Doctor Visit

- **Find out why you're there.** Confirm the reason for the appointment and/or the name of the test when signing in and also when the doctor or technician enters the room.
- **Be prepared to give information.** *Don't wait to be asked.* Start with an agenda rather than complaints. Say, "On my list for today are the following items." Address the most important issues first.
- **When the doctor talks, write down everything he or she says.** Ask permission first if you plan to record the session using a cassette recorder.
- **Make sure prescriptions are readable.** If the doctor's handwriting is unreadable, the pharmacist might not be able to read it, either. If the prescription is submitted electronically, ask for a copy.

PLAN FIVE

Ask questions and understand answers.

Good communication enhances care. During the doctor's appointment, keep encouraging your elders to stay involved by asking questions.

DOCTOR APPOINTMENT CHECKLIST

(This form is also available online at www.elderindustry.com)

Elder's Name: _____

Date of Appointment: _____

Doctor's Name: _____

Doctor's Contact Information: _____

OBTAIN QUALITY CARE

- Ask what unfamiliar words mean.
- Keep asking questions until what is being said is understood.
- Repeat what the doctor says in your own words to uncover any misunderstandings.
- Ask for copies of medical records, charts, and test results.
- Ask if there is a choice in hospitals if surgery is recommended.
- Ask about the cost if that is of concern.

ASK QUESTIONS ABOUT THE ILLNESS

- Does this illness have a name?
- What caused this illness?
- Do you personally have experience treating this illness or will you be recommending a specialist?
- What are the treatment options and related risks?
- Is this illness or pain likely to go away, get worse, or recur?
- What is your track record/success rate in treating similar cases?
- What long-term lifestyle changes are expected?

ASK QUESTIONS IF A TEST HAS BEEN RECOMMENDED

- What specifically do you hope to accomplish with this test?
- What are the risks involved with taking this test?
- What is the procedure?
- What are the chances of inaccurate test results?
- What happens if the test is not taken?
- What preparations are necessary ahead of time?
- Will personal assistance be necessary after the test?
- How long will it take to learn the test results?
- How will I be notified of the test results?

PLAN SIX

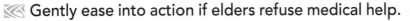 Gently ease into action if elders refuse medical help.

There are many deep-seated reasons why people don't seek medical attention. Waiting until something "bad" happens before taking action is not an uncommon strategy. Besides, a visit to the doctor can be a potentially traumatic experience. The question then becomes, how *bad* does it have to get before a visit to the doctor is inevitable? Here are some reasons why your elder may be avoiding medical attention.

- Your elder fears the worst.
- He or she does not want to spend the money.
- Your elder does not have an advocate to help navigate the complex health-care system.
- He or she has difficulty understanding medical jargon and is not willing to ask clarifying questions.
- Your elder is convinced there is no cure.
- He or she does not want to be cured.
- Your elder distrusts people in the medical profession.
- He or she is being influenced or intimidated by someone.
- He or she is reluctant to undergo the scrutiny of a medical team.
- Your elder has a fear of pain.
- Your elder has privacy issues about his or her body.
- He or she does not want to leave the house.

Compassion, combined with "soft-sell" conversation techniques, may be the answer to getting resistant elders to seek medical attention sooner rather than not at all. Try these tactics.

- Suggest a visit to a less-threatening medical environment, such as shopping-mall health fairs and drugstore testing sites for cholesterol and blood pressure.
- Optical shops offer glaucoma tests. Suggest a new and more fashionable pair of eyeglasses; then make an appointment for an eye exam.
- Make an appointment for teeth cleaning.
- Find a physician who is willing to do an initial home visit.
- Hire a social worker to visit and arrange for a geriatrician home visit.
- Attend a fitness or yoga class together.
- Get a pedicure together. You'll be able to see for yourself if there are any serious foot problems.
- Visit a health food store together. The person behind the counter is knowledgeable about preventive medicine.
- Is the current doctor the problem? Perhaps your elder is willing to switch doctors.

PLAN SEVEN

Pay attention to dental care.

We've reminded children over and over again to "Brush your teeth," and "Don't forget to floss!" Now these same words are being echoed to our elders. According to the American Dental Association, overseeing our elders' dental hygiene is a critical caregiving task.

Medical studies have found strong links between poor oral health and heart disease and stroke. Older adults with severely inflamed gums are more likely to suffer from unintended weight loss, which increases their risk for health complications. Nearly 75 percent of American adults suffer from various forms of periodontal (gum) disease and don't know it.[2] If left untreated, periodontal disease—more commonly known as gum disease—can lead to tooth loss and receding gums.

The first defense against periodontal disease is to brush and floss regularly. For arthritis sufferers, these movements can be difficult or painful. Speak to the dentist about dental products designed for arthritis sufferers. An electric toothbrush and fluoride rinses and gels may be an option. Contact the Arthritis Foundation (www.arthritis.org) for additional product suggestions.

PLAN EIGHT

Let technology lead the way.

Technology for personal use is gaining momentum, and no matter what ails our elders, there's an in-home health-care device that will make our life easier and foster their independence and dignity.

Many of the items suggested below can be purchased at pharmacies and discount stores. Look in the Yellow Pages under "Medical Equipment and Supplies" to find local retail stores. To hunt for gadgets on the Internet, type "independent living products" in your browser search engine. Also check out the home-safety products listed in chapter 10, "Safe and Secure," starting on page 206 in *The Complete Eldercare Planner.*

REMINDER DEVICES. Automated pill dispensers with talking, vibrating, beeping, or flashing lights remind people to take medicines. Watches, bracelets, and necklaces come with sound and vibration options to help elders remember specific tasks.

NONHUMAN "CAREGIVERS." Robots offer practical help. Family members caring for dementia patients understandably become frustrated repeating one phrase numerous times. A robot can say, "Please take your medicine," twenty times without flinching. A robot also can record and send information to a family member's computer or a doctor's office.

TELEMEDICINE. Patients take their own vital signs using standard equipment, and can transmit them electronically to the health-care team that is monitoring the results. People who suffer from chronic diseases such as diabetes, congestive heart failure, hypertension, or asthma can learn if their medical condition is potentially dangerous, and they can then initiate appropriate action.

E-MAIL AND ONLINE SHARING. If the plan is to communicate with physicians by e-mail, ask how privacy issues are addressed. Ask the hospital or care community if private websites for patients and family caregivers are available.

PHARMACY HEALTH-MONITORING SERVICE. Track data like blood pressure and medications use, and transmit information via the Web. Find out what online services are available through the local pharmacy.

KEEP AN EYE ON THE FUTURE. Online "medicine cabinets" monitor vital signs and share information via the Internet; adaptive clothing embedded with sensors transmit data to the doctor; interactive personal diagnosis systems monitor health and send messages and reminders through home computers and televisions.

PLAN NINE

Create a Medical History.

Becoming a more active participant in the health-care setting requires taking the time to create a *written* medical history. The more accurately a patient can describe symptoms, use of medications, and prioritize health concerns, the better the doctor can diagnose and treat the problem. For best results, bring a copy of the Medical History to *every* doctor's appointment and update it on the spot.

Keep copies of the Medical History with you at all times. Also distribute copies to other family members who are or could be involved in your elder's medical care. Update as needed.

MEDICAL HISTORY

(This form is also available online at www.elderindustry.com)

Today's Date: _____

MEDICAL HISTORY

Patient's full name/maiden name _____

Date of birth _____

Birthplace _____

Blood type_____

Allergies_____

Food allergies _____

Previous attending physicians_____

Current attending physicians_____

Pregnancies and miscarriages_____

Immunizations _____

Causes and dates of past physical illness_____

Existing health problems _____

Causes and dates of accidents _____

Surgeries and dates performed _____

Reasons and dates of hospitalizations _____

Reasons and dates of doctors' office visits_____

Reasons and dates of rehabilitation treatments _____

Negative reactions to medical treatments _____

Lab test results _____

Current use of eyeglasses, hearing aids, walking devices, wheelchairs, and others

_____

Current use of bathroom accessories, such as grab bars and raised toilet seats

_____

Recent changes in bodily functions _____

Existing mental-health problems_____

Personal stress and family problems _____

Mother's and father's dates and causes of death_____

Grandparents' cause of death _____

DENTAL HISTORY

Previous dentist_____

Current dentist_____

Past problems_____

Current problems_____

Negative reactions to dental treatments _____

Lab test results _____

Current use of dentures, etc. _____

MEDICATIONS

Current Use of Prescription Medications

Drug name and purpose _____

Quantity _____

Timing and manner of administering doses_____

Side effects (if any) _____

Current Use of Over-the-Counter Drugs and Alternative Remedies

Vitamins_____

Supplements _____

Herbs _____

Topical ointments _____

> **History of Drug Side Effects**
>
> _____
>
> _____

PLAN TEN

Keep tabs on personal medical records.

Making the effort now to organize and properly store medical-related documents and creating instant access to your elder's current health-care status, will save you time and improve the quality of medical attention.

WHAT TO STORE

Medical history (see Plan Nine in this chapter)

Current medications and dosages

Social Security number

Physician contacts (there may be many, so also note their specialties)

Emergency phone numbers (see page 5 of The Complete Eldercare Planner_)_

Proof of health and long-term care insurance

Living will and/or medical power of attorney and advance directives (see chapter 7, "Legal Matters")

Organ donation authorization

Vision and dental records

Family medical history

Permission forms for release of private medical information (HIPAA)

Recent medical test results and surgeries

Pictures and medical images (request a CD-ROM of images from the doctor)

Correspondence with health-care providers

Discharge summary from each hospitalization

Medical Web links and other education materials

Invoices and expense reports

The debate is on for privacy and information control in the health-care industry regarding patient medical records. Every storage system has limitations of one kind or another when it comes to updating and organizing patient-related data. To help avert medical information mishaps, health-care consumers are always better off when they **proactively control how they store their personal medical records** and keep the information up to date. Consider the following storage options.

ORGANIZING SYSTEMS. Store medical-related documentation in one convenient place—portable file containers, three-ring binders, and large, tear-resistant envelopes do the trick.

PHYSICIAN WEBSITES. Find out if the doctor's office offers patients access to their website. Medical practices may store patient information and records online. Ask if there are costs involved with this service.

ONLINE MEDICAL RECORD KEEPING. If we can retrieve cash and maintain bank records from our bank account anywhere in the world, we can do the same with personal medical data. Some websites are free; others charge. Type "personal health record" in your Internet search browser to access websites that offer this service.

PORTABLE MEDICAL RECORDS. Purchase computer software that offers the necessary forms needed to document, organize, store, update, and retrieve the medical and billing payment history. When the forms are completed, information can be downloaded onto a personal digital assistant (PDA), a wallet-size CD, or flash drives kept handy on a key chain or a necklace.

PLAN ELEVEN
Manage medical bills.

The process of assisting others with health-care expenses includes budgeting and bill paying, filing medical insurance claims, and managing bill disputes. Since this is an extremely time-consuming and complex task, you might want to purchase a medical expense manager software program and complete the task on your computer. Here are a few other tips for managing medical bills.

REQUEST ITEMIZED STATEMENTS. Most medical invoices contain errors because bills often reflect someone's memory. Look over *every* invoice and be sure that each charge reflects an actual item provided or procedure performed. If errors are found, call the manager of the department and ask him or her to explain the charges. Ask that wrongly billed charges be promptly removed or fees to be waived.

SPEAK WITH A PATIENT ADVOCATE. Ask if there is a staff member who might be able to translate any difficult medical abbreviations and/or someone to talk with about the bill.

ENLIST THE DOCTOR'S HELP. Doctors are used to dealing with health insurance issues. Ask the doctor to write a letter of "medical necessity" about the treatment or medication in question to submit to the insurance company. When contacting the health insurance company, ask to speak to the medical director who is reviewing the case.

Patient Care: Is Spirituality Good Medicine?

Nothing jump-starts the process of spiritual reflection and thoughts about God like the onset of chronic pain, a sudden injury, a serious operation, or a terminal illness. When a loved one becomes ill, thoughts begin to race: *Why is this happening? I don't understand why God is letting him suffer like this. What good can being spiritual do her now? I feel that God has abandoned me. It's now in the hands of God.* While your heart may be breaking and there's no hope in sight, the search for understanding about what is happening intensifies. The truth is, people hate illness, or at least resent it. At times you'll feel terrified and enraged, and at other times you may deny your feelings and mask them as a way to cope. Nevertheless, people long for their physicians as well as their families and friends to sit with them and console them as they struggle.[3]

For centuries, medicine and religion were intertwined. In the Middle Ages, priests in monasteries learned about anatomy and, at the same time, learned the pharmacology of plants—the first hospitals were attached to churches. Since the latter part of the nineteenth century, scientific medicine has led to a division between the priest and "the medicine man."

Medical ethicists have reminded us that religion and spirituality form the basis of meaning and purpose for many people.[4] One of the challenges physicians face is to help people find meaning and acceptance in the midst of suffering and chronic illness.[5] It is difficult for doctors to know what to say; there are no real answers.

Media attention on the links between spirituality and health has increased in recent years. Despite claims and research that spirituality enhances the physical and emotional healing process, the medical community remains divided. Either medical professionals laud studies on the subject as significant, compelling, and groundbreaking, or they condemn them as deeply flawed, quackery, nonscience, and harmful to patient well-being.

Complicating matters further, in our culture of religious pluralism, there is a range of beliefs ranging from atheism and agnosticism to a wide assortment of organized religions. In other words, patients, their family members, and the professionals who care for them could represent every culture, religion, and belief system imaginable.

This section of *The Complete Eldercare Planner* acknowledges the powerful influence and existing controversy regarding the relationship between spirituality and medical practices. Throughout this chapter, you will be encouraged to assume personal responsibility for your own spiritual beliefs—or lack thereof—as you address the medical issues of your elders.

PATIENT CARE: IS SPIRITUALITY GOOD MEDICINE?

- A survey of a stratified random sample of two thousand practicing U.S. physicians reported that 55 percent of physicians say their religious beliefs influence their practice of medicine, are likely to consider themselves *spiritual* but not *religious* (20 percent), and are likely to cope with major problems in life without relying on God (61 percent).[6]

- A survey of 456 patients revealed two-thirds felt that physicians should be aware of their religious or spiritual beliefs and that patient agreement with physician spiritual interaction increased strongly with the severity of the illness setting.[7]

- According to the American Association of Homes and Services for the Aging, three-quarters of the country's twenty-one hundred continuing-care retirement communities are run by faith-based organizations.

Whether you agree or disagree, be prepared to be questioned about your elders' spiritual and religious preferences in the health-care setting.

OBJECTIVES

After completing **"Patient Care: Is Spirituality Good Medicine?"** *you will be able to:*

Identify spiritual and/or religious preferences.

Complete a spiritual history.

Access spiritual resources in the health-care setting.

Consider continuing education classes on spirituality.

Offer spiritual practices.

PLAN ONE

Honor your elders' religious and spiritual preferences.

Spirituality is a slippery concept—the term has a variety of different meanings, not all of them having any formal connection to organized religion. People describe spirituality as having to do with such things as the search for meaning, hope, connection, value, and purpose. For others, the quest for spirituality is expressed in more specific religious and cultural terms and events.

Not only is the subject slowly moving up the research agendas of the health-care professions, patients also say they are relying on religious preferences to guide their medical decision making. According to a Harvard Medical School survey of two thousand Americans, one-third used prayer to address health concerns, 75 percent prayed for general wellness, 22 percent prayed for help with a specific medical condition such as cancer, and 69 percent said prayer was helpful. At the same time, there is no clinical evidence that prayer improves health.[8]

While the practice of spiritual and religious rituals may come naturally to some, not all people go that route—some elders have no strong sense of the sacred and may even find mention of the subject a source of extreme emotional discomfort. Adding to the complexity of the interaction of health care and spirituality is the fact that religious and cultural differences often exist between the patient and his or her own family members; and the belief systems of the physicians themselves can sometimes be interposed to add to the confusion.

Whose life is it, anyway? The principle of respect for the patient's own individual beliefs should transcend the ideology of all others. *There is no right or wrong here.* When a person is ill, the message should be perfectly clear.

> *Patients have the right to express and practice spiritual and cultural preferences, and find support for them.*
>
> *Patients have the right to reject any and all spiritual and religious invitations.*
>
> *Family members, physicians, and hospital staff, including clergy, must not impose religious, cultural, or spiritually based rituals on a patient without first considering whether such practices might be resented rather than appreciated.*

PLAN TWO
Prepare a spiritual history.

Enter any hospital, nursing home, outpatient clinic, or long-term-care facility and chances are your elder will be quizzed about his/her spiritual and or religious preferences. According to the Joint Commission, an independent, not-for-profit organization whose mission is to certify health-care organizations and improve the safety and quality of care provided to the public, a spiritual assessment is to be performed on every patient and "at a minimum determine the patient's denomination, beliefs, and what spiritual practices are important to the patient. This information would assist in determining the impact of spirituality, if any, on the care/services being provided and will identify if any further assessment is needed." The standards on spiritual assessment can be found in the Joint Commission's Comprehensive Accreditation Manual for Home Care (CAMHC).

There are no steadfast rules as to who will initiate the conversation in the health-care setting and how and when the subject will eventually come to light. A spiritual history can be taken orally or by way of a written questionnaire, and includes the process of gathering relevant information from the patient's perspective regarding spiritual values, religious beliefs, spiritual needs and concerns, and whatever gives the patient's life and illness meaning. The process may also include questions about how religion, spirituality, and culture affect their health, whether they have specific and immediate spiritual concerns and whether they have a spiritual counselor upon whom to call.

More often than not, the process of taking a spiritual inventory is incorporated under these circumstances:

- into the work-up of all new patients
- when a new diagnosis is given or a severe illness is present
- upon arrival of ambulance/paramedic personnel in the home setting
- at the onset of chronic pain or illness
- when there are addiction issues
- in the context of domestic violence or abuse
- during terminal-care planning
- addressing end-of-life issues

Preparing your elder for the possibility of providing a spiritual self-assessment is important; the line between assessment and intervention is blurred. Inquiring about a subject such as religious or spiritual coping may be interpreted by your elder as an opening for further exploration and validation of the importance of this experience, or can be perceived as intrusive and distressing. Because emotions can go either way when the subject is initiated, it's best to know his or her spiritual preferences and to talk about them *now* to avert emotional distress later on. **If your elder says no to wanting spiritual assistance in the health-care setting, and will not welcome any questioning about his or her spiritual preferences regarding medical care, put this declaration in writing to ensure that it will be honored**.

The **"Spiritual History Questionnaire"** on page 262 incorporates the kinds of questions typically asked by the medical staff. Discussing these issues and questions now provides an opportunity for you and your elder to confront and reflect upon these profound concerns at a time when life-threatening pressures are not upon you. If you want to ensure that his/her views will be respected, put your elder's responses in writing. Follow these guidelines.

- Attach a copy of the spiritual history to your elder's medical/medications history.
- Distribute copies to other family members.
- Ask the doctor's office to file a copy with his or her medical records.
- Attach a copy to all medical charts when entering a health-care facility.

PLAN THREE

Access spiritual resources in the health-care setting.

If spiritual and religious practices are important to your elder, the following resources will help fulfill their needs.

SPIRITUAL HISTORY QUESTIONNAIRE

(This form is also available online at www.elderindustry.com)

BELIEFS AND PRACTICES

Is spirituality, faith, and/or religion important to you?

Are you a member of a particular religious organization or spiritual community? If yes, which one?

Name the particular individual counselor or member of the clergy you would want to be contacted.

TREATMENT OF ILLNESS

Do you hold any spiritual or religious beliefs that might interfere with or impact your medical care? If yes, what are they?

Do you engage in any cultural practices that might interfere or conflict with your medical care? If yes, what are they?

How would you like your health-care provider to address your spiritual, religious, and/or cultural practices?

In the face of a terminal illness, how do your beliefs and culture influence end-of-life medical issues and decisions?

SUPPORT SYSTEMS

What are your main religious and/or spiritual support systems?

What activities do you participate in to help you maintain your religious and/or spiritual practices?

Do you have a group of like-minded friends who can serve as your support system?

What religious and/or spiritual support would you like right now?

Clergy

A patient's own cleric is a major source of comfort and reassurance and is typically welcomed at the hospital and long-term-care facility.

Hospital Chaplain

When hospitalized patients do not have their own minister or spiritual counselor readily available, the hospital chaplain on staff can be an important spiritual resource. The Joint

Commission has recognized the influence of spirituality on hospitalized patients by requiring a hospital chaplain, or at least access to pastoral services, in their standards for accreditation of all hospitals. Look to the hospital directory for the hospital chaplain's contact information.

The hospital chaplain is a skilled listener with a deep sense of caring to whom the patient can discuss his or her feelings about being sick, frightened by the prospect of invasive diagnostic procedures and the possibility of painful treatment and death. The chaplain is also a helpful resource in providing and arranging for certain rituals that are important for patients under particular circumstances. For example, some patients may wish to hear the assurances of Scripture; others may want the chaplain to lead them in prayer; still others may wish for the sacraments of Communion, baptism, anointing, or the last rites, depending upon their faith system. The chaplain may provide these direct services for the patient, or may act as a liaison with the patient's designated clergyperson.

Community Clergy and Lay Volunteers

While a hospital chaplain's role is to tend to the spiritual needs of the entire health-care community, the clergy represents the patient's particular faith and congregation. Hospitals and long-term-care facilities have access to a network of community clergy, counselors, and lay volunteers from a variety of organized religions who provide patients and families pastoral and spiritual care, sacramental ministries, advanced directive consultation, and other support services.

Interfaith Chapel

Most hospitals and long-term-care facilities offer interfaith chapels for private prayer and meditation. Chapels are typically open twenty-four hours a day.

Religious Services

Most hospitals and long-term-care facilities offer religious and prayer services at specified times and locations within the facility. Transportation might also be supplied to local community religious services.

Parish Nurse

Parish nurses provide community congregations with services such as health screenings, education and prevention programs, home visits to the sick, and community resource referrals. They also make home visits when someone is discharged from a hospital and help explain physicians' orders and aftercare. Call your elder's congregation and inquire about their parish nurse program. Also, request a nurse who speaks the patient's native language.

Seminars and Support Groups

Illness and a hospital stay are emotional experiences for anyone. Regardless of the reason for seeking health-care services, being in the hands of medical personnel may trigger feelings of discouragement, fear, loss, anxiety, grief, and loneliness. Most care facilities offer seminars and/or support groups, providing patients and their family members a safe place to vent and release emotions.

Palliative Care and Hospice

There may be overwhelming sadness, anger, or fear at life's end—not only for the patient, but also for loved ones. When a person is living with an advanced illness for which there is no effective medical treatment or cure, **palliative medical care** attempts to minimize the patient's pain, and physical and emotional discomfort. Concern for the entire family is what makes this kind of care different from traditional health care. For a more in-depth look at hospice care, refer to chapter 14, "Death and Dying," on page 301.

Physician

In most instances, physicians often leave in-depth religious counseling to the trained clergy: hospital chaplains, pastoral and hospice counselors, and support groups. However, physicians shouldn't be ruled out as a possible source of spiritual comfort.

Low-Cost and Free Resources

Hospitals, medical centers, and research centers may offer **geriatric medical assessments**. If your elder is an eligible veteran, some veterans' hospitals offer screenings at no cost. Contact the local agency on aging for program availability.

Registered complaints and disciplinary histories of any doctor are available by contacting the **state medical licensing board.** Basic information on physicians is contained in the *Official ABMS Directory of Board Certified Medical Specialists*, found at the local public library. Type the following keywords in your Internet search engine: "American Board of Medical Specialists," "American Medical Association," and the "Federation of State Medical Boards."

A **parish nurse** is a certified nurse who is committed to the healing ministry of the local church and helps parishioners meet their physical and spiritual needs. Type the keywords "parish nurse" in your Internet search engine for more information.

Hospitals and adult education centers offer **basic nursing programs** to family caregivers who are providing home health services for their elders.

The local dental school may offer **reduced-cost dental treatments** and may be a good source for second opinions. Also contact the state or local health department to find out what dental services are offered at a discount. Medicaid dental coverage is available by contacting the local Medicare office.

If a **dietitian** is not part of your elder's health-care team, a hospital dietitian, a home economist, or a nutrition instructor at the local community college or weight-loss clinic may be able to provide a free consultation about proper eating habits.

Local **specialized organizations** can be found in the White Pages of the telephone book and by typing keywords of the information you are seeking in your Internet search engine browser. Helpful organizations include the Alzheimer's Association, the American Cancer Society, the American Diabetes Association, the American Dietetic Association, the American Heart Association, the Arthritis Foundation, the American Foundation for AIDS Research, Mental Health America, the National Osteoporosis Foundation, the National Pain Foundation, the National Parkinson Foundation, the National Stroke Association, and the Simon Foundation for Continence.

ORGANIZATIONS AND WEB RESOURCES

AGS Foundation for Health in Aging
Website: www.healthinaging.org

All About Vision
(Medical exams for eligible seniors)
Toll-free: (800) 222-3937
Website: www.allaboutvision.com

American Cancer Society
Toll-free: (800) 227-2345; TTY: (866)
     228-4327
Website: www.cancer.org

American Chronic Pain Association
PO Box 850
Rocklin, CA 95677
Toll-free: (800) 533-3231
Website: www.theacpa.org

American Geriatrics Society
Website: www.americangeriatrics.org

American Health Assistance Foundation
22512 Gateway Center Drive
Clarksburg, MD 20871
(301) 948-3244; toll-free: (800) 437-2423;
     fax: (301) 258-9454
Website: www.ahaf.org

American Health Care Association
1201 L Street, NW
Washington, DC 20005
(202) 842-4444
Website: www.ahca.org

American Health Quality Association
(Working to improve health-care quality and
     patient safety)
1155 21st Street, NW
Washington, DC 20036
(202) 331-5790; fax: (202) 331-9334
Website: www.ahqa.org

American Medical Association
(Online doctor finder)
Website: www.ama-assn.org

American Podiatric Medical Association
(Online podiatrist finder)
Website: www.apma.org

Canadian Health Network
Jeanne Mance Building, 10th Floor
Tunney's Pasture, A.L. 1910B
Ottawa, ON K1A 0K9
Canada
Website: www.canadianhealthnetwork.ca

Health Privacy Project
1120 19th Street, NW, 8th Floor
Washington, DC 20036
(202) 721-5614
Website: www.healthprivacy.org

Hearing Loss Association of America
7910 Woodmont Avenue, Suite 1200
Bethesda, MD 20814
(301) 657-2248; V-TTY: (301) 913-9413;
     fax: (301) 657-2248
Website: www.hearingloss.org

Lighthouse International
(Features the Geriatric Center of Excellence)
Website: www.lighthouse.org

Mental Health America
2000 N. Beauregard Street, 6th Floor
Alexandria, VA 22311
(703) 684-7722; toll-free: (800) 969-6642;
    TTY: (800) 433-5959
Website: www.nmha.org

**National Center for Complementary
    and Alternative Medicine**
National Institutes of Health
9000 Rockville Pike
Bethesda, MD 20892
Website: www.nccam.nih.gov

**National Citizens' Coalition for
    Nursing Home Reform**
1828 L Street, NW, Suite 801
Washington, DC 20036
(202) 332-2276; fax: (202) 332-2949
Website: www.nccnhr.org

National Health Information Center
(Health information referral service)
Website: www.health.gov/nhic

National Institute on Aging
Building 31, Room 5C27
31 Center Drive, MSC 2292
Bethesda, MD 20892
(301) 496-1752; TTY: (800) 222-4225
Website: www.nia.nih.gov

National Institutes of Health
9000 Rockville Pike
Bethesda, MD 20892
(301) 496-4000; TTY: (301) 402-9612
Website: www.nihseniorhealth.gov

**National Long Term Care Ombudsman
    Resource Center**
(To resolve nursing-home and
    assisted-living issues)
1828 L Street, NW, Suite 801
Washington, DC 20036
(202) 332-2275
Website: www.ltcombudsman.org

National PACE Association
(Health-care assistance for people on limited
    incomes)
Toll-free: (800) 633-4227;
    TTY: (877) 486-2048
Website: www.npaonline.org

Patient Advocate Foundation
(Medical expenses mediation and
    negotiation on behalf of patients)
700 Thimble Shoals Boulevard, Suite 200
Newport News, VA 23606
Toll-free: (800) 532-5274
Website: www.patientadvocate.org

People's Medical Society
Website: www.peoplesmed.org

**U.S. Department of Health and Human
    Services**
200 Independence Avenue, SW
Washington, DC 20201
(202) 619-0257; toll-free: (877) 696-6775
Website: www.hhs.gov

U.S. Department of Veterans Affairs
810 Vermont Avenue, NW
Washington, DC 20420
(202) 273-5771; toll-free: (800) 827-1000;
    fax: (202) 273-5716
Health-care benefits toll-free: (877) 222-8387
Website: www.va.gov

Visiting Nurse Associations of America
99 Summer Street, Suite 1700
Boston, MA 02110
(617) 737-3200
Website: www.vnaa.org

WebMD
Website: www.webmd.com

Spirituality

Center for Spirituality and Health
University of Florida
Website: www.spiritualityandhealth.ufl.edu

Center for Spirituality, Theology and Health
Box 3825 Duke University Medical Center
Busse Building, Suite 0507
Durham, NC 27710
(919) 660-7556
Website: www.dukespiritualityandhealth.org

George Washington Institute for Spirituality and Health
George Washington University
Warwick Building, Suite 313
2300 K Street, NW
Washington, DC 20037
(202) 994-6220
Website: www.gwish.org

University of Pennsylvania Health System—Pastoral Care
Website: www.uphs.upenn.edu/pastoral

MANAGING MEDICAL CARE ACTION CHECKLIST

(This worksheet is also available online at www.elderindustry.com)

PARTNERSHIP FOR QUALITY HEALTH CARE	To Do By	Completed
Create a plan if your elder refuses medical help	_____	☐
Get HIPAA authorization from elder	_____	☐
Become familiar with health-care professions	_____	☐
Take active role in health care for better service		
Help elders track the pain	_____	☐
Put everything in writing	_____	☐
Prioritize health issues	_____	☐
Conduct research	_____	☐
Check medical staff board certifications and licenses	_____	☐
Make plans to accompany elders to medical appointments	_____	☐
Prepare for doctors' appointments		
medical history	_____	☐
dental history	_____	☐
medication history	_____	☐
Verify appointment in advance	_____	☐
Consider a second opinion when applicable	_____	☐
Switch doctors if unsatisfied	_____	☐
Consider technology to assist with in-home health care	_____	☐
Pay attention to elderly dental care	_____	☐
Gather and store personal medical records	_____	☐

Manage medical bills _____ ❏

Obtain contact information for

    doctor _____ ❏

    dentist _____ ❏

    health-care providers _____ ❏

    emergency contact information _____ ❏

    pharmacy _____ ❏

    hospital _____ ❏

    health insurance _____ ❏

**Keep important phone numbers
immediately accessible** _____ ❏

**Distribute phone numbers to key
family members** _____ ❏

**PATIENT CARE: IS SPIRITUALITY
GOOD MEDICINE?**

**Assume personal responsibility for
own spiritual beliefs and
professional practices** _____ ❏

**Know the spiritual and religious
rights of elderly patients** _____ ❏

**Identify your elder's spiritual
and/or religious preferences** _____ ❏

**Help your elder to complete the
"Spiritual History Questionnaire"**

    attach a copy of the document to your
        elder's medical/medications history _____ ❏

    distribute copies to other family
        members _____ ❏

    ask the doctor's office to file a copy
        with your elder's medical records _____ ❏

    attach a copy to all medical charts
        when entering a health-care facility _____ ❏

**Put your elder's spiritual and
religious preferences in writing** _____ ❏

**Access spiritual resources in the
health-care setting**

clergy _____ ❏
hospital chaplain _____ ❏
community clergy and lay volunteers _____ ❏
interfaith chapel _____ ❏
religious services _____ ❏
parish nurse _____ ❏
seminars and support groups _____ ❏
palliative care and hospice _____ ❏
physician _____ ❏

13

Quality of Life

What's Age for, Anyway?

Everybody ages differently. The evidence is everywhere: There are older adults who use a cane to walk, watch hours of television, and pretty much keep to themselves, and there are people of the same generation running marathons, buying Harleys, and dating online. In addition to genetics, diet, and exercise, the later years are also influenced by a lifetime of experiences and belief systems. *And if life suddenly offers a more generous gift of time, how might we decide to spend it?* While some people welcome challenges and opportunities for learning new things, others shy away from trying anything different. While some are social and eager to reach out to help those in need, others isolate themselves from the rest of the world.

Anyone who uses their own chronological age as a measuring stick is seriously diminishing opportunities for finding contentment and a life of purpose in later years. We have numerous role models to look upon for inspiration: Benjamin Franklin helped to write the United States Constitution at 81; Albert Schweitzer ran a hospital in Africa at 89; Coco Chanel was at the helm of her design firm at 85; Giuseppe Verdi wrote the opera *Falstaff* in his late seventies; Golda Meir worked up to twenty hours a day in her late seventies; Helena Rubinstein led her cosmetic company until age 94; Winston Churchill published *A History of the English-Speaking Peoples* at 82; and Pablo Picasso painted well into his nineties.

Is anything stopping us as we age? The experts say no. An important goal of this section of *The Complete Eldercare Planner* is to help **break the vicious cycle of loneliness, neediness, depression, and self-centeredness** among the older people in our lives and in return lessen their demands and dependence on family caregivers. From establishing social networks, taking classes, sharing special talents and skills, giving back, and pursuing new careers, your elders can awaken to the infinite possibilities and adventures the world has to offer. It may be just what they need to feel renewed, fulfilled, and positive about redefining their seniorhood.

WHAT'S AGE FOR, ANYWAY?

- Elderly people can be just as misinformed and prejudiced about "old people" as any other generation.
- Centenarians share a remarkable number of habits and traits that gerontologists associate with longevity: strong social networks, staying close to extended families, and keeping their minds and bodies active on a regular basis.
- Older people tell us they don't want to be a burden; they may think about suicide as a way to make things easier on everyone else.
- Though no one has an exact count, it's probable that 10 million or more older Americans are enduring the torment of depression.[1]

The experience of old, old age is changing. Americans are living longer and healthier lives due to improvements in health care, nutrition, and overall standard of living.

OBJECTIVES

After completing "What's Age for, Anyway?" you will be able to:

Be alert to issues of physical pain and depression.

Encourage your elders to engage in life-enriching activities.

Offer specific activity ideas that foster learning and connection to others.

Tap into resources that cater to older adults.

PLAN ONE

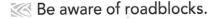 Be aware of roadblocks.

We all know what it's like to experience ongoing physical pain. Think of a time when your feet hurt because your shoes were too tight or when you experienced a toothache. When you are in pain, you can think of nothing else. **Unrelieved physical pain** produces adverse consequences, such as irritability, loss of appetite, movement impairment, fatigue, anxiety, and sleeplessness.

Sinking into periods of **regret or depression** is another kind of pain. When doctors talk about depression, they aren't talking about the occasional "blues" that all of us experience at one time or another. They are referring to a group of symptoms that persist consistently for several weeks or more. People with depressive symptoms have a significantly higher likelihood of needing help with daily tasks such as dressing, bathing, cooking, and taking medications. When everyone and everything stops being enjoyable and feelings of helplessness and hopelessness prevail, there is little quality of life to speak of.

Engaging in conversations with your elders about doing new things and living a more active and rewarding lifestyle will probably go nowhere unless you are willing to address any physical and mental obstacles that are emotionally wearing them down. Better recognition and treatment of pain and depression is what is needed. You'll find many resources listed at the end of this chapter for managing physical pain and late-life depression. Here are a few additional suggestions.

Pain Management

DON'T ACCEPT PAIN AS INEVITABLE. People tolerate physical pain for many reasons: They expect to live in pain as they grow older, they expect that any malady they have is supposed to be painful, they grew up valuing the ability to "grin and bear it," they don't want to make a fuss, they prefer pain in lieu of being under the influence of any drug that will alter their ability to think clearly, and they fear addiction to powerful painkillers.

TALK TO THE DOCTOR. If you are unaware that your elder is in pain, do you think that the doctor is also unaware? Step one is to consult the doctor and work as a team to help get rid of the elder's pain.

INSIST ON MORE ALTERNATIVES IF PAIN PERSISTS. If pain is not relieved by normal remedies (regardless of the doctor's expectations), continue the search for other ways to manage and alleviate the pain. The person in pain is the one usually in the best position to judge which pain management approach is right, rather than the doctor. The right "prescription" relieves pain throughout the day and night without unacceptable side effects.

Late-Life Depression

Is it illness, medication, depression? The signs of depression in older adults are not always easy to identify. Weight loss, losing interest in activities they once enjoyed, and sleeping too little or too much may be a few of the clues of depression.

Taking time to ask questions allows the opportunity to explore what's on our elder's minds. *Are they worried about finances? Are they dealing with a newly diagnosed disease? Are they upset about urinary incontinence issues? Are they sad or angry about where they live?* If the depression is brought on by a particular medicine, the good news is that a medication substitution could be the cure. Among the nondrug therapies the National Institute of Mental Health endorses are talk therapy, support groups, cognitive therapy, and exercise. Depression is treatable and is something that nobody should ever have to live with without putting up a fight.

National Institute of Mental Health data suggest that women attempt suicide three times more often than men do, often as a cry for help, but men are four times more likely to finish the job. The single highest suicide completion rate for any demographic group in the United States is older white males. Most suicide attempts are expressions of extreme distress, not harmless bids for attention. A person who appears suicidal should not be left alone and needs immediate mental-health treatment.[2] While emotional experiences of sadness, grief, response to loss, and temporary "blue" moods are normal, persistent depression, which interferes significantly with the ability to function, is not.[3]

People who are contemplating suicide might say, "I'd be better off dead," or "My family would be better off without me." Risk factors for homicide-suicide include: the husband is a caregiver and the wife has Alzheimer's disease or a similar disorder; the health status of one spouse is changing; a move to a nursing home is pending; the couple is talking of divorce.

If you believe there is a risk of suicide or homicide-suicide, call a suicide crisis center, a suicide hotline, a physician, a hospital emergency room, or the local mental health clinic. Also, if there is a gun in the house, remove it. Local agency on aging social workers are also trained to talk to older adults who are at risk of committing suicide.

WATCH FOR ALCOHOLISM. Studies reveal that millions of older adults drink heavily. Even drinkers who have not overindulged over the course of their lives are abusing alcohol late in life as a way to cope with emotional and physical difficulties and losses. For help, look under "Alcohol & Drug Testing" in your local telephone directory and call the local alcohol treatment center for advice and additional resources.

PLAN TWO

Retire retirement.

Older adults are redefining "retirement." Instead of using the later years as a time to "take it easy," they are creating everyday opportunities to live with vitality and purpose. There are no age limits for improving the quality of life. **The process of aging can be a pursuit of growing and learning of all kinds**—physically, intellectually, occupationally, emotionally, spiritually, and socially.

Encouraging your elders to pursue a more productive and engaged lifestyle begins by asking them the kinds of questions that will help get them out of a rut. The idea is to empower them in a direction that fosters independence and reaching potential. Perhaps the following questions will rekindle their zest for living a meaningful life.

What interests you?

What is important for you to do right now?

Is there anything you would like to learn?

Is there a special talent that you can teach someone else?

Can you think of anyone who can use your help right now?

Would you like to pursue any unfulfilled dreams?

Who is alone and lonely whom you can visit?

Would you like to get back in touch with former friends?

Have you restored any strained relationships?

Have you traveled to all the places you wanted to visit?

Do you have an interest in visiting your hometown?

Have you considered volunteering for a cause that's important to you?

PLAN THREE

⧖ Add life to years, not years to life.

There's no magic recipe for living a long and happy life. While some people who eat well and exercise throughout their lives die relatively young, others break all the rules, indulge in vices like smoking and drinking, and live well into their nineties. Genes and luck are big factors—*and out of our control.* Yet scientists and people who work with older people say that some tricks seem to work in favor of a long and healthy life. **Number one among the tricks? Positive thinking.** The confidence to cope with loss and maintain optimism whether it's losing driving privileges or burying family members or friends, people who age successfully accept the fact that people and things they love come and go.

What do satisfied older people do during the day? Most are busy with hobbies or chores; others have jobs or engage in volunteer efforts; others play bridge and bingo and enjoy their leisure time. Having a purpose in life and staying mentally active gives individuals good reason to get out of bed in the morning, in spite of their aches and pains.

Having a close network of family and friends is equally important. Unfortunately, recent studies indicate that Americans report fewer close friends and confidants than they did just two decades ago. For most people, their only close confidant is their spouse, and many others report having no close confidant—a sign that people may be living lonelier, more isolated lives than in the past.[4]

Relief from loneliness and isolation requires investing in others and patience until that investment results in real and sincere relationships. Perhaps any one of these activities will cultivate new interests and create opportunities for learning and connecting with others:

acting and modeling	fitness clubs and walking groups
babysitting	games and puzzles
Bible study	gardening
bird-watching groups	handicrafts and sewing
book club	inventing
caring for animals	journal writing
computer	knitting and quilting circles
cooking and baking	learning a foreign language
creative writing	letter writing
cultural pursuits	photography
drawing and painting	playing a musical instrument
employment	pottery

reading to others
singing and dancing
spiritual and religious activities
stamp or coin collecting
storytelling

taking a class
teaching
telephoning shut-ins
traveling
volunteering

PLAN FOUR

Focus on "senior-friendly" resources.

The aging of the population is creating an increasing demand for products and services tailored to older adults. When discussing life-enhancing activities and opportunities, steer your elders in the direction of **resources that cater to their unique needs.** Here are a few examples.

Travel

All one has to do is type "senior travel" in their Internet browser to find a world of adventure waiting for the older traveler. A variety of factors make a **travel destination senior-friendly,** and seniors who have "been there, done that, seen it" will find innovative ideas for new travel experiences: history, culture, nature, music, walking and biking tours, volunteering, culinary arts, crafts, and classroom cruises.

Travel tips for people with special needs can be found in chapter 11, "Transportation and Mobility," of *The Complete Eldercare Planner*. Also refer to the Yellow Pages of the telephone directory under the following headings for more ideas about senior-friendly travel destinations:

Amusement
Auto Club
Bed and Breakfast
Chamber of Commerce
Cruises
Elderhostel
Guest Ranch

Historic Places
Resorts
Retreats
Sightseeing
Tours
Travel Agencies
University Tours

Learning Centers

The learning and growing process never ends, and places of inspiration and education come in all shapes, sizes, and prices. **Adult education classes are geared to help keep older minds stimulated**—without the stress and worry of grades. Class locations include:

adult education centers
churches
clubs

community centers
community colleges
elderhostels

hospitals	retreat centers
nursing homes	semester at sea
public libraries	universities
retail outlets	YMCAs

Fitness Centers

There's so much to love about working out and being physically fit. There's so much to hate about those twenty-four-hour fitness clubs with all those young, beautiful bodies, not to mention complicated machinery and triathlon-level workouts. No wonder so many elderly people refuse to step inside the neighborhood gym. They can't relate.

Now there's an alternative for older adults. Fitness clubs for people fifty and over are sprouting up all over the country. Over the past fifteen years, the defining characteristic of industry change has been the growth in the population of older health club members. In 2005, there were 8 million health club members over the age of fifty-five, an increase of 314 percent over 1990.[5] No loud music or spandex. The fitness experts have thought of everything to keep the older body (and mind) ticking—yoga, tai chi, strength training, and "brain gyms" with memory-enhancing computer games. Some clubs even offer driving simulation courses. Workouts are geared for people who are not only out of shape but also suffer from joint problems and other common ailments. There's nutrition counseling, too.

Fitness clubs, gym boutiques, the local community center, and the YMCA may offer the SilverSneakers Fitness Program (www.silversneakers.com) or similar programs. Better yet, senior fitness programs may be covered by Medicare. Be sure elders check with their doctor before starting an exercise regime.

PLAN FIVE

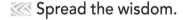 Spread the wisdom.

Our elders have much to offer in terms of time and talent, and are usually willing to share their know-how and experience when invited to do so. **Volunteering and sharing special skills and talents** provide opportunities for making new friends, staying connected to others, and becoming a positive influence in someone else's life.

Volunteer Resources

adult day-services centers	charity groups
adult education outlets	child day care
adult literacy programs	church ministries
animal shelters	city gardening initiatives
associations	community centers

community theaters	pen pals
consultants	preschools
court watchers	public and private libraries
family service agencies	reading to the blind
grade schools	religious groups
homebound meal delivery	schools
hospitals	senior advocacy groups
hotlines	Senior Olympics and Special Olympics
medical transportation	soup kitchens
museum/park/zoo docents	special interest groups
nursing homes	tour guides
online support groups	tutor
orphanages	youth groups

Employment Options

To be elderly, gifted, and employed is not so rare anymore. A retiree may go back to work for any number of reasons, ranging from financial hardship to the simple desire for more active and social interactions.

Employment opportunities for older workers are plentiful. People are working full-time, part-time, under contract for defined projects, job-sharing, and in seasonal jobs. An income-producing employment status, however, may affect Social Security entitlements. Before starting any job, your elder should seek advice from the local Social Security office.

A number of creative approaches are being designed by people who want to remain employed. People living in motor homes and RVs are traveling and working as they go. According to Workamper (www.workamper.com), a website source of job opportunities for RVers, singles and couples are constantly in demand at campgrounds, resorts, national parks, marinas, forests, theme parks, lodges, state parks, ski resorts, youth camps, wildlife preserves, RV parks, guest ranches, canoe outfitters, circuses, racetracks, and more.

Ideas for employment opportunities are listed in the classified section of the newspaper, on the Internet, and at employment agencies. Work options include:

activity director	consultant
actor	day care
babysitter	doorman
bookkeeper	editor
butler/valet	food service
cashier	gardener
chauffeur	golf course attendant
companion	handyman
concierge	hostess

housekeeper	pet sitter
house sitter	proofreader
magician	receptionist
mail sorter	retail
model	security guard
musician	tour guide
parking-lot attendant	tutor

PLAN SIX

Facilitate spiritual and religious needs.

Spiritual and religious rituals and traditions can provide a source of support when the going gets rough as well as offer direction toward a life of purpose. Importantly, do older family members have access to a clergyperson or a spiritual director? Additional information about addressing your elders spiritual needs can be found on pages 258–264 in the "Managing Medical Care" chapter of *The Complete Eldercare Planner*. Religious and spiritual groups have much to offer in terms of programs, including:

Bible study

choir clubs

counseling

education

prayer groups

retreats

volunteer opportunities

PLAN SEVEN

Love them, love their pets.

Pets play an important role in the lives of older adults, and the bond between the two can help ease the family caregiver's load. Animals make no distinction between the sick and the healthy or the young and the old, and their love is unconditional; elders transfer much of their love and attention to their pets as a way of dealing with natural losses in their lives. A study in the *Journal of the American Geriatric Society* looked at nearly a thousand men and women (average age: seventy-three years) and found that owning a cat or dog helped maintain or even slightly enhanced their Activities of Daily Living score.[6]

Though we may not share our elder's enthusiasm for his or her pet, it's important to recognize the depth of their emotional attachment to the animal and the benefits that the animal provides.

- Pets provide constant companionship.
- Caring for pets offers a sense of purpose.
- Larger animals, such as dogs, may make them feel more safe and protected.
- Watching fish in an aquarium or stroking a furry animal has been known to reduce stress and lower blood pressure.
- Birds make music they enjoy listening to.
- Training pets to do tricks offers a sense of accomplishment.
- Taking the animal for a walk offers daily exercise.

Pet care comes at a cost. Pet food, special diets, and medications can be overwhelmingly expensive, especially for large and active animals. Vet bills, accessories like cages, leashes, and toys, obedience training, and pet-sitting services can be costly. While pets can be great company for people of all ages, there are considerations regarding the cost of pet care. On the other hand, people who can't care for an animal at home might enjoy volunteering and interacting with dogs and cats at the local animal shelter. And your elder might enjoy receiving a soft, furry teddy bear–type stuffed animal to cuddle and stroke.

Family Power

You do a lot for your older family members. You arrange for various services, check in with them to make sure everything is okay, respond to emergencies, worry about what's going to happen to them. You talk things over, you argue, you laugh and cry, you care for them when they're sick and unpleasant to be around. You get tired but help anyway, and you keep on giving. Caring for family members is hard work. Unquestionably, the ups and downs of the family caregiving experience will have a profound effect on your life in ways that may not be obvious right now.

What are the rewards for caring for your elders? Seasoned family caregivers will tell you about the unique perspective they have gained on the process of aging itself, making better choices for themselves later in their own lives based on what they have witnessed firsthand. Family caregivers also have the advantage of being the recipients of the lessons their elders have to share. Older family members are teachers who can offer guidance to the younger generation. To reap the benefits of family caregiving, it's up to you to set the stage for your elders to tell their stories, bequeath family traditions, teach cultural rituals, and share special talents with those they leave behind.

Family members are finding ways to maintain relationships in spite of the miles that may separate them. And while sticking together through thick and thin isn't easy, the ability to stay connected has improved with the use of the Internet and technology. This section of *The Complete Eldercare Planner* offers ideas and numerous resources that strengthen family ties, including exploring family genealogy, preserving family traditions, and accessing organizations that address the unique needs of diverse cultures. Imagine how delighted your elders will be when you put them in touch with others who can speak with them in their native language. This section also gives valuable tips on gift giving. Who isn't stumped when it comes to giving gifts to older people who seem to have everything they need? Beyond the hackneyed scarves and neckties that ultimately end up on the closet shelf, this is the section of the book you'll rely on again and again when holidays, birthdays, and anniversaries dictate that only a special gift will do.

FAMILY POWER

- The experience of family shifts over time, and socializing across the ages is vital to all generations.
- It's up to family members to maintain the quality of life of the family, because there is no social system to guarantee it.
- Making the commitment to move from "me" to "we" improves family effectiveness.

Making a family work well takes cooperation, maturity, and an acknowledgment of values, traditions, and culture.

OBJECTIVES

*After completing **"Family Power,"** you will be able to:*

Become more aware of positive caregiving moments.

Set the stage to capture family lore and history.

Preserve family customs, traditions, and rituals.

Give more meaningful and memorable gifts.

Create opportunities for elders to contribute back to the family.

PLAN ONE

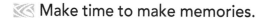 Make time to make memories.

What will you remember about your caregiving days after your elders are gone? It's impossible to know the answer right now. Sometimes something small and insignificant happens during the course of a typical day and you may never consider the possibility that you'll remember that moment for the rest of your life. You may also remember stories your elders tell you about the good old days, and time may stand still when you recognize their unmistakable handwriting on cancelled checks and recipes.

Give yourself as many positive memories as possible. The moments you remember may ultimately become the foundation of stories you choose to share when you become an elder. Here are a few ways to set the stage to create special memories.

LISTEN UP. Pick up the phone and call your elders with no agenda other than to say hello. Listen to the sound of their voices as they speak. Tell a funny story and hear the sound of their laughter. If they leave you an endearing message on your voice mail, save it.

SPEND TIME TOGETHER. Share meals, take a "Sunday" drive, celebrate birthdays, anniversaries, and special occasions, go shopping, sit on the porch and listen to the rain, play games, listen to music and sing along, attend religious services, take walks, or plan a family vacation.

GATHER THE CLAN. Organizing a family reunion has never been easier with the use of family websites and e-mail. Use software programs that make the planning of a family reunion almost as much fun as the event itself. The public library and the Internet offer how-to books and information on family reunions.

JUST DO IT. Life is short. Offer forgiveness, or ask forgiveness. Say, "I love you," before it's too late.

PLAN TWO

Reminiscing: Capture the gift of a lifetime.

Older people want what everyone wants—recognition and respect—and one of the ways to validate a lifetime is to walk elders down memory lane. *What will be lost if your elders' stories, traditions, recipes, and philosophies are never told?* Ignoring and dishonoring your predecessors forfeits the opportunity to make a difference in the lives of younger generations.

Recording their stories is an act of love. While the task of memorializing a person's past is not to be underestimated, the end result is priceless: to reveal one's values and dreams, to allow younger family members the opportunity to bear witness to a life and to preserve ethnicity and traditions.

Time spent talking with your elders about the past not only benefits them but you, as well. Older people are "living answers." They've been through the worst and best that life has to offer. Asking questions such as *"What did you want to be when you grew up?"* and *"Looking back, what would you have done differently?"* and *"What was the most memorable day of your life?"* offers valuable insights. Once conversations are under way, suddenly, everything seems to slow down. Solutions to your own present-day problems may be revealed through new perspectives and leave you feeling more confident and hopeful about your ability to navigate through your lifetime.

"When I have time" is memory's burial ground. If parents, grandparents, aunts and uncles, godparents, and mentors are available for a reminiscing session, act now. Laugh together. Be sad together. But do it together.

Make a Plan to Start

Reminiscing techniques range from informal question and answer sessions over a cup of coffee to hiring a professional family historian. Choose the communication method that feels most natural to you; the more relaxed you are the better. There are hundreds of books written on the topic of reminiscing and even more information available on the Internet. If they don't welcome the idea of communicating face-to-face with anyone about their life experiences, perhaps encouraging your elders to write a personal letter or keep a journal—to be read later on or not—could be a more positively received idea.

For the most part, the process of reminiscing with older people is a positive experience for them and for you, but sometimes the opposite can be true. Not all memories are meant to be shared. Throughout conversations, be on the lookout for clues that the topic of the moment may be off-limits: If he or she immediately expresses the desire to change the subject, if he or she looks upset or agitated, if he or she suddenly stands up and starts pacing or walking around the room it's probably a good idea to change the subject. At the same time, you may feel as though they are opening up far too much, and you may learn something that is disturbing or you might be stricken with embarrassment. Anything goes, so be prepared.

Bring Life to Memories

Sometimes the process of showing them simple objects will help jog their memory. Here are a few suggestions that may encourage hours of discussions and help bring memories back to life:

> *jewelry such as wedding bands, watches, and brooches*
> *hats and interesting articles of clothing*
> *awards and trophies*
> *paintings and artwork*
> *photo albums*
> *newspaper clippings*
> *personal letters*
> *diaries*
> *postcards*
> *theater ticket stubs*
> *maps*
> *passports*
> *marriage certificates*
> *school degrees*
> *songs*
> *home movies*

Plan for Engaging Conversations

Initiate a dialogue that focuses on a single topic with special relevance or meaning for that particular person. Since memories are often recalled layer by layer, there's no need to "rush" conversations. Also, go with the flow even if you know what they are saying is inaccurate and untrue. As long as what is being reconstructed gives meaning to them, let them talk. Subjects that evoke sharing and reminiscing include:

family traditions

cultural rituals

radio and television programs

school activities

career choices

historical events

holidays

family recipes

childhood games

home remedies

family pets

seasons and unusual weather conditions

hometown events

Remember to Remember

There are a number of ways to capture the stories our elders have to tell. Deciding how you want to store the documentation you are gathering should also include a plan for how you will ultimately distribute the information to future generations. Fortunately, the Internet will greatly assist in the process: Computing resources, journaling software, digital photos, video clips, family-history-gathering Web services, and scanning images will help create a rich and valuable historical family archive. Remembering devices include:

photo albums

scrapbooks

family websites

family newsletters

Internet photo services

Internet video websites

journals

audiotapes

digital camcorders

video cameras

shadow boxes

picture frames

diaries

heirloom hardbound books

binders with plastic sleeves for storage

home movies, slides, and photos transferred to newer technologies (CD-ROM and DVD)

PLAN THREE

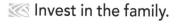 Invest in the family.

A strong family has a commitment to one another. **Keeping family customs, traditions, and rituals alive** nourishes family roots, bridges generations, and provides a sense of continuity, understanding, and closeness when feeling disconnected. From the food you eat together to the things you do during the holidays, customs, traditions, and rituals are the threads of life that bind a family together.

If they haven't done so already, ask older family members to share as much information as possible about family customs, traditions, and rituals. Put what they say in writing since there's a chance that their words may be forgotten and other family members may not be willing participants in carrying on certain family traditions at all times.

PLAN FOUR

Get to know *you.*

Reminiscing with your elders and learning more about family traditions may spark an interest in searching for your family roots. **Genealogy** is a popular pastime, and with the use of the Internet it can be easy to locate family records, gather photos and historical documents, and share the results with family and friends. For more information on genealogy, review the resources listed at the end of this chapter. Here are some basic tips on getting started.

DRAW A FAMILY TREE. Create a chart that shows how family members are related. Computer software programs will help simplify this process.

CHECK OUT THE LIBRARY. Public and private libraries offer valuable family data, such as obituaries, maps, local history books, historical property deeds, private letters, and legal documents.

SEARCH FAMILY RECORDS. Birth and death certificates, marriage licenses, divorce decrees, citizenship papers, wills, deeds, and medical histories are available for viewing at the county clerk's office, state vital statistics bureaus, and state health departments.

CONDUCT INTERVIEWS. Find people who can add depth to family stories. Create a list of questions to ask ahead of time. Write down the answers and use a tape recorder as a backup. Offer photographs to jog memories. Ask family members to name people in photographs, how they are related to the family, the date of the photo, and where it was taken.

ASK QUESTIONS ABOUT POSSESSIONS. Antiques, collectibles, vintage clothing and jewelry, and heirlooms have a story to tell. Find out the circumstances of how or when such items were acquired.

EXPLORE ATTICS. Look for forgotten items such as newspaper clippings, letters, report cards, invitations, passports, autograph books, costumes, musical instruments, dolls, diplomas, diaries, yearbooks, scrapbooks, baby books, trophies, maps, and photographs.

GO HOME. Make arrangements to take your elders back to the place where they were born and where they spent their childhood.

PLAN FIVE

Give the special gift of undivided attention.

With decades of birthdays and holidays gone by, *who isn't stumped when it comes to knowing what gifts to buy older family members?* By now, they've received their fair share of neckties and slippers, and there's a good chance they already have what they want and need. Time is a precious commodity; few of us can afford to spend hours of shopping for the perfect gift, and overspending on unwanted and unneeded items.

What is treasured most by older people is spending quality time together and gifts that relay loving messages that they are special and thought of and cared about each day. To touch the heart and soul of the people who mean so much to you, here are a few gift ideas that are sure to make that happen.

GO BACK TO SCHOOL. Learning something new is twice the fun when you do it together. Adult education classes offer a variety of learning opportunities—from exploring ancient history and learning the computer or a new language to arts and crafts. Spend time together taking a class.

PICTURE THIS. Offer to organize your elders' photograph collection. Buy new photo albums and photo boxes, and spend a few afternoons looking at the photos together as you put them in order.

WRITE ON. Give a small decorative box of stationery cards and stamped envelopes, and offer to be their personal secretary. Let them dictate letters to friends and family as you write down their thoughts and mail the letters in their behalf.

SING-ALONG. Attend sing-along events, at movie theaters, community events, and college musical venues. Singing and harmony are always fun. If they are homebound, buy or rent a karaoke system.

LEAD THE WAY. Offer to chauffeur your elders down memory lane by driving them around neighborhood streets and familiar places that hold special meaning for them. Pack a healthy picnic basket and enjoy the sights as you munch away.

PLUG THEM IN. Watch your elders' faces light up when they receive their first e-mail. Presto sends e-mails without a computer. Plug the printing mailbox into any electric outlet to receive e-mail, digital photos, subscriptions to newsletters, and more. The Presto mailbox makes a wonderful and unique gift. (For more information, go to www.presto.com.)

GET COZY WITH COMPOSERS. Do they like musicals, new age, classical, jazz, or blues? Research the life of a composer and create a biography to read aloud. Listen to the music together while sipping coffee or tea. Giving them beautiful new coffee mugs and tea cups will remind them of this special visit.

LET THE BEAT GO ON. If you think there's a chance your elders want to resurrect an instrument they formerly played, offer to pay for music classes. If singing is their thing, offer to pay for voice lessons. Offer to drive them to class and take them out to eat afterwards to hear about their experience.

BOOK IT. Go to your local photocopy shop to create a beautifully bound book of your elder's poetry, photographs, short stories, and works of art. Seeing his or her creations in print will delight your elder.

TAKE THEM BACK. Invite your elders to journey back to their hometown. This is truly a gift of a lifetime. Creating a scrapbook of the trip will bring joy for years to come.

SHOW OFF. Never underestimate the power of giving your elders credit for all they've done for you. A home video reminds them of how they have positively influenced your life. Show off your cooking skills or perform a magic trick or tap dance (all of the talents you got from Mom or Dad, of course). If grandchildren are featured, have them recite a poem, play a musical instrument, or show off their bowling or baseball abilities. End the video with a heartfelt message or song. Transfer the video to DVD for easy viewing.

FRAME IT. Daily reminders of how special they are can give them an instant pick-me-up. Words like "We love you, Mom" and "I'm thinking about you, Aunt Betty" placed in a beautiful picture frame will inevitably make them smile.

MAKE TIME STAND STILL. Celebrate the years of being a family by creating a timeline greeting card. Fold a legal piece of paper (construction weight) into five panels. Gather five photos of yourself—from infancy to childhood to teen years to young adult and now. Arrange one photo per panel and write a brief story under each photograph.

THROW A CARD PARTY. Invite friends and family members to send your elders a greeting card and include any remembrance about them: a funny story, a photograph, a poem. Ask young grandchildren to draw a picture. Everyone loves to get mail, and for days they will be thrilled at getting lots of mail and cards with funny, endearing, and touching notes. Place the cards in a beautiful scrapbook.

SING PRAISES. Treat your elders to a special dinner at their favorite restaurant. Present a fragrant orchid or lapel carnation to wear. Have everyone at the table stand up and offer a special toast for the guest of honor. Invite local city officials such as the mayor to compose a letter of recognition to be read at the dinner table. Videotape the occasion and transfer to DVD for easy viewing.

MAKE A WISH. Do your elders long to fulfill a dream? Make their wish come true.

COOK UP A STORM. Beyond learning how to create nutritious meals, cooking classes are naturally fun and entertaining. Offer to attend classes together. Don't forget the camera.

BLOOM THE ROOM. A beautiful vase filled with an arrangement of silk flowers will bring happiness and a sense of the outdoors into any room, and also remind them of you.

TAKE IT PERSONALLY. Composing a personal letter will touch your elders on many levels. Perhaps a note of thanks is in order explaining why you are grateful for them and how they blessed your life. Perhaps the letter is one of forgiveness for long-standing disputes that can now be put to rest. Remind your elders to reread the letter often to remind them of how much they are loved and appreciated.

TURN UP THE VOLUME. Satellite radio offers hundreds of stations and twenty-four-hour continuous entertainment: music from the 1940s, radio programs from the 1930s, 1940s, and 1950s featuring Lucille Ball, Jack Benny, and other favorites, the Suspense series, the Lone Ranger, and much more. Satellite radio subscriptions are modestly priced. Spend time reminiscing and listening together.

INVITE ART. Color-by-number, finger painting, stencil place mats—the ideas are endless when you visit your local arts and craft store. The fun continues when the final product is on display for all to admire.

PLAY BALL. Taking an older baseball fan to the ballpark can be a memorable outing. Senior citizen discount day is only one of many reasons why sitting in the stands, eating hot dogs, and cheering for the home team will put a smile on any elder's face. They're sure to start telling you stories of old-time players they used to watch. If you want to go the extra mile, inquire in advance about having a personalized message displayed on the scoreboard. Bring the camera and create a day-at-the-ballpark photo album.

KEEP IT GREEN. Tending to plants and gardening is a favorite pastime for many older gardeners; don't let physical impairments like arthritis put an end to tending to plants. Raised flower beds and window boxes are ideal for gardeners who find going outdoors difficult. A child's wagon or wheelbarrow makes an attractive movable garden. Purchase modified gardening tools that are especially designed to assist those who have difficulty with grasping, cutting, and digging motions. Place heavy container potted plants on wheeled wooden palates for easy mobility.

SPRUCE UP. Offer to give the bathroom a safety makeover. Install grab bars for the bathtub and toilet, nonslip pads for the tub, door grippers, and a nonskid bath mat. For a special touch, purchase a decorative night-light that displays a photograph of family, friends, pets, or a favorite place.

FEED THE BIRDS. Place bird feeders and birdbaths in visible locations around the yard, deck, or patio or attached to the outside of a picture window to make it easy for them to enjoy from their favorite chair. Spend time discussing the different types of birds you are most likely to see. Purchase a bird reference guide to help identify each species.

STAY IN TOUCH. Create a personalized telephone directory. Practical and caring, this is a gift that reminds your elders that family and friends are always nearby. Purchase a small three-ring binder. In large type, list the contact information for family, friends, and service providers, such as the beauty shop operator and local movie theater. Customize the cover of the binder and use colorful index tabs to separate the information. Display emergency contacts and telephone numbers in the front of the book. Update the information as needed.

TIME IT RIGHT. You've heard of Book-of-the-Month; now there's YOU once a month. Decide on something you can realistically do for your elders on a monthly basis—from washing the car and organizing the closet to computer lessons and a night at the movies. Make a beautiful card and insert twelve coupons with promises of special activities for the year ahead.

PHONE HOME. Budget-conscious elders love receiving long-distance phone cards to call family and friends as often as they like. What a great way to stay in touch and to take away the guilt of spending money for long-distance calls.

TALK ABOUT IT. Start a book-discussion group that meets monthly at your elder's house. Invite friends and neighbors. Beyond books, the group can discuss poems, short stories, movies, and Bible verses. If reading books is difficult, check out books on tape and videos from the local library.

PLAY AT WORK. Work sites come alive when parents accompany their children to work. Why not share this important part of your life with older family members? Won't they beam with pride as you introduce them to coworkers? Keep the visit short, perhaps during lunch hour, since spending the entire day may be too tiresome for both of you. Take pictures of this memorable outing.

SET THE TABLE. Purchase brightly colored dishes, drinking glasses, coordinating place mats, and flatware, and every time they sit down to eat they'll be reminded of you.

SHAPE UP. Fifty-and-over fitness centers make working out together more enjoyable, since programs and services are tailored to meet the needs of the older mind and body. Purchase a joint membership and attend classes together on a regular basis.

HAM IT UP. Performing together in a community theater production is nothing less than fun and invigorating. From auditioning and attending rehearsals to opening night, this is one experience that will be talked about for years to come. Ask someone to videotape the play and transfer to DVD for easy viewing.

WORK IT OUT. Do you have a work conference coming up in your near future? Consider taking your elder with you. These days, juggling work-life responsibilities is not easy, and employers are beginning to see the benefits of encouraging employees to combine work travel with family vacations. They know how difficult it may be for you to get away, and bringing your favorite family members with you might be a win-win solution. While you're off to a workshop, loved ones can shop or relax by the pool.

PLAN SIX

⚒ Foster *grand* grandparenting.

Grandparents and grandchildren are a magical combination. While grandparents help channel the energy and enthusiasm of youth in productive ways and transmit family values down the family tree, grandchildren can have an equally positive influence on grandparents. Who but a grandchild could convince Grandpa to give up smoking or have the patience to teach Grandma how to use the computer? *There is indeed a special warmth and wonder in this family bond.*

At the same time, an increasing number of older adults are finding themselves in the unplanned role of parent to their grandchildren. Nationally, millions of children are living in grandparent-headed households. Grandparents step in when the parent can't take care of the children due to substance abuse, divorce, or a variety of other circumstances. Support groups and special programs for grandfamilies are plentiful. Review the "Grandparent as Parents" resources listed at the end of this chapter.

Keeping the connection strong between grandparents and grandchildren also helps lighten our load as family caregivers. Great-grandparents, grandparents, and grandchildren who live a long distance from each other can stay in touch in a variety of ways. Here are some suggestions.

SEE AND HEAR. Video cams allow grandparents and grandchildren to see and hear each other when they talk on the phone or the computer. Place cameras on the tops of computer and television monitors and other places in the home where it's convenient to make telephone calls.

NO E-MAIL? NO PROBLEM. The process of e-mailing comes naturally to grandchildren, and when grandparents resist using a computer, grandchildren's communication methods are seriously impaired. There's a simple way to get around this through the use of a computerless e-mail system. Presto.com is a service that sends e-mails without a computer. Plug the printing mailbox into any electric outlet and grandparents can receive e-mails, digital photos, and subscriptions to newsletters. E-mail messages are printed on standard plain paper.

VIDEOS. Grandparents can tell stories, give a guided tour of their home and neighborhood, and ask questions about school projects. Grandchildren can act out nursery rhymes, sing and dance, recite a poem, and play a musical instrument. Anything recorded on video offers ample opportunities to remember voices and faces.

PHOTOGRAPHS. Recent photographs of family, friends, family pets, and places of interest keep everyone up to date. Post photos on family websites and create family photo albums.

SPECIAL DELIVERY. Family members young and old love to receive personal letters in the mail. Younger children enjoy cards filled with stickers, comic strips, word games, and animal pictures. Grandparents often enjoy children's drawings, penmanship worksheets, and family photos.

BEDTIME STORIES. Ask grandparents to purchase a bedtime storybook and read the stories aloud while recording their voices on a cassette player. Send the book and audiotape to the grandchild. As the young child "reads" the book, he or she can play the cassette and listen to Grandma or Grandpa read the stories to them.

SLEEPOVERS. For many families, visiting grandparents is a ritual of summer and holidays. It's a time of making root beer floats, cooking dinner, pulling weeds and gardening, watching parades, taking walks, singing songs, and visiting the public library. Spare rooms can become the grandchild's second home and opens the way for even more significant and decades-long relationships between grandparents and grandchildren.

VACATIONS. Sharing of knowledge and interests while vacationing together cements intergenerational bonds. From renting a beach house to camping out in a national park, when the parents stay home and it's just the grandparents and grandchildren together on vacation, it can be a wonderful experience. Grandparents should insist on sharing responsibilities with the grandchildren, including the planning of the trip, choosing destinations, taking photographs, and keeping a trip journal.

SIMPLE GIFTS. Never underestimate the value of baggy shirts for girls of all ages. Grandpa's faded old baggy shirt with long sleeves and extra-large pockets may be the perfect thing to wear on moving day, during a pregnancy, and cold winter days. Grandma's stamp collection might spark an interest in younger generations. Encourage grandparents to give something they own, however simple, to their grandchildren. As a bonus, the ceremony of giving grandchildren the item personally is often just as special as the gift itself.

HOMEWORK. Working on a school project together can be a fun learning experience for both of the participants. While the grandchild might conduct research for assignments online, grandparents can offer additional information found at the public library and other resources.

EXTEND THE FAMILY. If there are no grandchildren in the immediate family, encouraging them to participate in neighborhood intergenerational programs may be the next best thing. Foster programs that link older adults and children together can be found at local community centers, religious centers, and child day-care centers.

PLAN SEVEN

Encourage elders to give back.

One of the hardest things about caregiving is the temptation to do *too much* for our elders; we love them and love doing things that show how much we care. However, to live a dignified life of their own, **we must keep them in the driver's seat as long as possible.**

They may move slowly, so a task that takes us minutes to complete may take them an hour. Stacking and restacking the dishwasher, for example, could take the better part of a day. Rest assured that nothing dreadful will happen if a task takes twice as long to complete. Much as you adjust to the rhythms of young children, so must you readjust to the pace of your elders. The most important thing you can give them is your patience and tolerance.

There is little question that older people are happiest when they feel needed and respected. Finding them jobs to do within the family is important. Trading household tasks may suit their current capabilities and create a sense of equal partnership. Exchange the task of bill paying for plant sitting, or cooking for folding the laundry.

The best classroom in the world is at the feet of an older person. What is it that they have to teach? Perhaps lessons in knitting, cooking, Bible studies, card games, or a foreign language, to name just a few of the possibilities.

The following may help keep older family members engaged and involved:

babysitting	light housekeeping
brushing pets	office work
cooking	organizing
fund-raising	pet sitting/walking
gardening	researching
home repairs	running errands
house-sitting	sewing

Low-Cost and Free Resources

Pet adoption discounts may be available. Contact the local humane society. Conduct an Internet keyword search and include the city and state where your elder resides. Keywords include "canine partners," "animal shelter," "pet rescue," "pet cemetery," "pet stores," "humane society," "pet adoption," "assistance dog," "hearing dogs," "guide dogs," and "pet therapy."

For a wealth of information on **activities for seniors,** conduct an Internet search using the following keywords: "older workers," "senior travel," "volunteer," "senior," "retirement," and "assistive technology."

State bureaus of tourism, state historical societies, state parks, and state chamber of commerce offices supply **free information and maps for travelers.**

The local agency on aging has information on programs and support groups for **grandparents who are raising grandchildren.**

Colleges and **universities** have back-to-school programs for seniors. This often means free or low-cost tuition and special housing rates.

Community centers and **YMCAs** give people a sense of belonging and opportunities to make a difference to others. Comprehensive centers provide nutrition, recreation, and social and educational services, as well as fitness activities and Internet training. Contact the local agency on aging for the nearest location.

Computer software programs and Internet searches offer a multitude of **intergenerational family activities** and **reminiscing techniques.** Type the following keywords in the Internet search engine browser: "genealogy," "ancestry," "family tree," "scrapbook," "personal historian," "family history," and "family traditions." The local public library offers books on the subject of reminiscing and genealogy.

Sources for **volunteer organizations** include the local Yellow Pages under the "Social Services Organizations" listing. Additional listings can be found in the classified section of community newspapers, the public library, the agency on aging, and the local chamber of commerce. Search the Internet by typing "senior volunteer" in the search engine browser.

There are unique values, rituals, and traditions within cultures and populations. Special populations include African Americans, Latinos/Hispanics, Asian/Pacific Islanders, and Native Americans. **Help elders connect with people who understand their culture and speak their native language.** Internet search keywords include "Coalition of Limited English Speaking Elderly," "National Asian Pacific Center on Aging," "National Resource Center on Native American Aging," "National Caucus and Center on Black Aged," and "National Hispanic Council on Aging."

ORGANIZATIONS AND WEB RESOURCES

International Council on Active Aging
3307 Trutch Street
Vancouver, BC V6L-2T3
Canada
(604) 734-4466; toll-free:
    (866) 335-9777
Website: www.icaa.cc

National Council on Aging
1901 L Street, NW, 4th Floor
Washington, DC 20036
(202) 479-1200; TDD:
    (202) 479-6674
Website: www.ncoa.org

**National Library Service for the Blind and
    Physically Handicapped**
(To connect to a local library)
Toll-free: (888) 657-7323
Website: www.loc.gov/nls

Ontario Seniors' Secretariat
(Canadian quality-of-life resources)
Website: www.culture.gov.on.ca/seniors

Computer

SeniorNet
(Computer access and education for older
    adults)
Website: www.seniornet.org

Travel

Elderhostel
(Adventures in lifelong learning)
Website: www.elderhostel.org

Work and Volunteering

AARP
(Click on the "Money and Work" tab)
601 E Street, NW
Washington, DC 20049
Toll-free: (888) 687-2277
Website: www.aarp.org

Administration on Aging
(Select "Volunteer Opportunities" in the
    search box)
Website: www.aoa.gov

**Corporation for National and
    Community Service**
1201 New York Avenue, NW
Washington, DC 20525
(202) 606-5000; TDD: (202) 634-9256
Website: www.cns.gov
Website: www.seniorcorps.org

Elder Wisdom Circle
Website: www.elderwisdomcircle.org

OASIS
(Enriching the lives of mature adults)
Website: www.oasisnet.org

Retired Brains
(Helping older workers find jobs)
Website: www.retiredbrains.com

Senior Corps
1201 New York Avenue, NW
Washington, DC 20525
(202) 606-5000; TTY: (202) 606-3472
Website: www.seniorcorps.gov

Senior Service America
(Training and employment opportunities for
    older adults)
8403 Colesville Road
Silver Spring, MD 20910
(301) 578-8900
Website: www.seniorserviceamerica.org

Spiritual and Religious Quests

Beliefnet
Website: www.beliefnet.com

Pain Management and Later-Life Depression

American Association for Geriatric Psychiatry
7910 Woodmont Avenue, Suite
    1050
Bethesda, MD 20814-3004

(301) 654-7850; fax: (301)
    654-4137
Website: www.aagpogpa.org

American Chronic Pain Association
PO Box 850
Rocklin, CA 95677
Toll-free: (800) 533-3231
Website: www.theacpa.org

American Pain Society
Website: www.ampainsoc.org

National Pain Foundation
Website: www.nationalpainfoundation.org

Family

Family Search
(Tools to explore and document your family
    history)
Website: www.familysearch.org

Generations United
Website: www.gu.org

**National Archives and Records
    Administration**
8601 Adelphi Road
College Park, MD 20740-6001
Toll-free: (866) 272-6272
Website: www.archives.gov

Grandparents as Parents

AARP Foundation Grandparent Information Center
601 E Street, NW
Washington, DC 20049
Toll-free: (888) 687-2277
Website: www.aarp.org/families/grandparents

GrandsPlace
Website: www.grandsplace.org

National Center on Grandparents Raising Grandchildren
Georgia State University
140 Decatur Street
Atlanta, Georgia 30303
(404) 651-1049

Pets

Canine Companions for Independence
Toll-free: (866) 224-3647
Website: www.caninecompanions.org

QUALITY OF LIFE ACTION CHECKLIST

(This worksheet is also available online at www.elderindustry.com)

WHAT'S AGE FOR, ANYWAY?	To Do By	Completed
Be aware of roadblocks to quality of life		
chronic pain	_____	☐
depression	_____	☐
illness	_____	☐
alcohol abuse	_____	☐
medication and drug abuse	_____	☐
suicidal tendencies	_____	☐
Ask life-enriching questions	_____	☐
Tap into senior-friendly resources		
travel	_____	☐
learning centers	_____	☐
fitness centers	_____	☐
Suggest employment options and volunteer opportunities	_____	☐
Facilitate spiritual and religious needs	_____	☐
Plan for pets	_____	☐
Know the locations of the local		
community centers	_____	☐
adult education centers	_____	☐
religious congregations	_____	☐
support groups	_____	☐
FAMILY POWER		
Plan to capture special caregiving moments	_____	☐
Create opportunities for reminiscing	_____	☐
Research family history	_____	☐
Make good use of remembering techniques and devices	_____	☐

Keep family customs, traditions, and rituals alive _____ ❑

Learn more about your family roots

   draw a family tree _____ ❑

   conduct library research _____ ❑

   search family records _____ ❑

   conduct interviews _____ ❑

   inquire about possessions _____ ❑

   explore attics _____ ❑

   accompany your elders back to their hometowns _____ ❑

Plan on giving meaningful and memorable gifts _____ ❑

Foster the grandparent and grandchild connection _____ ❑

Create opportunities for elders to contribute back to the family _____ ❑

14

Death and Dying

Saying Good-bye

Something wonderful happens when loved ones begin the process of letting go. Not giving up on life or hope, and not resignation or despair—but separating themselves from people and objects that hold memories in preparation of a peaceful death.

The process of helping a person die well can begin early. When you notice Mom isn't keeping up the house like she used to or Dad suddenly quits driving, you'll hire housekeeping services and find transportation alternatives. Everything seems fine for a while. And if your loved ones need more help, you give more help—but then the laws of nature take over and there's a different kind of help that's needed now. You sit together and are present to them. This is how you will give the people you love a good death.

Robert Hellenga wrote in his book *The Sixteen Pleasures*, "Death was a lens that would reveal things as they really were: what was important would assume its true importance, what was unimportant would recede into the shadows."[1] Witnessing the death and dying process of someone you love is a profound event. You may feel adrift in the world; strange, anomalous, and sometimes just plain weird. A zombie-like numbness overcomes you. You may feel helpless, as you have no control over the dying process and can't solve this "problem."

Intellectually, you know that the caregiving experience ends with the death of the care receiver, and yet you have no way of preparing yourself emotionally when the time comes. For some, the death may feel like a blessing, especially if the elder suffered a great deal of physical pain. Others may find the finality of their elder's death particularly traumatic. Feelings of sadness, anger, emptiness, shock, confusion, and guilt are normal.

This section of *The Complete Eldercare Planner* offers insights into the dying process and attempts to demystify the stage of caregiving you may fear the most—the death of your elder. Learning how to comfort the dying and offer final farewells allows loved ones to die a dignified, peaceful death.

SAYING GOOD-BYE

- When you move beyond the fear of talking about death, and accept the realization that life is valuable *because* it is limited, the knowledge that your elders won't live forever may be just what is needed for you to live with more purpose and joy.
- While people say they want to go quickly, in their sleep, the fact is only 10 percent of us die suddenly. The more common process is a slow decline periodically associated with life-threatening crises.[2]
- Bearing witness to the aging of your elders and watching helplessly as they walk through death's door is a rite of passage in caregiving.
- Only 24.9 percent of Americans die at home, although more than 70 percent say that is their wish.[3]

The dying process of someone we love can be a turning point in our life when we make the effort to exchange heartfelt words and offer acts of forgiveness.

OBJECTIVES

*After completing **"Saying Good-bye,"** you will be able to:*

Become more present to the needs of the dying.

Mend fences and move relationships to a better place.

Create quality final moments.

PLAN ONE

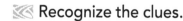 Recognize the clues.

There is no template for how a good death should happen. Death comes in its own way, and with no apparent timetable or predictability. The dying process is not one process, but many, and is unique to each individual. The dying process can take five years, five weeks, or five minutes. Emotionally, the dying become "an island unto themselves," and they begin the separation process in ways that are meaningful to *them*.

Helping loved ones die well is both an experience and a process. The rewards of giving in to the laws of nature and coming to terms with the fact that they will eventually leave us are priceless. Here are a few ways that we can become more present to our loved ones' impending death.

Letting Go

"I'll see you next month, God willing. I hope I'm still around to make it to your party." "I'd like you to have this bracelet to remember me by when I'm gone." Statements such as these are clues that our elders have begun to contemplate their own death. The thought of them leaving us is not something we like to think about. Their words may startle and jolt us, and in response we might say, "Nothing's going to happen to you. I'll see you next month," or "Let's not do this now. You can give me your bracelet later, okay?"

Acknowledging statements that reference the subject of death and dying and graciously accepting gifts and tokens of love validates what they are preparing to do—and that is to die in peace. While death may not be happening any time soon, what you've been given is a **window of opportunity** to acknowledge what is important to your elders.

Telling your elders you would miss them lets them know *now* how much they are loved. Saying thank you for the item you are about to receive and asking questions, such as where it came from and what special memories the object holds, brings joy to gift givers. Allow time *now* for them to tell their stories.

Attaining Goals

Although there's scant research explaining how **people can seemingly time their deaths,** families and health-care professionals have been aware of the phenomenon for centuries. Older people may speak of attaining an important goal such as celebrating a milestone anniversary and expressing a strong desire to attend the wedding of a grandchild.

Hospital chaplains talk of having prayed with people who asked God for a few more hours, enough time for a son, a daughter, or a spouse to make it to the hospital and say goodbye. While doctors can't explain the link, it's a common occurrence among the dying; having something special to look forward to seems to keep death at bay.

Withdrawing

Are your elders becoming less interested in what is happening around them? Have they greatly reduced their interactions with others? Are they planning a trip in spite of being ill? *(Some people physically vacate familiar surroundings in order to die. This was the situation with my own father.)* Are they extremely short-tempered and unapproachable? Do they sleep more? Eat less?

These and other clues may be signs of **quieting the mind, lessening heartfelt experiences, and reaching inward.** They may be aware that they are pulling away, or they may not—it doesn't much matter. This is a journey that they are going alone. Do not take their actions and words personally. Their withdrawal is not a rejection, nor does it mean that you are unloved or unimportant; it means your role as family caregiver is coming to an end.

Respecting Wishes

Most people do not fear death as much as they do the process of dying. If you haven't done so already, make time to **talk about last rites, funerals, and last wishes.** Review the next section of this chapter, "Managing Death's Details" for additional insights. Also be sure that legal and important documents, such as the power of attorney for health care, physician directives, and power of attorney for finances, are in place. Reviewing the "Legal Matters" chapter of *The Complete Eldercare Planner* will be most helpful.

You will want to honor their final requests, whether out of love or duty. If they are dying in a hospital setting and want to go home, you may want to make that happen. A dying person's wishes should always be respected.

PLAN TWO

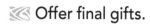 Offer final gifts.

The simple truth about the dying is this: They want their lives validated, and they don't want to die alone. Strive to fill those needs. What does a dying person really need? **The final gift you can give someone is to journey with them unafraid.** There are professionals who can be of great help to *you* at this time. Call upon the assistance of a clergyperson, a social worker, or a hospice nurse. They have extensive experience in the death and dying process and can lend guidance when it comes to *how* to interact with the dying. You will be the final judge on what's best for *you* as your elder nears death.

Validate the Death

During this time, you may wonder if you should be masking your grief around dying loved ones in order to keep their spirits up or to prevent letting your emotions show. Some hospice experts recommend that you honestly acknowledge to your loved one that you're sorry you're losing them. The belief is that sharing your grief is healthy for all concerned and tears can break through layers of isolation. Other experts recommend taking the lead from the person who is dying.

People who are dying may have difficulty talking about death, even if they would like to. If a person did not normally talk candidly about his or her feelings, the likelihood of opening up on a deathbed isn't great; but **the unmistakable message from a dying person is "Don't abandon me."** Let your loved one know that you will be with him or her to the end.

Spend Quality Time

When there is no cure, the best medicine is gifts of presence, comfort, and dignity. Spend time together doing simple things. Sit and look out the window. Talk about what's going on with work and current events. Every conversation with the dying is a privilege, bringing us closer to who *you* are and making you wiser in ways that will be revealed to you over time. Encourage happy reminiscences. It's okay to laugh. Allow for silence. **Your presence alone is valuable.**

Being together offers opportunities to exchange words of meaning and relevance. Words of thanks and love go a long way. You might take a moment to reassure them that whatever happens *you* will be all right. They may want to give you further instructions on what they want for you after they're gone. Being together gives them the chance to say good-bye *to you*.

Soften the Journey

When you know your elders are comfortable and content, you'll feel good. Though the dying are dying, they do enjoy moments of pleasure. And never are they more entitled to joy than now. They may want real butter, not margarine; they may want to go to the park; they may want to have this light off and that light on, a window open, another blanket. **By being allowed their choices, however small, they can count themselves among the living.**

A warm, supportive atmosphere conveys comfort and care: Soft lighting, soothing music, holding hands, and simply sitting bedside are gifts of love. If your elder is in a comatose state, speak as though he or she can hear you (in many cases, he or she can). When you speak to others, speak as though your loved one is present in the room; do not refer to him or her as if he or she were already dead. If there is a need to discuss funeral plans, leave the room.

A dying person has the same physical needs as any other person—to be kept clean, comfortable, and free from pain. When you ask your dying loved ones if there is anything you can do to make them more comfortable, you are giving them the attention they deserve as human beings. When they die, they will know that somebody cared.

Choose Higher Ground

If your relationship with your elder has been turbulent and you now **want to mend fences about any past grievances,** seek the assistance of hospice professionals and social workers who have completed a training program offered by the American Hospice Foundation called "Caregiving at Life's End." It may help you to resolve issues and move the relationship with your elder to a better place. Experts agree that putting closure on strained relationships helps make the bereavement process less complicated.

Speak of Spiritual Quests

The spiritual aspect for the dying may be important, but they may not ask for spiritual guidance outright. Ask loved ones what they want. Do they want to pray? Do they seek spiritual or religious direction?

There are also **spiritual quests in the death and dying process for those who do not have a conventional religious belief.** The need to cope with death and mortality and the pain of loss and separation is universal, yet we must lay aside the assumption that the only real comfort for the dying is through a religious belief system. Again, the best approach is to ask loved ones what they want.

Permission to Let Go

When the dying cling to life and try to stay alive beyond what seems medically possible, a loved one can assist them by offering the ultimate, unselfish parting gift: words that give them permission to let go. Until then, the dying may attempt to sustain life until they are assured that those who are left behind will be in good hands.

We may be able to release them of their concerns by saying, *"Don't worry about Sally, we promise to watch over her,"* or, *"I will be fine, Mom, and well taken care of,"* and *"Dad, if you don't want to be here anymore, you can go now. It's okay."*

PLAN THREE

Ease the way at life's end.

Far too often, people don't discuss death with their doctor or their family, and leave it to others to make gut-wrenching decisions about their end of life. In the hospital setting, **professional counselors** will provide advice and moral support for family members of terminally ill patients. If your elder has already empowered you legally to be the decision maker regarding medical care in the final stages, be sure that his or her wishes have been communicated to the medical staff.

For patients who are receiving institutionalized medical care, the **Federal Patient Self-Determination Act** requires that all hospitals, skilled nursing and assisted-living facilities, home health agencies, providers of home health care (and for Medicaid purposes, providers of personal-care services), and hospices give patients information regarding their right to accept or decline any kind of medical treatment, including life support. A patient can also elect to wear an **armband** that directs staff not to resuscitate if he or she so wishes.

Pain Management

Pain management is a family affair because people in great pain may not necessarily speak up for themselves, and **family members are encouraged to become advocates for loved ones who may be suffering in silence.**

First, ask your loved one if he or she is in pain. If the answer is yes, ask the doctor what else can be done to alleviate the pain. If the doctor is unwilling to address the issue of pain to your satisfaction, ask a hospice nurse to speak with the doctor on your elder's behalf. Everyone is entitled to proper pain control, so continue to ask for alternatives.

The Wonders of Hospice

Hospice is a philosophy of care that is based on the belief that every person with a life-limiting illness, no matter what age, is entitled to be as free of pain and symptoms as possible.

Concern for the entire family is what makes this kind of care different from traditional health care.

Care is provided by an interdisciplinary team that includes physicians, nurses, home health hospice aides, social workers, chaplains, therapists, dietary counselors, and trained volunteers. The decision to choose hospice, by law, is the patient's. Hospice services are available when specific criteria are met.

- The patient's doctor and the hospice medical director agree that the patient has a life expectancy of six months or less.
- The patient and family agree with the hospice philosophy.
- The patient and family are seeking supportive services rather than curative medical treatment.

The emotional support the family receives through hospice is invaluable. In spite of doing everything possible, when you arrive at this stage in the caregiving process, you may feel as though you've failed. Hospice volunteers and chaplains understand the emotional landscape of death and dying. Chaplains are ecumenical, and experienced with religious beliefs and spiritual quests of all kinds when it comes to terminal illness.

Hospice care is available at home, in the hospital setting, in nursing homes, in hospice centers, and in assisted-living residential communities. Private insurance companies and Medicare and Medicaid may cover the costs of hospice services.

The Dying Person's Bill of Rights*

I have the right to be treated as a living human being until I die.

I have the right to maintain a sense of hopefulness, however changing its focus may be.

I have the right to be cared for by those who can maintain a sense of hopefulness, however changing this might be.

I have the right to express my feelings and emotions about my approaching death, in my own way.

I have the right to participate in medical decisions.

I have the right to expect continuing medical and nursing attention, even when "cure" goals must be changed to "comfort" goals.

I have the right to not die alone.

I have the right to be free from pain.

I have the right to have my questions answered honestly.

I have the right not to be deceived.

I have the right to have help from and for my family in accepting my death.

---

* "The Dying Person's Bill of Rights" was created at a workshop titled "Terminally Ill Patient and the Helping Person" in Lansing, Michigan. The workshop was sponsored by the Southwest Michigan Inservice Education Council and conducted by Amelia J. Barbus, associate professor of nursing at Wayne State University.

I have the right to die in peace and dignity.

I have the right to retain my individuality and not be judged for my decisions, which may be contrary to the beliefs of others.

I have the right to discuss and enlarge my religious and/or spiritual experiences, regardless of what they may mean to others.

I have the right to expect that my body will be respected after death.

I have the right to be cared for by caring, sensitive, knowledgeable people who will attempt to understand my needs and who will be able to gain some satisfaction in helping me face my death.

Managing Death's Details

Preplanning a funeral and/or memorial service for oneself makes sense, and people feel a huge sense of relief once they have made their decisions. In most cases, however, grieving family members are left to make arrangements just prior to or immediately following the death of a loved one, when heads are unclear and hearts are overburdened.

Typically, there are several decision makers in the family involved in the planning of a funeral, and coming to a consensus is an experience unto itself: Someone wants to spend a lot of money; someone wants to spend as little money as possible; someone tries to second-guess what the person who has died would have wanted.

Knowing up front what is entailed in managing death's details will, it is hoped, inspire a conversation with your elders about making funeral arrangements ahead of time. A funeral and a memorial service is a celebration of the life of a person, and giving your elders every opportunity to be involved in their own planning is a gift they can give loved ones now. Before bringing up the subject, you may want to review the talking tips offered in the "Communicaring" chapter of *The Complete Eldercare Planner*, starting on page 86. To the extent that you're able to make any headway at all, and if you're one of the lucky few whose elders have already completed their own planning, consider yourself ahead of the game.

This section of *The Planner* discusses the business side of the consequences of a death. From planning a funeral or a memorial service to writing an obituary, from dividing up the estate to seeking bereavement support, the action plans provide a comprehensive list of suggestions and may provide some relief and peace during these emotionally trying times.

PLAN ONE

Make arrangements ahead of time.

To help relieve families of making decisions upon a person's death, an increasing number of people are planning their own funerals and making arrangements for memorial services as an extension of their will and estate planning. If the opportunity exists to plan ahead for services, put your elder's preferences in writing. Ask an attorney to review all agreements if

---

MANAGING DEATH'S DETAILS

- People are updating traditions when it comes to funerals and memorial services, making them less formal and more personalized.
- Former caregivers of spouses with Alzheimer's or other forms of dementia can still show levels of depression and loneliness years after caregiving ends.[4]

Preplanning a funeral and a memorial service may reduce costs considerably.

OBJECTIVES

After completing "Managing Death's Details," you will be able to:

Plan a funeral and a memorial service.

Locate missing documents.

Settle the deceased's financial affairs.

Identify sources of bereavement support.

---

signatures are required. Prepayment plans should be guaranteed, provide for inflation, and trigger little or no penalty for cancellation.

Store death-related documents in a handy place and make a record of the location of the paperwork listed throughout **"The Document Locator"** chapter of *The Complete Eldercare Planner* on page 327. Avoid storing paperwork in a safe-deposit box in the event that funeral services have to be arranged on a weekend or holiday. Distribute copies of any death-related documents to family members.

The decision to preplan does not necessarily include paying in advance. Prices can go up and down, businesses may close, ownership may change, and the deceased may have moved to a different city. Some funeral directors will simply keep a person's wishes on file. Encourage your elders to review their funeral plans yearly and revise if desired.

PLAN TWO

Gather important documents.

You will need to supply proof of the following vital statistics in order to make funeral arrangements and also to settle financial affairs later on:

- full legal name and maiden name
- current residence

- former place of residence
- date of birth
- birthplace
- citizenship
- Social Security number
- military records
- marital status
- spouse's name (maiden name)
- legal heirs
- father's name
- father's birthplace
- mother's maiden name
- mother's birthplace
- marriage certificate
- divorce certificate
- employment record

PLAN THREE

Decide on a final resting place.

Planning for death-related services requires a decision as to where the deceased's remains will be buried, entombed, or scattered. There are a number of disposition options.

- **Burial.** The deceased is placed in a casket and set in a grave. Burial occurs after a ceremony or service, or without any service. Burial at sea also is an option.
- **Entombment.** The deceased is placed in a casket and laid to rest aboveground in a tomb, mausoleum, or crypt.
- **Cremation.** The deceased is taken to a crematorium, where a heating process reduces the remains to ashes and bone particles. The cremated remains are placed in a container that can be buried or stored in a vault, or retained in a decorative memorial urn, or the ashes may be scattered in a location that would be meaningful to the deceased and/or loved ones.
- **Whole body donation.** The deceased may have made arrangements ahead of time to donate his or her body to a medical school for research. Donations can occur after a service. The cremation option remains available after the school has completed its use of the body.
- **Simple disposition.** The deceased is taken directly to a cemetery or crematory. A memorial service may take place afterward.

PLAN FOUR

Ask the experts.

While people are not legally required to use a funeral home to plan and conduct a funeral, funeral directors can serve as a valuable consultant during these difficult times. Ask professionals to assist with the following details:

- funeral services
- cemetery services
- disposition of the remains
- memorial services
- religious services
- transportation and shipping needs
- stationery needs
- gifts in memory of the deceased
- legal paperwork, such as death certificates and burial permits
- organ donations
- writing services, such as eulogies, death notices, and obituaries
- compliance with local, state, and federal regulations

PLAN FIVE

Celebrate the life of the deceased.

When it comes to celebrating the life of a loved one, just about anything goes. Customized services are simply a matter of preference and budget. You may even consider consulting an event-planning professional. The idea is to provide a loving and positive remembrance of the deceased. Here are a few ideas to keep in mind in the planning process:

- services from traditional to highly customized events
- settings from funeral homes and marinas to baseball stadiums
- symbolic gestures and parting gifts
- memory bulletin boards, including photographs and memorabilia
- videos of the deceased
- religious and cultural considerations
- military honors
- food and refreshments
- speakers and musicians
- resting-place services

- environmentally friendly burials, including biodegradable caskets and urns and other "green" products
- cremation-scattering services
- online services (videos, real-time live Internet viewing of the visitation at the funeral home, Internet photo albums, online death notices and guest books), which allow mourners at a distance to participate in the grieving ceremony when they cannot attend in person
- death anniversary events

PLAN SIX

Don't make an emotional loss a financial loss.

As callous as this may sound, *"How much is this going to cost?"* is a legitimate question to ask. People who are used to haggling with car dealers over the price of a car feel uncomfortable comparing prices or negotiating the cost of a funeral and memorial service. Compounding this discomfort is the fact that some people "overspend" because they feel that the event is a reflection of their feelings for the deceased. Services can cost thousands of dollars; grief and guilt can add thousands more.

Be aware of the following federal rules while keeping these savvy buying tips in mind.

- When working with a funeral director, get a **written itemized list** of charges up front *(it's the law)*. Be sure the list includes food service, and the use of common areas like restrooms and parking lots.
- Many funeral providers offer "packages" of commonly selected goods and services. You have the **right to buy individual goods and services** and can reject items offered in a package.
- **Shop around** for funeral homes and related merchandise. Prices vary. You are not locked in to purchasing merchandise from the funeral home.
- Funeral homes are **not allowed to charge a handling fee** for products purchased elsewhere.
- People who wish to be cremated are not required to buy a casket.
- A funeral provider that offers cremations must **make a range of containers for the remains available and at different price points**.
- If the funeral director tells you, "The state requires . . . ," **request written proof of the law**.

Ways to pay for the services include:
prepayment plans
Social Security benefits
veterans benefits

life insurance policies

burial trusts

savings accounts

proceeds from the sale of the residential real estate

People who die while traveling may have purchased trip insurance. Airlines, cruise lines, and travel outfitters offer insurance policies that may cover the cost of transporting the deceased's body back home, emergency travel expenses of family members, and medical care the traveler may have received on the trip. *When family members make trip plans in the future, ask them to purchase trip insurance for this purpose.*

PLAN SEVEN

Notify others of the death.

Family, longtime friends, neighbors, coworkers, and local merchants with whom the deceased had frequent contact will want to be informed of the death. You may find the task of figuring out who to notify a little easier by reviewing the contacts listed in your elder's personal address book and computer e-mail address book.

The death notification process also may include submitting a death notice to local and national newspapers, alumni and membership organizations, and former employers. Include a photo. A death notice typically offers the following information:

age	funeral or memorial services
cause of death	maiden name
deceased's full name	nickname
donation requests	survivors

An obituary is another way to inform people of a death. Be as creative as you like. Ask friends and coworkers of the deceased to supplement the obituary with interesting biographical details. Submit a photo and include information such as:

amusing anecdotes	hobbies and interests
awards	military honors
club and union memberships	offices held
degrees earned	quotations
educational background	religious affiliations
employment	social and civic accomplishments
family history	special achievements

PLAN EIGHT

⧛ Gather important and legal paperwork.

Filing claims, closing accounts, transferring titles, paying final bills, submitting tax reports, and resolving debts are some of the many responsibilities associated with settling the affairs of the deceased. For starters, you'll need ***certified* copies of the death certificate and proof that you are the beneficiary to file insurance and other financial claims.** Obtain at least a dozen certified copies of the death certificate because you will most likely be asked for proof of death from each entity you contact. The doctor, the hospital, the funeral consultant, or the nursing-home director can provide copies of the death certificate for you.

When people die, they leave behind documentation of their personal and financial history. Putting all the pieces of the puzzle together in order to "settle up" is no easy task; the process can take years to complete. There are numerous and complex legal requirements and pitfalls involved in the settling of someone's final affairs, and the laws governing death-related proceedings vary from state to state. Seek legal advice at your earliest opportunity.

Sift through *every* box, drawer, file cabinet, and nook and cranny in your elder's house. You are on the hunt for any and all papers that refer to financial transactions and statements, as well as personal memos and instructions. You don't want any surprises later on. In addition to using the following list as a prompter to locate important and legal documents, also review whatever notations you had already made in "The Documents Locator," starting on page 327 of *The Complete Eldercare Planner*.

The paperwork you are searching for may include:

- will
- trusts
- letters of instruction
- life insurance policies
- Social Security benefits and death benefits
- certified death certificates
- Social Security number
- citizenship papers
- birth certificate
- adoption papers
- company pension records
- bank records
- bank power of attorney
- power of attorney
- safe-deposit-box records
- marriage license
- divorce decree

- military records
- property deeds and titles
- mortgage and loan documents
- credit-card statements and applications
- personal and business contracts and agreements
- income tax returns and backup records
- vehicle titles
- stocks and bonds certificates
- paid invoices
- receipts for valuables and collectibles
- proof of debts paid
- proof of money owed to the deceased

PLAN NINE

⫸ Don't leave cash on the table.

Explore whatever **cash on hand** your elder may have left behind. There may be cash sitting in checking and savings accounts and security deposit boxes. If he or she did not authorize anyone to have entry privileges to the safe-deposit box, the bank, by law, may not allow access to the box. If that is the case, ask the bank what they require from you to gain access.

Also look for cash in wallets, purses, a safe, and "hiding places" in the house. Review insurance policies to file claims. Locate receipts for new and unused items and return them to the store for a refund.

Funds for distribution can also come from **less-obvious sources**. Travel clubs, airline mileage awards, and credit-card companies, among others, may offer entitlements upon death of members. Be on the lookout for membership handbooks and other documentation that spell out death benefits. Read the fine print.

Ask about survivors benefits from the following sources, where applicable:

Social Security office
life insurance policies
annuities
retirement accounts
tax refunds
veterans benefits
railroad retirement benefits
teachers retirement benefits
civil service benefits
union benefits
company pensions

PLAN TEN

⚡ **Follow the rules.**

The transfer of property upon death will happen in a variety of ways, including the deceased's last will and testament, joint ownership, beneficiary trust designations, and life insurance policies.

Property owned solely by the deceased undergoes a **probate** process that identifies and pays heirs and creditors, and determines taxes. This legal process will take a minimum of six months, and can easily extend much longer. If elders leave a will, it will have appointed an executor to carry out their instructions and property transfers. If they die without a will (the legal term is *intestate*), family members designate an individual to act as the administrator of the estate, or the court will appoint one.

Before banks and other financial institutions will legally permit withdrawals or transfers of assets of the deceased, **letters of office** issued by the probate court or a legal affidavit must be obtained.

After the process of securing funds is completed, the deceased's final bills will have to be paid. But there something important you should remember: ***Family members are under no obligation to pay the bills of the deceased out of their own pocket unless the bills are also in their name.*** In other words, you cannot inherit debt. Maintain detailed notes and files on *all* financial transactions and decisions. You may be questioned later on, and you will need concise records to back you up.

PLAN ELEVEN

⚡ **Locate missing links.**

In a perfect world, your elders would have maintained a neatly organized file of important information and paperwork and left explicit instructions on where to find the documents in the event of their death. Unfortunately, this is rarely the case. You may search for months for papers and clues as to what was happening in their lives, and you may not find everything in spite of your efforts.

Playing detective comes with the territory of settling someone else's affairs. The good news is this: The process of locating missing information is easier than you think and will cost practically nothing (except your time and energy, of course).

Here are some suggestions on how to find important information and documents.

- Review "The Documents Locator" chapter of *The Complete Eldercare Planner*, which starts on page 327. The papers listed in this chapter will serve as a guideline for important documents to have on hand.
- If you want to learn about important people in your elder's life, look to his or her **personal address book** and computer e-mail address book for clues.

- **Checkbooks** and **canceled checks** will reveal a history of important relationships and also tell you of payment patterns, including whom your elder gave money to and who gave money to him or her.
- Look for **paid invoices** to reveal where your elder spent his or her money.
- **Credit-card agreements** may turn up additional insurance coverage.
- Conduct a **thorough search**—at home and at work. Look in storage areas, drawers, cabinets, closets, attics, the refrigerator, and under the mattress. Move furniture away from the wall, lift rugs and carpets, and check the floor and the ceiling for lose tiles. Open safes.
- Look for **payments of storage rentals and safe-deposit-box rentals** in checkbooks, paid bills, credit-card statements, and bank statements.
- **Copies of filed tax returns** will reveal a history of financial and employment status and may lead to the discovery of bank/investment accounts.
- Locate **Social Security** documents for a work and income history.
- **Employers** will provide documentation regarding company pensions, life insurance policies, retirement savings, and union memberships.
- If you believe the deceased had a will and you have searched unsuccessfully among his or her personal effects, check the local **probate court** to see if a will has been filed.
- Advertise in the **classified section** of the local newspaper and local bar association publication to inquire about the existence of a will. If many months pass and no will is found, it is safe to assume that one does not exist.
- Obtain copies of marriage licenses and birth and death certificates at the **office of the county clerk** where the license was issued. Divorce decrees or any legal guardianship documents will be found at the **county courthouse.**
- To gather veteran information, including obtaining a certificate of honorable discharge, contact the local **Veterans Affairs** office.
- Search the state's **unclaimed property division,** located within the department of revenue or treasury.
- If designer clothes, expensive handbags, and fur coats are missing from your elder's inventory, check the local **consignment shop** to see if your elder placed them up for sale. **Pawnshops** may also be housing your elder's valuables.

PLAN TWELVE

Tie up loose ends.

Working through the final details of a loved one's death includes clearing the house of the deceased's belongings and coming to a consensus with other family members on what to keep, what to give away, what to sell, what to auction off, and what to donate.

Take as much time as needed to make decisions and complete the following tasks.

- Notify the post office of the death and provide a forward mailing address.
- Cancel credit cards.
- Cancel newspaper and magazine subscriptions.
- Cancel club and union memberships.
- Cancel insurance when properties are sold or transferred.
- Cancel utility services, telephone, and cable television.
- Review bank statements for the existence of any automatic deductions and cancel payments.
- If your elder rented an apartment or home, ask the landlord for the return of the security deposit. Depending on the laws and statutes of the particular jurisdiction, landlords may be required to return the security deposit within a certain number of days, with interest. This usually applies only to multiunit apartment buildings.
- File a final tax return.
- Transfer vehicle titles.
- Keep property and vehicles locked and secure to protect against accidents and claims against the estate until such property is sold.
- Send acknowledgment cards to those who sent flowers and donations. You are not obligated to send cards to everyone who sent sympathy cards or attended funeral services unless you want to.

PLAN THIRTEEN

 Grieve and heal.

Carrying out the responsibilities of funeral planning and settling affairs will keep you busy and perhaps temporarily distracted from dealing with the loss of your loved one. Once things have settled down, however, you will come to grips with the loss one way or another; no two people will respond the same way.

The following are just *some* of the feelings and manifestations people experience during the grieving stages.

- tears and expressions of deep feelings
- diminished appetite or loss of weight
- periods of helplessness and despair
- vivid dreams of the recently deceased
- guilt and regret
- anger directed at the person who died, God, the family doctor, and others

Watch for excessive behavior patterns, such as:

- poor self-care, not exercising or not eating right
- isolating oneself from contact with others
- speaking of the dead in the present tense in ways that are not healthy
- severe depression, nonstop crying, thoughts of suicide
- abuse of alcohol or drugs

Each of us deals with loss differently. Sometimes friends and family are an important source of strength during times of grief. Make use of other bereavement support resources, as well, including:

- religious groups
- spiritual director
- hospice nurse
- family therapist
- bereavement support group
- individual bereavement counseling

PLAN FOURTEEN

Carry on after a loved one dies.

You did your best to be helpful and loving when your elders needed you. You may have struggled through difficult end-of-life care decisions, resulting in an even deeper commitment to your elder. But now all that has changed. The one you cared for has died, and your caregiving role has ended.

Repair Damaged Relationships and Create New Ones

Sadly, some **families are torn apart** in the eldercare process, and the family member who did the bulk of the care may find that once-close relationships have suffered or, worse yet, disappeared.

Caregiving sometimes carries with it the by-product of **losing your friends**. Your life was hectic due to the demands of eldercare, and the discomfort friends felt with the situation may have resulted in them avoiding you and the situation altogether. This experience is not unique. It can be hard to face up to the fact that the people you thought were your real friends did not stand by you in your time of need.

Discuss your feelings of alienation with family and friends. Seek the services of a therapist to help you work through the situation. Get closer to family and friends who never left your side and thank them for their support.

Create a New Purpose in Life

Caregiving may have been your full-time job. In the end, you may question, *"Who am I now? Do I remember how to have a life of my own?"* You will slowly come to the realization that life as you once knew it will never be the same. You may feel lost and even depressed now that you have extra time on your hands.

Former caregivers may need **psychological help** and **support** even though their caregiving duties are over. Caregiving, especially for a spouse with dementia, is very difficult, and the effects can linger for years. To get back on track, you may want to join a support group and seek the advice of a therapist.

Get Affairs in Order

In the midst of caregiving tasks, you may have wondered, "Who will take care of *me* when the time comes?" Take note of the lessons you learned—financially and otherwise—as a result of family caregiving and make plans today to provide for your own long-term care and quality of life as you age. *Who would you want to make health-care decisions for you if you could not make them for yourself? What legal documents should be prepared now? Are there steps you can take now to make things easier and smoother for your caregivers and advocates-to-be?*

Make a Difference in the Lives of Other Caregivers

People everywhere are talking about their own personal eldercare experiences—at work, at social gatherings, on the Internet—and you can't help but chime in the moment others describe themselves as caregivers. You've been there. You know what they're going through. Do you have tips to share with those who are or will be caring for their elders?

Capture Memories

While spending time with your elder is still fresh in your mind, look to the "Family Power" section of chapter 13, "Quality of Life," starting on page 272, for ideas on the many wonderful and creative ways to keep his or her memory alive.

Low-Cost and Free Resources

People who wish to make an **anatomical gift** or **organ donation** must make such arrangements in advance. Contact organ banks, a hospital, a medical school, the department of motor vehicles, and the local agency on aging for further information.

All **veterans** are entitled to a free burial in a national cemetery and a grave marker. This eligibility also extends to some civilians who have provided military-related service and some Public Health Service personnel. Spouses and dependent children also are entitled to a lot and marker when buried in a national cemetery. Contact the regional Veterans Affairs office for details.

To lower funeral expenses, you can **buy a casket or urn directly from the manufacturer**. Look in the Yellow Pages and on the Internet under "casket companies."

Funerals and Memorial Services

**Cremation Association of
    North America**
401 N. Michigan Avenue
Chicago, IL 60611
(312) 245-1077
Website: www.cremationassociation.org

Federal Trade Commission
(Regulates the funeral industry; keyword:
    "funerals")
Website: www.ftc.gov

Funeral Consumers Alliance
(To file a complaint)
33 Patchen Road
South Burlington, VT 05403
Toll-free: (800) 765-0107
Website: www.funerals.org

**International Cemetery Creation and
    Funeral Association**
107 Carpenter Drive, Suite 100
Sterling, VA 20164
(703) 391-8400; Toll-free: (800) 645-7700
Website: www.icfa.org

End of Life and Grief Support

Aging with Dignity
820 E. Park Avenue, Suite D100
Tallahassee, FL 32301-2600
Toll-free: (888) 594-7437
Website: www.agingwithdignity.org

Americans for Better Care of the Dying
1700 Diagonal Road, Suite 635
Alexandria, VA 22314
(703) 647-8505
Website: www.abcd-caring.org

Caring Connections
Website: www.caringinfo.org

Compassion and Choices
Toll-free counselor assistance: (800) 247-7421
Website: www.compassionandchoices.org

Forgiveness Web
Website: www.forgivenessweb.com

Get Palliative Care
Website: www.getpalliativecare.org

Growth House
(End of life resources)
Website: www.growthhouse.org

Hospice Foundation of America
12000 Biscayne Boulevard, Suite 505
Miami Beach, FL 33181
(305) 981-2522; toll-free: (800) 854-3402
Website: www.hospicefoundation.org

Hospice Net
Website: www.hospicenet.org

Hospice Patients Alliance
Website: www.hospicepatients.org

**National Association for Home
   Care & Hospice**
228 7th Street, SE
Washington, DC 20003
(202) 547-7424; fax: (202) 547-3540
Website: www.nahc.org

National Association of Social Workers
750 First Street, NE, Suite 700
Washington, DC 20002-4241
(202) 408-8600
Website: www.socialworkers.org

**National Hospice and Palliative Care
   Organization**
1700 Diagonal Road, Suite 625
Alexandria, VA 22314
(703) 837-1500
Website: www.nhpco.org

ShareTheCare
(How to organize a group to care for someone
   who is seriously ill)
Website: www.sharethecare.org

Social Workers
Website: www.helpstartshere.org

To Locate Missing Documents

**National Association of Unclaimed Property
   Administrators**
(Keeps a state database of unclaimed
   property)
Website: www.unclaimed.org

DEATH AND DYING ACTION CHECKLIST

(This worksheet is also available online at www.elderindustry.com)

SAYING GOOD-BYE	To Do By	Completed
Recognize the clues of letting go	_____	❏
Be aware of your elder's goal to reach milestones		
family events	_____	❏
important projects	_____	❏
personal goals	_____	❏
Spend quality time	_____	❏
Seek professional counseling	_____	❏
Discuss end-of-life directives		
nutritional and respiratory life support decisions	_____	❏
funeral arrangements	_____	❏
memorial services arrangements	_____	❏
power of attorney for health care	_____	❏
physician directives	_____	❏
review "Managing Death's Details" section	_____	❏
review "Legal Matters" chapter	_____	❏
Get legal papers in order	_____	❏
Fulfill last wishes	_____	❏
Manage pain issues	_____	❏
Consider hospice services	_____	❏
Review "The Dying Person's Bill of Rights"	_____	❏

MANAGING DEATH'S DETAILS

**Seek professional advice for
funeral planning** _____ ❑

**Review "Communicaring" chapter
before talking about funerals** _____ ❑

**Incorporate plans as part of letter
of instruction in your elder's will** _____ ❑

**Shop around for funeral merchandise
and services** _____ ❑

Tap into sources to pay for funeral

Social Security _____ ❑
Veterans Affairs _____ ❑
prepayment plans _____ ❑
life insurance policies _____ ❑
burial trusts _____ ❑
savings accounts _____ ❑
travel insurance _____ ❑
house sale _____ ❑

Notify others of the death

telephone calls _____ ❑
death notice _____ ❑
obituary _____ ❑

**Gather legal and important
documents** _____ ❑

Retain attorney _____ ❑

Obtain copies of death certificates _____ ❑

**Review "The Documents Locator"
chapter** _____ ❑

Explore sources of leftover cash _____ ❑

Inquire about survivors benefits _____ ❑

Review travel insurance policies _____ ❑

Understand transfer of property
regulations _____ ❏

Begin probate process _____ ❏

Obtain letters of office _____ ❏

Settle financial affairs _____ ❏

Search for missing information and
documents _____ ❏

Tie up loose ends

distribution of items _____ ❏
lock up property _____ ❏
keep record of all transitions _____ ❏

Grieve and heal

watch for excessive behavior patterns _____ ❏
consider bereavement support _____ ❏

Carry on after a loved one dies

repair damaged relationships _____ ❏
create new relationships _____ ❏
seek a new purpose in life _____ ❏
get affairs in order _____ ❏
make a difference in the lives of other
caregivers _____ ❏
capture your elder's memories _____ ❏

15

The Documents Locator

Taming the Task of Gathering Information

Quick: *What's Dad's Social Security number? Where does Mom keep the title documents to the house? Do they have a will? Has power of attorney been established? Does Aunt Betty have long-term care insurance? What are the passwords for retrieving voice messages and e-mail?* Discovering what documents already exist, knowing where important information is stored, and then producing information on demand is an inevitable responsibility in the caregiving process.

"The Documents Locator" is an invaluable planning tool, and making the effort now to complete the information in this section of the book will help you to avoid the trauma, expense, and inconvenience of having to scramble for important papers under stressful emergency conditions, especially in unfortunate cases when our elders may be incapacitated and unable to advise us of any answers.

The list of important documents in this section of *The Complete Eldercare Planner* is extensive. *The task of gathering this information will take longer than you think.* An easy way to get started is to photocopy the contents of your elder's wallet. In a matter of minutes, you'll have copies of his or her driver's license, proof of health insurance, Social Security number, credit cards, membership cards, and more.

If you are the gatekeeper of important original documents, store them in a safe location that is accessible 24/7. You will also find "The Documents Locator" online at www .elderindustry.com. Complete the information in the spaces offered and download onto a flash drive or CD-ROM for easy access. As you complete sections of this chapter, make copies and distribute to key family members, including your elders, so they will also know how to find the documents in a pinch. Update information as needed.

PIN NUMBERS / ACCESS CODES

*Bank by phone*_____

*Bank online*_____

*Debit cards*_____

*Cash station*_____

*Telephone voice mail*_____

*Cell phone*_____

*Personal digital assistant (PDA)*_____

*Property*_____

COMPUTER & INTERNET USAGE

*Computer access password*_____

*Wireless security code*_____

*E-mail address*_____

*E-mail access code*_____

*Important websites & passwords*_____

*Location of CD-ROMs & flash drive backup files*_____

PERSONAL BANK ACCOUNTS

*Account name and number*_____

*Name(s) on account*_____

*Bank*_____

*Telephone*_____

*Type of account*_____

*Location of account documents*_____

*Second signature*_____

*Power of attorney*_____

AUTOMATIC BILL PAYING

*Name of store and service*_____

*Contact name*_____

*Telephone*_____

*Date payment deducted*_____

*Bank and account number*_____

*Name of store/service*_____

*Contact name*_____

*Telephone*_____

*Date payment deducted*_____

*Bank and account number*_____

ELECTRONIC FUNDS TRANSFER ACCOUNT (ETA)

*Account name and number*_____

*Name(s) on account*_____

*Bank*_____

*Telephone*_____

PERSONAL LOAN

*Name(s) on loan*_____

*Loan number*_____

*Bank*_____

*Telephone*_____

*Type of loan*_____

*Location of loan papers*_____

OUTSTANDING LIEN AGAINST PROPERTY

*Name(s) on loan*_____

*Loan number*_____

*Bank*_____

*Telephone*_____

*Location of loan papers*_____

PAID LIENS AGAINST PROPERTY

*Name(s) on loan*_____

*Loan number*_____

*Bank*_____

*Telephone*_____

*Location of proof of payment papers*_____

INSTALLMENT LOAN

*Name(s) on loan*_____

*Loan number*_____

*Bank*_____

*Telephone*_____

*Location of loan papers*_____

BUSINESS BANK ACCOUNT

Bank_____

Telephone_____

Location of account documents_____

Business name on account_____

Account number_____

Type of account_____

Second signature_____

Power of attorney_____

BUSINESS LOAN

Name(s) on loan_____

Loan number_____

Type of loan_____

Bank_____

Telephone_____

Location of loan papers_____

CREDIT UNION

Union name_____

Telephone_____

Name on account_____

Type of account_____

Account number_____

Location of documents_____

FOREIGN BANK ACCOUNT

Name(s) on account_____

Account number_____

Type of account_____

Bank_____

Telephone_____

Location of account papers_____

COMPANY PENSION

Name on pension_____

Reference number_____

*Dates of employment*_____

*Company name*_____

*Telephone*_____

*Location of pension papers*_____

RETIREMENT ACCOUNT

*Name on account*_____

*Account reference number*_____

*Type of account*_____

*Bank*_____

*Telephone*_____

*Location of account documents*_____

SAVINGS CERTIFICATE

*Depositor*_____

*Certificate number*_____

*Bank*_____

*Telephone*_____

*Location of certificate*_____

SAVINGS BOND

*Bond held by*_____

*Type of bond*_____

*Bond series number*_____

*Location of bond*_____

STOCK CERTIFICATE

*Stockholder(s)*_____

*Stock name*_____

*Stock number*_____

*Broker*_____

*Telephone*_____

*Location of stock documents*_____

SAFE-DEPOSIT BOX

*Box holder*_____

*Has access to box*_____

*Telephone number*_____

*Box number*_____

*Bank*_____

*Telephone*_____

*Key location*_____

CASH-ON-HAND

*Location*_____

HOME SAFE

*Has access to safe*_____

*Telephone*_____

*Location of combination or key*_____

BUSINESS SAFE

People with access to safe _____

*Telephone*_____

*Location of safe*_____

Location of combination or key _____

WILL

*Will of*_____

*Attorney*_____

*Telephone*_____

*Location of original will papers*_____

*People with copies of will papers*_____

*Telephone*_____

TRUST

*Established by*_____

*Trust for*_____

*Attorney*_____

*Telephone*_____

*Location of original trust papers*_____

*People with copies of trust papers*_____

LIVING WILL

Will of _____

*Attorney*_____

*Telephone*_____

*Location of original living will*_____

*People with copies of living will*_____

*Telephone*_____

POWER OF ATTORNEY FOR PROPERTY

*Given to*_____

*Telephone*_____

*Attorney*_____

*Telephone*_____

*Location of original document*_____

*People with copies of papers*_____

POWER OF ATTORNEY FOR HEALTH CARE

*Location of original document*_____

*People with copies of the document*_____

*Agent*_____

*Telephone*_____

*Agent*_____

*Telephone*_____

*Agent*_____

*Telephone*_____

LETTERS OF INSTRUCTION

Written by _____

Telephone _____

People with copies of documents _____

Telephone _____

Location of original documents _____

FUNERAL INSTRUCTIONS / MEMORIAL SERVICES

*Arranged by*_____

*Funeral home*_____

*Telephone*_____

*Location of instruction papers*_____

*People with copies of instructions*_____

*Telephone*_____

DONOR ARRANGEMENT
Location of documentation _____

AUTOPSY PERMISSION
Location of documentation _____

SOCIAL SECURITY
Social Security number _____
Location of Social Security card _____

MILITARY DISCHARGE PAPERS
Veteran's name _____
Service number _____
Discharge papers location _____

INCOME TAX FILINGS
Name of taxpayer _____
Tax identification number _____
Tax adviser _____
Telephone _____
Location of tax records _____

PASSPORT
Name on passport _____
Passport number _____
Location of passport _____

DRIVER'S LICENSE
Name on license _____
License number _____
State license issued _____
License renewal date _____

CREDIT CARDS / CHARGE ACCOUNTS
Account name(s) _____
Account number _____
Name on account _____
Location of card _____

MEDICARE

Name _____

Number _____

Effective date _____

MEDICAID

Name _____

Number _____

Effective date _____

HEALTH-CARE INSURANCE

Subscriber's name _____

Contract number _____

Group number _____

Insurance company _____

Telephone _____

LONG-TERM CARE INSURANCE

Name on policy _____

Policy number _____

Insurance company _____

Insurance agent _____

Telephone _____

Location of policy _____

LIFE INSURANCE

Name on policy _____

Policy number _____

Insurance company _____

Insurance agent _____

Telephone _____

Location of policy _____

ANNUITY

Name on annuity _____

Insurance company _____

Contract number _____

Location of papers _____

DISABILITY INSURANCE
Name on policy _____
Policy number _____
Insurance company _____
Insurance agent _____
Telephone _____
Location of policy _____

HOMEOWNERS INSURANCE
Name(s) on policy _____
Policy number _____
Insurance company _____
Insurance agent _____
Telephone _____
Location of policy _____

REAL-ESTATE INVESTMENT INSURANCE
Name(s) on policy _____
Policy number _____
Insurance company _____
Insurance agent _____
Telephone _____
Location of policy _____

RENTERS INSURANCE
Name(s) on policy _____
Policy number _____
Insurance company _____
Insurance agent _____
Telephone _____
Location of policy _____

BUSINESS INSURANCE
Business named on policy _____
Policy number _____
Insurance company _____
Insurance agent _____

Telephone _____

Location of policy _____

LIABILITY INSURANCE

Name on policy _____

Policy number _____

Insurance company _____

Insurance agent _____

Telephone _____

Location of policy _____

VEHICLE INSURANCE

Policyholder _____

Vehicle insured _____

Vehicle registration number _____

Insurance company _____

Insurance agent _____

Telephone _____

Location of title _____

VEHICLE

Vehicle _____

Make and model _____

Serial number _____

Where purchased _____

Telephone _____

Name on title _____

Location of title papers _____

Location of electronic toll collection system _____

VALUABLES INSURANCE

Policyholder _____

Item insured _____

Policy number _____

Insurance company _____

Insurance agent _____

Telephone _____

Location of policy _____

REAL-ESTATE OWNERSHIP DOCUMENTS

Property address _____

Owner _____

Telephone _____

Co-owner _____

Telephone _____

Bank or mortgage company _____

Telephone _____

Location of documents _____

CEMETERY PLOT

Owner _____

Plot intended for _____

Cemetery _____

Plot location _____

Telephone _____

Location of plot deeds _____

SUBSCRIPTIONS

Name of publication _____

Sent to _____

Name of publication _____

Sent to _____

Name of publication _____

Sent to _____

CLUB MEMBERSHIPS

Organization _____

Telephone _____

Organization _____

Telephone _____

MEMBERSHIP / SMART CARDS

Account name _____

Account number _____

Name on account _____

Location of card _____

RELIGIOUS AFFILIATION

*Place of worship*_____

Address _____

Clergyperson _____

Telephone _____

RELIGIOUS RITES AND CEREMONIES

*Event*_____

*Event date*_____

*Place of event*_____

Records storage location _____

ITEMS IN STORAGE

Stored in name of _____

What is being stored _____

Storage company _____

Telephone _____

Location of storage documents _____

ITEMS—REPAIRED/RESTORED/CLEANED

Item owner _____

Item description _____

*Shop name*_____

Telephone _____

Claim ticket location _____

ITEMS BORROWED

Item description _____

Lent to _____

Telephone _____

ITEMS ON ORDER

Ordered for _____

Item description _____

Order reference number _____

*Shop name*_____

Telephone _____

*Expected order date*_____

Location of paperwork _____

PERSONAL CONTRACTS / AGREEMENTS

Name(s) on contract _____

Telephone _____

Nature of agreement _____

Location of paperwork _____

MEDICAL HISTORY

History of _____

*Birth date*_____

Location of records _____

BIRTH RECORD

Name at birth _____

*Birth date*_____

Place of birth _____

Birth certificate location _____

ADOPTION PAPERS

Adoption name _____

Adopted by _____

State of adoption _____

Adoption agency _____

Telephone _____

Location of paperwork _____

NATURALIZATION PAPERS

Citizen name _____

*Place of naturalization*_____

*Location of papers*_____

MARRIAGE LICENSE

*Names on license*_____

Marriage date _____

State license issued _____

*License location*_____

DIVORCE DECREE

Names on decree _____

Divorce date _____

State divorce granted _____

Decree location _____

SCHOOL RECORDS

Student name _____

School _____

School location _____

Telephone _____

Dates attended _____

Graduation date _____

Diploma location _____

EMPLOYMENT HISTORY

Employee name _____

Dates of employment _____

Company _____

Company address _____

Telephone _____

MOTHER'S HISTORY

Mother's name at birth _____

Date of birth _____

Place of birth _____

Birth certificate location _____

Mother's name at death _____

Cause of death _____

Date of death _____

Location of death _____

Burial location _____

Death certificate location _____

FATHER'S HISTORY

Father's name at birth _____

Date of birth _____

Place of birth _____

Birth certificate location _____

Father's name at death _____

Cause of death _____

Date of death _____

Location of death _____

Burial location _____

Death certificate location _____

DEPENDENTS

Name _____

Date of birth _____

Location of birth certificate _____

GROWN CHILDREN—NO LONGER DEPENDENTS

Name _____

Date of birth _____

Address _____

City/State/Zip _____

Telephone _____

PETS

Name of pet _____

Breed _____

Date of birth _____

Sex _____

Animal hospital _____

Telephone _____

Breeder _____

Is promised to _____

HOME INVENTORY (FIXTURES, FURNITURE, EQUIPMENT, APPLIANCES)

Item description _____

Model number _____

Purchase price _____

Value of item today _____

Location of receipt _____

Location of warranty _____

*Location of item instructions*_____

Is promised to _____

PERSONAL-ITEMS INVENTORY (CLOTHES, BOOKS, PHOTOS, MEMENTOS)

Item description _____

Purchase price _____

Value of item today _____

Location of receipt _____

Is promised to _____

VALUABLES INVENTORY (COLLECTIONS, JEWELRY, ARTWORK, ANTIQUES)

Item description _____

Serial number _____

Purchase price _____

Value of item today _____

Location of receipt _____

Is promised to _____

BUSINESS INVENTORY (FIXTURES, FURNITURE, EQUIPMENT, APPLIANCES)

Item description _____

*Model number*_____

Purchase price _____

Value of item today _____

Location of receipt _____

*Location of warranty*_____

*Location of item instructions*_____

Is promised to _____

THE DOCUMENTS LOCATOR ACTION CHECKLIST

(This worksheet is also available online at www.elderindustry.com)

THE DOCUMENTS LOCATOR	To Do By	Completed
Complete "The Documents Locator"	_____	❑
Make copies of original documents	_____	❑
Store original documents in safe place	_____	❑
Maintain twenty-four-hour access to original documents	_____	❑
Back up "Documents Locator" information on a flash drive	_____	❑
Keep in safe-deposit box		
stock certificates	_____	❑
securities and bonds	_____	❑
certificates of deposit	_____	❑
titles to property and vehicles	_____	❑
deeds	_____	❑
bills of sale—major purchases and valuables	_____	❑
appraisals of property and valuables	_____	❑
retirement bank account records	_____	❑
company pension records	_____	❑
contracts and legal agreements	_____	❑
naturalization papers	_____	❑
Duplicate and distribute copies of these documents to key family members and family attorney		
proof of insurance	_____	❑
letters of instruction	_____	❑
power of attorney for property	_____	❑
power of attorney for health care	_____	❑
living will	_____	❑
"The Documents Locator"	_____	❑

Keep in fireproof box at home

birth certificates _____ ❑

death certificates _____ ❑

marriage licenses _____ ❑

divorce decrees _____ ❑

financial records _____ ❑

passports _____ ❑

insurance policies _____ ❑

wills _____ ❑

letters of instruction _____ ❑

power of attorney for property _____ ❑

power of attorney for health care _____ ❑

military discharge papers _____ ❑

income tax returns for past six years _____ ❑

property tax receipts _____ ❑

warranties _____ ❑

THE READING ROOM

Here are some of my favorite books as a supplement to *The Complete Eldercare Planner.*

Caregiving: The Spiritual Journey of Love, Loss, and Renewal, by Beth Witrogen McLeod (Wiley)

Caring in Remembered Ways: The Fruit of Seeing Deeply, by Maggie Steincrohn Davis (Heartsong)

Control Theory: A New Explanation of How We Control Our Lives, by William Glasses, MD (Perennial Library)

Coping with Your Difficult Older Parent: A Guide for Stressed-Out Children, by Grace Lebow and Barbara Kane (Avon Paperback)

Elder Rage, or Take My Father . . . Please! How to Survive Caring for Aging Parents, by Jacqueline Marcell (Impressive Press, 2nd ed.)

The Four Agreements: A Practical Guide to Personal Freedom, a Toltec Wisdom Book, by Don Miguel Ruiz (Amber-Allen)

How to Be an Adult: A Handbook on Psychological and Spiritual Integration, by David Richo (Paulist Press)

How to Say It to Seniors: Closing the Communication Gap with Our Elders, by David Solie (Prentice Hall)

A Journey of Work-Life Renewal: The Power to Recharge & Rekindle Passion in Your Life, by Bonnie Michaels and Michael Seef (Managing Work & Family)

Managing Anger: A Handbook of Proven Techniques, by Mitchell H. Messer, MA, LPC (Anger Institute)

Relocation 101 and *Home Away from Home,* by Beverly Roman (BR Anchor Publishing; available at www.branchor.com)

Senior Housing 101: Your Basic Field Guide to Understanding Today's Complex Senior Housing Market, by Randalym Kaye and Gabriel Gloege (Elder-Transitions, LLC)

Simple Truths, by Kent Nerburn (NewWorld)

Stretching, by Bob Anderson (Shelter Publications)

Successful Aging, by John W. Rowe, MD, and Robert Kahn, PhD (DTP Health)

The 36-Hour Day: A Family Guide to Caring for People with Alzheimer Disease, Other Dementias, and Memory Loss in Later Life, by Nancy L. Mace and Peter V. Rabins (Johns Hopkins Press, 4th ed.)

What Are Old People For? How Elders Will Save the World, by William H. Thomas, MD (V & B)

ORGANIZATIONS INDEX

American Bar Association
321 N. Clark Street
Chicago, IL 60610
Toll-free: (800) 285-2221

American Cancer Society
Toll-free: (800) 227-2345;
    TTY: (866) 228-4327

American Chronic Pain Association
PO Box 850
Rocklin, CA 95677
Toll-free: (800) 533-3231

American Health Assistance Foundation
22512 Gateway Center Drive
Clarksburg, MD 20871
(301) 948-3244; toll-free: (800) 437-2423;
    fax: (301) 258-9454

American Health Care Association
1201 L Street, NW
Washington, DC 20005
(202) 842-4444

American Health Quality Association
1155 21st Street, NW
Washington, DC 20036
(202) 331-5790; fax: (202) 331-9334

American Heart Association
7272 Greenville Avenue
Dallas, TX 75231
Toll-free: (800) 242-8721

**American Institute of Certified Public
    Accountants**
1211 Avenue of the Americas
New York, NY 10036-8775
(212) 596-6200

American Institute of Financial Gerontology
1525 NW 3rd Street, Suite 8
Deerfield Beach, FL 33442
(954) 421-1403; toll-free:
    (888) 367-8470

American Seniors Housing Association
5100 Wisconsin Avenue, NW, Suite 307
Washington, DC 20016
(202) 237-0900; fax: (202) 237-1616

Americans for Better Care of the Dying
1700 Diagonal Road, Suite 635
Alexandria, VA 22314
(703) 647-8505

America's Health Insurance Plans
601 Pennsylvania Avenue, NW, South Building,
    Suite 500
Washington, DC 20004
(202) 778-3200

Anger Clinic
29 S. La Salle
Chicago, IL 60603-1507
(312) 263-0035
Mitch H. Messer, Director

Assisted Living Federation of America
1650 King Street, Suite 602
Alexandria, VA 22314-2747
(703) 894-1805; fax: (703) 894-1831

Association for Conflict Resolution
1015 18th Street, NW, Suite 1150
Washington, DC 20036
(202) 464-9700; fax: (202) 464-9720

BenefitsLink
1298 Minnesota Avenue, Suite H
Winter Park, FL 32789
(407) 644-4146

Better Business Bureau—Canada
2 St. Clair Avenue E., Suite 800
Toronto, ON M4T 2T5
Canada
(416) 644-4936

Better Business Bureau—United States
4200 Wilson Boulevard, Suite 800
Arlington, VA 22203-1838
(703) 276-0100

BR Anchor
4596 Capital Dome Drive
Jacksonville, FL 32246
(904) 641-1140

Canadian Health Network
Jeanne Mance Building, 10th Floor
Tunney's Pasture, A.L. 1910B
Ottawa, ON K1A 0K9
Canada

Canine Companions for Independence
Toll-free: (866) 224-3647

Center for Medicare Advocacy
PO Box 350
Willimantic, CT 06226
(860) 456-7790

Center for Social Gerontology
2307 Shelby Avenue
Ann Arbor, MI 48103
(734) 665-1126; fax: (734) 665-2071

Center for Spirituality, Theology and Health
Box 3825 Duke University Medical Center
Busse Building, Suite 0507
Durham, NC 27710
(919) 660-7556

Centers for Medicare and Medicaid Services
Medicare Service Center:
 (800) 633-4227
Medicare Service Center TTY:
 (877) 486-2048
Report Medicare Fraud and Abuse:
 (800) 447-8477

Children of Aging Parents
PO Box 167
Richboro, PA 18954
Toll-free: (800) 227-7294

Compassion and Choices
Toll-free counselor assistance:
 (800) 247-7421

Consumer Coalition for Quality Health Care
1101 Vermont Avenue, NW, Suite 1001
Washington, DC 20005
(202) 789-3606; fax: (202) 898-2389

Consumer Health Information Corporation
8300 Greensboro Drive, Suite 1220
McLean, VA 22102-3604
(703) 734-0650; fax: (703) 734-1459

Corporation for National and Community Service
1201 New York Avenue, NW
Washington, DC 20525
(202) 606-5000; TDD: (202) 634-9256

Cremation Association of North America
401 N. Michigan Avenue
Chicago, IL 60611
(312) 245-1077

Direct Marketing Association
Do Not Call Registry: (888) 382-1222

Easter Seals
230 West Monroe Street, Suite 1800
Chicago, IL 60606
(312) 726-6200; toll-free:
 (800) 221-6827
Website: www.easterseals.com

ElderCare Rights Alliance
2626 E. 82nd Street, Suite 230
Bloomington, MN 55425
(952) 854-7304; toll-free: (800) 893-4055;
 fax: (952) 854-8535

Elder Cohousing Network
1460 Quince Avenue, Suite 102
Boulder, CO 80304
(303) 413-8066; fax: (303) 413-8067

Faith in Action
Wake Forest University School
 of Medicine
Medical Center Boulevard

Winston-Salem, NC 27157
(336) 716-0101; toll-free (877) 324-8411;
    fax: (336) 777-3284

Families and Work Institute
267 5th Avenue, Floor 2
New York, NY 10016
(212) 465-2044

Federal Trade Commission
Toll-free: (877) 382-4357

Financial Planning Association
1600 K Street, NW, Suite 201
Washington, DC 20006
Toll-free: (800) 322-4237

Funeral Consumers Alliance
33 Patchen Road
South Burlington, VT 05403
Toll-free: (800) 765-0107

**George Washington Institute for
    Spirituality and Health**
George Washington University
Warwick Building, Suite 313
2300 K Street, NW
Washington, DC 20037
(202) 994-6220

Global Action on Aging
777 UN Plaza, Suite 6J
New York, NY 11017
(212) 557-3163

Gray Panthers—National Office
1612 K Street, NW, Suite 300
Washington, DC 20006
(202) 737-6637; toll-free: (800) 280-5362;
    fax: (202) 737-1160

Health Privacy Project
1120 19th Street, NW, 8th Floor
Washington, DC 20036
(202) 721-5614

Hearing Loss Association of America
7910 Woodmont Avenue, Suite 1200
Bethesda, MD 20814
(301) 657-2248; V-TTY: (301) 913-9413; fax
    (301) 657-2248

Hospice Foundation of America
12000 Biscayne Boulevard, Suite 505
Miami Beach, FL 33181
(305) 981-2522; toll-free: (800) 854-3402

Institute for the Future of Aging Services
2519 Connecticut Avenue, NW
Washington, DC 20008
(202) 508-1208; fax: (202) 783-4266

Insurance Information Institute
111 William Street
New York, NY 10038
(212) 346-5500

Internal Revenue Service
Toll-free: (800) 829-1040; TDD:
    (800) 829-4059

**International Association of Homes and
    Services for the Ageing**
2519 Connecticut Avenue, NW
Washington, DC 20008
(202) 508-9468; fax: (202) 220-0041

**International Cemetery, Cremation and
    Funeral Association**
107 Carpenter Drive, Suite 100
Sterling, VA 20164
(703) 391-8400; toll-free: (800) 645-7700

International Council on Active Aging
3307 Trutch Street
Vancouver, BC V6L-2T3
Canada
(604) 734-4466; toll-free: (866) 335-9777

Medicare Rights Center
Toll-free: (888) 466-9050

Mental Health America
2000 N. Beauregard Street, 6th Floor
Alexandria, VA 22311
(703) 684-7722; toll-free: (800) 969-6642;
    TTY: (800) 433-5959

Mobility International USA
132 E. Broadway, Suite 343
Eugene, OR 97401
(541) 343-1284 (Tel. and TTY)

National Academy of Elder Law Attorneys
1604 N. Country Club Road
Tucson, AZ 85716
(520) 881-4005; fax: (520) 325-7925

National Adult Day Services Association
2519 Connecticut Avenue, NW
Washington, DC 20008
Toll-free: (800) 558-5301

National Aging in Place Council
1400 16th Street, NW, Suite 420
Washington, DC 20036
(202) 939-1784; fax: (202) 265-4435

National Archives and Records Administration
8601 Adelphi Road
College Park, MD 20740-6001
Toll-free: (866) 272-6272

National Association for Home Care & Hospice
228 7th Street, SE
Washington, DC 20003
(202) 547-7424; fax: (202) 547-3540

National Association of Area Agencies on Aging
1730 Rhode Island Avenue, NW, Suite 1200
Washington, DC 20036
(202) 872-0888; fax: (202) 872-0057

**National Association of Insurance
    Commissioners**
2301 McGee Street, Suite 800
Kansas City, MO 64108-2662
(816) 842-3600; fax: (816) 783-8175

**National Association of Professional Geriatric
    Care Managers**
1604 N. Country Club Road
Tucson, AZ 85716
(520) 881-8008; fax: (520) 325-7925

**National Center for Complementary and
    Alternative Medicine**
National Institutes of Health
9000 Rockville Pike
Bethesda, MD 20892
Toll-free: (888) 644-6226;
    (301) 519-3153

National Center on Elder Abuse
1201 15th Street, NW, Suite 350
Washington, DC 20005
(202) 898-2586

**National Center on Grandparents Raising
    Grandchildren**
Georgia State University
140 Decatur Street
Atlanta, Georgia 30303
(404) 651-1049

National Center on Senior Transportation
1425 K Street, NW, Suite 200
Washington, DC 20005
Toll-free: (866) 528-6278; TDD:
    (202) 347-7385

**National Citizens' Coalition for
    Nursing Home Reform**
1828 L Street, NW, Suite 801
Washington, DC 20036
(202) 332-2276; fax: (202) 332-2949

**National Committee for Quality
    Assurance**
2000 L Street, NW, Suite 500
Washington, DC 20036
(202) 955-3500; toll-free: (888) 275-7585;
    fax: (202) 955-3599

National Committee for the Prevention of Elder Abuse
1612 K Street, NW
Washington, DC 20006
(202) 682-4140

National Committee to Preserve Social Security and Medicare
10 G Street, NE, Suite 600
Washington, DC 20004
(202) 216-0420; toll-free: (800) 966-1935;
  fax: (202) 216-0451

National Conference of State Legislatures
444 North Capitol Street, NW, Suite 515
Washington, DC 20001
(202) 624-5400; fax: (202) 737-1069

National Consumers League
1701 K Street, NW, Suite 1200
Washington, DC 20006
(202) 835-3323

National Council on Aging
1901 L Street, NW, 4th Floor
Washington, DC 20036
(202) 479-1200; TDD: (202) 479-6674

National Council on Patient Information and Education
4915 Saint Elmo Avenue, Suite 505
Bethesda, MD 20814-6053
(301) 656-8565; fax: (301) 656-4464

National Crime Prevention Council
1000 Connecticut Avenue, NW, 13th Floor
Washington, DC 20036
(202) 466-6272

National Domestic Violence Hotline
Toll-free: (800) 799-7233

National Family Caregivers Association
10400 Connecticut Avenue, Suite 500
Kensington, MD 20895-3944
(301) 942-6430; toll-free:
  (800) 896-3650

National Foundation for Credit Counseling
801 Roeder Road, Suite 900
Silver Spring, MD 20910
(301) 589-5600; toll-free: (800) 388-2227

National Fraud Information Center
Toll-free: (800) 876-7060

National Guardianship Association
526 Brittany Drive
State College, PA 16803
(814) 238-3126; fax: (814) 238-7051

National Hospice and Palliative Care Organization
1700 Diagonal Road, Suite 625
Alexandria, VA 22314
(703) 837-1500

National Institute on Aging
Building 31, Room 5C27
31 Center Drive, MSC 2292
Bethesda, MD 20892
(301) 496-1752; TTY: (800) 222-4225

National Institutes of Health
9000 Rockville Pike
Bethesda, MD 20892
(301) 496-4000; TTY: (301) 402-9612

National Insurance Consumer Helpline
Toll-free: (800) 942-4242

National Library Service for the Blind and Physically Handicapped
Toll-free: (888) 657-7323

National Long Term Care Ombudsman Resource Center
1828 L Street, NW, Suite 801
Washington, DC 20036
(202) 332-2275

National Network of Estate Planning Attorneys
10831 Old Mill Road, Suite 400
Omaha, NE 68154
Toll-free: (800) 638-8681

National PACE Association
801 N. Fairfax Street, Suite 309
Alexandria, VA 22314
(703) 535-1565; toll-free: (800) 633-4227;
   TTY: (877) 486-2048

National Parkinson Foundation
1501 N.W. 9th Avenue / Bob Hope Road
Miami, FL 33136-1494
(305) 243-6666; toll-free: (800) 327-4545

**National Partnership for Women
   and Families**
1875 Connecticut Avenue, NW, Suite 650
Washington, DC 20009-5729
(202) 986-2600; fax: (202) 986-2539

National Private Duty Association
941 E. 86th Street, Suite 270
Indianapolis, IN 46240
(317) 663-3637

**National Rehabilitation Information
   Center**
8201 Corporate Drive, Suite 600
Landover, MD 20785
(301) 459-5900; toll-free: (800) 346-2742;
   TTY: (301) 459-5984

**National Resource Center on Supportive
   Housing and Home Modification**
Andrus Gerontology Center
University of Southern California
3715 McClintock Avenue
Los Angeles, CA 90089
(213) 740-1364

National Safety Council
1121 Spring Lake Drive
Itasca, IL 60143-3201
(630) 285-1121

National Senior Citizens Law Center
1101 14th Street, NW, Suite 400
Washington, DC 20005
(202) 289-6976; fax: (202) 289-7224

**Office of Disability, Aging, and Long-Term Care
   Policy**
U.S. Department of Health and Human Services
200 Independence Avenue, SW
Washington, DC 20201
(202) 690-6443

Older Women's League
3300 N. Fairfax Drive, Suite 218
Arlington, VA 22201
(703) 812-0687

Partnership for Prescription Assistance
Toll-free: (888) 477-2669

Patient Advocate Foundation
700 Thimble Shoals Boulevard, Suite 200
Newport News, VA 23606
Toll-free: (800) 532-5274

Pension Rights Center
1350 Connecticut Avenue, NW, Suite 206
Washington, DC 20036
(202) 296-3776; fax: (202) 833-2472

Rosalynn Carter Institute for Caregiving
800 GSW Drive
Georgia Southwestern State University
Americus, GA 31709-4379
(229) 928-1234

Rural Assistance Center
501 N. Columbia Road, Stop 9037
Grand Forks, ND 58202
Toll-free: (800) 270-1898

Rural Information Center
National Agricultural Library
10301 Baltimore Avenue
Beltsville, MD 20705-2351
Toll-free: (800) 633-7701

SAGE
305 7th Avenue, 16th Floor
New York, NY 10001
(212) 741-2247

Senior Corps
1201 New York Avenue, NW
Washington, DC 20525
(202) 606-5000; TTY: (202) 606-3472

Senior Service America
(Training and employment opportunities
for older adults)
8403 Colesville Road
Silver Spring, MD 20910
(301) 578-8900

Seniors Real Estate Specialists
Toll-free: (800) 500-4564

ShareTheCare
551 Fifth Avenue, 28th Floor
New York, NY 10176
(646) 467-8097

Social Security Administration
Toll-free: (800) 772-1213;
TDD: (800) 325-0778

Society of Certified Senior Advisors
1777 S. Bellaire Street, Suite 230
Denver, CO 80222
Toll-free: (800) 653-1785

Society of Financial Service Professionals
17 Campus Boulevard, Suite 201
Newtown Square, PA 19073
(610) 526-2500

**U.S. Department of Agriculture Rural
Development**
(202) 690-1533; toll-free TTY: (800) 877-8339

U.S. Department of Health and Human Services
200 Independence Avenue, SW
Washington, DC 20201
(202) 619-0257; toll-free: (877) 696-6775

**U.S. Department of Housing and Urban
Development**
Toll-free: (800) 569-4287

U.S. Department of Veterans Affairs
810 Vermont Avenue, NW
Washington, DC 20420
(202) 273-5771; toll-free: (800) 827-1000;
fax: (202) 273-5716
Health-care benefits toll-free:
(877) 222-8387

U.S. Food and Drug Administration
5600 Fishers Lane
Rockville, MD 20857-0001
Toll-free: (888) 463-6332

U.S. Securities and Exchange Commission
Toll-free: (800) 732-0330

Visiting Nurse Associations of America
99 Summer Street, Suite 1700
Boston, MA 02110
(617) 737-3200

Volunteers of America
1660 Duke Street
Alexandria, VA 22314
(703) 341-5000; toll-free:
(800) 899-0089

Wayne E. Oates Institute
1733 Bardstown Road
Louisville, KY 40205
(502) 459-2370

Well Spouse Association
63 W. Main Street, Suite H
Freehold, NJ 07728
Toll-free: (800) 838-0879

WFC Resources
5197 Beachside Drive
Minnetonka, MN 55343
(952) 936-7898; toll-free: (800) 487-7898

Women's Institute for a Secure Retirement
1725 K Street, NW, Suite 201
Washington, DC 20006
(202) 393-5452

WEBSITE INDEX

American Cancer Society
www.cancer.org

American Chronic Pain Association
www.theacpa.org

American Geriatrics Society
www.americangeriatrics.org

American Health Assistance Foundation
www.ahaf.org

American Health Care Association
www.ahca.org

American Health Quality Association
www.ahqa.org

American Heart Association
www.americanheart.org

American Institute of Certified Public Accountants
www.aicpa.org

American Institute of Financial Gerontology
www.aifg.org

American Medical Association
www.ama-assn.org

American Pain Foundation
www.painfoundation.org

American Pain Society
www.ampainsoc.org

American Podiatric Medical Association
www.apma.org

American Public Transportation Association
www.apta.com

American Seniors Housing Association
www.seniorshousing.org

Americans for Better Care of the Dying
www.abcd-caring.org

Americans with Disabilities Act
www.ada.gov

Anger Clinic
www.angerclinic.com

Assisted Living Federation of America
www.alfa.org

Association for Conflict Resolution
www.acrnet.org

Association for Driver Rehabilitation Specialists—Aging and Driving
www.driver-ed.org

Beliefnet
www.beliefnet.com

Benefits CheckUp
www.benefitscheckup.org

BenefitsLink
www.benefitslink.com

Better Business Bureau—Canada
www.bbb.org

Better Business Bureau—United States
www.bbb.org

BR Anchor
www.branchor.com

The Bright Side
www.the-bright-side.org

Call for Action
www.callforaction.org

Canadian Automobile Association
www.caa.ca/agingdrivers

Canadian Health Network
www.canadianhealthnetwork.ca

Canine Companions for Independence
www.caninecompanions.org

CareCommunity
www.mycarecommunity.org

Caregiver's Home Companion
www.caregivershome.com

Caregiving.com
www.caregiving.com

Caring Connections
www.caringinfo.org

Center for Aging Services Technologies
www.agingtech.org

Center for Social Gerontology
www.tcsg.org

Center for Spirituality and Health
www.spiritualityandhealth.ufl.edu

Center for Spirituality, Theology and Health
www.dukespiritualityandhealth.org

Centers for Medicare and Medicaid Services
www.cms.hhs.gov

Children of Aging Parents
www.caps4caregivers.org

**Commission on Accreditation of Rehabilitation
    Facilities (CARF)**
CARF International website: www.carf.org
CARF Canada website: www.carfcanada.ca

Commission on Law and Aging
www.abanet.org/aging

Compassion and Choices
www.compassionandchoices.org

The Complete Eldercare Planner
www.elderindustry.com

Consumer Consortium on Assisted Living
www.ccal.org

Consumer Health Information Corporation
www.consumer-health.com

Cremation Association of North America
www.cremationassociation.org

Direct Marketing Association
www.the-dma.org
www.donotcall.gov

DisabilityInfo.gov
www.disabilityinfo.gov

Eden Alternative
www.edenalt.com

Elder Abuse Foundation
www.elder-abuse-foundation.com

Eldercare Locator
www.eldercare.gov

ElderCare Online
www.ec-online.net

ElderCare Rights Alliance
www.eldercarerights.org

Elder Cohousing Network
www.eldercohousing.org

Elderhostel
www.elderhostel.org

ElderLawAnswers
www.elderlawanswers.com

ElderWeb
www.elderweb.com

Elder Wisdom Circle
www.elderwisdomcircle.org

Faith in Action
www.fiavolunteers.org

Families and Work Institute
www.familiesandwork.org

Families for Depression Awareness
www.familyaware.org

Family Caregiver Alliance
www.caregiver.org

**Family Caregiver Alliance / LGBT Caregiver
    Discussion Group**
www.caregiver.org

Family Search
www.familysearch.org

Federal Government Websites
White House: www.whitehouse.gov
U.S. House of Representatives: http://house.gov
U.S. Senate: http://senate.gov

Federal Trade Commission
www.ftc.gov

FedWorld
www.fedworld.gov

Financial Planning Association
www.fpanet.org/public

Financing Long Term Care
www.financinglongtermcare.umn.edu

Food Stamp Program
www.fns.usda.gov/fsp

Forgiveness Web
www.forgivenessweb.com

National Foundation for Credit Counseling
www.nfcc.org

National Fraud Information Center
www.fraud.org

National Governors Association
www.nga.org

National Guardianship Association
www.guardianship.org

National Health Information Center
www.health.gov/nhic

National Hopeline Network
www.hopeline.com

National Hospice and Palliative Care
  Organization
www.nhpco.org

National Institute on Aging
www.nia.nih.gov

National Library Service for the Blind and
  Physically Handicapped
www.loc.gov/nls

National Long Term Care Ombudsman
  Resource Center
www.ltcombudsman.org

National Network of Estate Planning
  Attorneys
www.netplanning.com

National PACE Association
www.npaonline.org

National Pain Foundation
www.nationalpainfoundation.org

National Parkinson Foundation
www.parkinson.org

National Partnership for Women and Families
www.nationalpartnership.org

National Private Duty Association
www.privatedutyhomecare.org

National Rehabilitation Information Center
www.naric.com

National Resource Center on Supportive
  Housing and Home Modification
www.homemods.org

National Respite Locator Service
www.respitelocator.org

National Safety Council
www.nsc.org

National Senior Citizens Law Center
www.nsclc.org

National Working Caregivers Resource Center
www.americanbusinesscares.net

NIH Senior Health
www.nihseniorhealth.gov

NORCS: An Aging in Place Initiative
www.norcs.org.

Nursing Home Abuse Resource
www.nursing-home-abuse-resource.com

OASIS
www.oasisnet.org

Office of Disability, Aging, and Long-Term
  Care Policy
http://aspe.hhs.gov/daltcp

Older Women's League
www.owl-national.org

Ontario Seniors' Secretariat
www.culture.gov.on.ca/seniors

Partnership for Advancing Technology
  in Housing
www.pathnet.org

Partnership for Prescription Assistance
www.pparx.org

Patient Advocate Foundation
www.patientadvocate.org

Pension Rights Center
www.pensionrights.org

People's Medical Society
www.peoplesmed.org

Women's Institute for a Secure Retirement
www.wiserwomen.org

WorkingCaregiver.com
www.workingcaregiver.com

WorkLife Law
www.worklifelaw.com

The Wright Stuff
www.thewright-stuff.com

SUBJECT INDEX

NOTES

Chapter 3. Be Kind to Yourself

1. P. M. Barnes, E. Powell-Griner, K. McFann, and R. L. Nahin, "Complementary and Alternative Medicine Use Among Adults: United States, 2002," CDC Advance Data Report #343, *Seminars in Integrative Medicine* 2, no. 2 (June 2004): pp. 54–71.

Chapter 5. Emergency Preparedness

1. "Take As Directed: A Prescription Not Followed," research conducted by Polling Company, National Community Pharmacists Association, December 15, 2006, retrieved on March 16, 2008, from http://www.talkaboutrx.org/documents/enhancing_prescription_medicine_adherence.pdf.
2. Michelle Meadows, "Preventing Serious Drug Interactions," *FDA Consumer* 38, no. 4 (July–August 2004), retrieved on March 16, 2008, from http://www.fda.gov/fdac/features/2004/404_drug.html.
3. Ibid.

Chapter 7. Legal Matters

1. Wan He, Manisha Sengupta, Victoria A. Velkoff, and Kimberly A. DeBarros, *65+ in the United States: 2005*, U.S. Census Bureau, Current Population Reports, P23-209 (Washington, D.C.: U.S. Government Printing Office, 2005), p. 15.
2. The National Health Care Anti-Fraud Association estimates that of the nation's annual health-care outlay, at least $51 billion in 2003 is lost to outright fraud. Other estimates by government and law enforcement agencies place the loss as high as $170 billion—each year. NHCAA White Paper on Fraud, *Health Care Fraud: A Serious and Costly Reality for All Americans*, February 22, 2006, p. 1, retrieved on March 16, 2008, from http://www.hcinsight.com/docs/papers/NHCAA%20White%20Paper%20on%20Fraud.pdf.
3. U.S. Administration on Aging, *America's Families Care: A Report on the Needs of America's Family Caregivers* (Fall 2000), retrieved on March 16, 2008, from http://www.aoa.gov/carenetwork/report.html.

Chapter 9. Housing

1. *Are Americans Talking with Their Parents about Independent Living: A 2007 Study Among Boomer Women* (November 2007), p. 2, data collected by ICR, report prepared by Laura Skufca, MA, AARP Knowledge Management, retrieved on March 16, 2008, from http://assets.aarp.org/rgcenter/il/boomer_women.pdf.

Chapter 10. Safe and Secure

1. P. Teaster, T. Dugar, M. Mendiondo, E. Abner, K. Cecil, and J. Otto, Graduate Center for Gerontology, University of Kentucky, National Committee for the Prevention of Elder Abuse, and National Adult Protective Services Association, prepared for National Center on Elder Abuse, *The 2004 Survey of State Adult Protective Services: Abuse of Adults 60 Years of Age and Older* (February 2006), p. 6.

Chapter 11. Transportation and Mobility

1. I. Potts, J. Stutts, R. Pfefer, T. Neuman, K. Slack, and K. Hardy, *Guidance for Implementation of the American Association of State Highway and Transportation Officials Strategic Highway Safety Plan; Volume 9: A Guide for Reducing Collisions Involving Older Drivers*, National Cooperative Highway Research Program Report 500, Transportation Research Board of the National Academies (Washington, D.C., 2004), p. I-1, retrieved on March 16, 2008, from http://onlinepubs.trb.org/onlinepubs/nchrp/nchrp_rpt_500v9.pdf.
2. Wan He, Manisha Sengupta, Victoria A. Velkoff, and Kimberly A. DeBarros, *65+ in the United States: 2005*, U.S. Census Bureau, Current Population Reports, P23-209 (Washington, D.C.: U.S. Government Printing Office, 2005), p. 15.

Chapter 12. Managing Medical Care

1. Ann Bookman and Mona Harrington, "Family Caregivers: A Shadow Workforce in the Geriatric Health Care System?" *Journal of Health Politics Policy and Law* 32 (December 2007): pp. 1005–1041.
2. Thomas Moloney, "Dealing with Gum Disease: A Life-Threatening Health Risk," American Dental Hygienists' Association, retrieved on March 16, 2008, from http://www.adha.org/downloads/2001_NDHM_poster.pdf, p. 1.
3. Christina M. Puchalski, MD, MS, "The Role of Spirituality in Health Care," George Washington Institute for Spirituality and Health, George Washington University Medical Center Departments of Medicine and Health Care Sciences, and George Washington University, Washington, D.C., presented at Baylor University Medical Center on February 28, 2001, Baylor University Medical Center *Proceedings* 14, no. 4: pp. 352–357, retrieved March 16, 2008, from http://www.pubmedcentral.nih.gov/picrender.fcgi?artid=1305900&blobtype=pdf.
4. J. P. Foglio and H. Brody, "Religion, Faith, and Family Medicine," *Journal of Family Practice* 27, (1988): pp. 473–474.
5. Puchalski, "Role of Spirituality in Health Care," pp. 352–357.
6. Farr A. Curlin, MD, John D. Lantos, MD, Chad J. Roach, BS, Sarah A. Sellergren, MA, and Marshall H. Chin, MD, MPH, "Religious Characteristics of U.S. Physicians: A National Survey," *Journal of General Internal Medicine* 20, no. 7 (July 2005): pp. 629–634, doi:10.1111/j.1525-1497.2005.0119.x.
7. Charles D. MacLean, MD, Beth Susi, MD, Nancy Phifer, MD, Linda Schultz, MD, Deborah Bynum, MD, Mark Franco, MD, Andria Klioze, MD, Michael Monroe, MD, Joanne Garrett, PhD, and Sam

Cykert, MD, "Patient Preference for Physician Discussion and Practice of Spirituality: Results from a Multicenter Patient Survey," *Journal of General Internal Medicine* no. 18, no. 1 (January 2003): pp. 38–43, doi:10.1046/j.1525-1497.2003.20403.x.

8. Anne M. McCaffrey, MD, David M. Eisenberg, MD, Anna T. R. Legedza, ScD, Roger B. Davis, ScD, and Russell S. Phillips, MD, "Prayer for Health Concerns: Results of a National Survey on Prevalence and Patterns of Use," *Archives of Internal Medicine* 164 (2004): pp. 858–862, retrieved on March 16, 2008, from http://archinte.ama-assn.org/cgi/content/full/164/8/858?SEARCHID= 1084721917699_899&hits=10&gca=archinte%3B164%2F8%2F858&FIRSTINDEX=0&FULL TEXT=Anne+M.+McCaffrey&.

Chapter 13. Quality of Life

1. Jim Thornton, "So Tough It Hurts," *AARP The Magazine,* (September–October 2005), retrieved on March 16, 2008, from http://www.aarp.org/health/conditions/articles/depression_in_men.html.
2. *Suicide in the U.S.: Statistics and Prevention,* NIH Publication No. 06-4594, page last reviewed on March 14, 2008, retrieved on March 16, 2008, from http://www.nimh.nih.gov/health/ publications/suicide-in-the-us-statistics-and-prevention.shtml#adults.
3. *Older Adults: Depression and Suicide Facts,* NIH Publication No. 4593, revised April 2007, page last reviewed on March 14, 2008, retrieved on March 16, 2008, from http://www.nimh.nih .gov/health/publications/older-adults-depression-and-suicide-facts.shtml.
4. Miller McPherson, Lynn Smith-Lovin, and Matthew E. Brashears, "Social Isolation in America: Changes in Core Discussion Networks over Two Decades," *American Sociological Review* 71 (June 2006): pp. 353–375, retrieved on March 16, 2008, from http://www.asanet.org/galleries/default-file/June06ASRFeature.pdf.
5. International Health, Racquet and Sportsclub Association, "U.S. Health Club Membership by Age," retrieved on March 16, 2008, from http://cms.ihrsa.org/index.cfm?fuseaction=Page.viewPage& pageId=18811&nodeID=15.
6. P. Raina, D. Waltner-Toews, B. Bonnett, et al., "Influence of Companion Animals on the Physical and Psychological Health of Older People: An Analysis of a One-Year Longitudinal Study," *Journal of the American Geriatric Society* 47 (1999): pp. 323–329.

Chapter 14. Death and Dying

1. Robert Hellenga, *The Sixteen Pleasures* (New York: Delta, 1995).
2. L. L. Emanuel, C. F. von Gunten, and F. D. Ferris, "Gaps in End-of-Life Care," *Archives of Family Medicine* 9, no. 10 (November 2000): pp. 1176–1180, retrieved on March 16, 2008, from http://arch-fami.ama-assn.org/cgi/content/abstract/9/10/1176?ijkey=fe24583b93a62db6e545e69de3a12 b957fd26595&keytype2=tf_ipsecsha.
3. *Means to a Better End: A Report on Dying in America Today* (Washington, D.C.: Last Acts National Program Office, November 2002), p. 13, retrieved on March 16, 2008, from http://www .rwjf.org/files/publications/other/meansbetterend.pdf.
4. S. Robinson-Whelen, Y. Tada, R. MacCallum, L. McGuire, and J. Kiecolt-Glaser, "Former Caregivers Still Show Psychological Ills Years After Caregiving Ends," *Journal of Abnormal Psychology* 110, no. 4 (December 2001): pp. 573–584, retrieved on March 16, 2008, from http://researchnews .osu.edu/archive/formcare.htm.

ACKNOWLEDGMENTS

This book began when I was fourteen years old, and carries with it the spirit of the seven people who welcomed me into their hearts one cold and rainy Thanksgiving morning. I walked into the nursing home as a young volunteer offering comfort and joy and walked away a person on a mission. For this life-altering experience, I am forever grateful to the Sinsinawa Dominican Sisters of Trinity High School, River Forest, Illinois.

I thank my husband and partner in life, David Schultz, for sharing the journey of this book with me. My respect for your composition and editing skills is immeasurable, and the experience of finding everlasting love is reflected in the inner peace I feel when I walk beside you.

To my daughter, Bonnie Blackburn, her husband, Joe, my grandchildren, Lanea and Henry, and also Jacqueline, Michael, Trinity, and Emily. To Jeff and Amy Schultz, and Greg, Kim, Sam, Ellie, and Jack Schultz—you are my foundation of family and my source of joy, balance, and infinite inspiration.

The foundation for writing a book of this nature comes from the unconditional love and attention I receive every day from my immediate family. To my incredibly wonderful mother, Alba, and her loving husband, Bill Wright: *Mom, you are my role model and taught me everything I know today about caring for loved ones.*

To my siblings James, Carol, Peter, and Linda (I love all of you so much), and also to Dominic DiFrisco, Orasa, Angelina, and Maria Loverde; Louis, Nicolas, and Louis Belpedio; the Frank and Bernice Nesti family; the Sergio and Iola Nesti family; Larry Mafia; the Frank and Margaret Loverde family; the Graziella and Natalino Pagni family; Nina, Pasquale, and Bob Mariano; Dr. Sal Termini; Nina Mottern; Lisa and Jeff Rich; Laura Loverde; the Robert and Ethel Stanton family; Shirley Fadim; the Herb and Maxine Weintraub family; Sharon Arkin and family; the Gardner Stern family; the Jamey and Melissa Fadim family; the Bunny and George Kennedy family; and the Howard and Ursula Dubin family.

To special people who in a very real sense reflect the choices I have made in life: Jill and Steve Morris, Bernice Pink, Mitch Messer, Kathryn Cunningham, Carl and Patty Sanders, Rick and Maureen Gilardi, Frank and Grace DeLuca, Joanne Desmond, Angie and John Thoburn, Gay Gelman, Clark Weber, Peter and Vicki Walker, and Rick and Roxanne Hunsicker.

This book is a reflection of insights on life because of the friendships I share with Sandra Neff; Bonnie Michaels and Michael Seef; Georgia Evans; Bob and Janet Ebel; Steve Harpo Wolski; Carol Marx; Jerry Kalish; Martha Kluk; Dr. Richard Ofstein; Deanna Schultz; Michael Scott; Deb Turner; Carmen Trombetta; Fred Gardaphe; Helen and Nick at Crystal Cleaners; Brent Kolhede; Fran Perry; Mary Dempsey; Becky Barclay; Debbie and Peter Berman; Jim Lodas; Diana Heliotes and Nunzio; Donna Matsie Berg and her wonderful parents, Bob and Mary; Diane and Jerry Hansen; Mark Zaragoza and Desiree Baines; Joan and Herb Bays; Beata Lundeen; Jan, Nancy, and Zach Rozen; Ellie and Wes Monty; Pati and Rick Saulig; Phil Kosanovich; Joyce Carpino; Joe Scandariato; John and Karen Pink; Michael and Sharon Pink; Paul and Karen Sullivan; Janet Marvin; Kurt and Mia Inderbitzen; Larry and Diana Fischer; Pamela Peterson; Ned and Peggy Rosenheim; Laura Amend; Patty McGarr DiMaria; Cecelia Clark; Leiah Bowden; Jimmy Damon; Leslie Glutzer; Sarah Lauzen; Marcal Souto; Marcia Cosentino; Karen Werner; Nina and David Feinberg; Paul, Elaine, and Alexis Cohen; Randy Schools; Paula Kahn; Riva and Alvin Blick; Ricky and Linda Silverman; Reggie and Kim Hill; Sue Gitleson; Teri Folisi; Scott Mies; and Ted and Sherri Pincus.

To my special men's senior baseball family: Dan and Tina, Michelle and Lou, Susan and Perry, Neal and Carol, Frankie and Nancy, Paul and Theresa, Andy and Linda, Dick and Linda, Jeff and Ellen, Jan and John, Tom and Vicki, Ricky and Bonnie, Jules and Bruce, Bart and Barbara, Steve Bradford, Sandy Weissent, Steve Obert, and Tommy Hynes. Play ball!

To the devoted eldercare advocates whose mission is to improve the quality of life for older adults and the people who care for them, I express my deepest appreciation and respect—especially to Dr. John W. Eberhard, who works tirelessly on behalf of older drivers. Thank you, again, for your generous contributions regarding the mobility issues addressed in this book. Thanks also to Robert B. Blancato, Dr. Roger Landry, Larry Landry, Mark Lichtenwalner and the team at Masterpiece Living, Dr. Robert Kahn, Rob Adams, Denise Brown, Jennifer Openshaw, Amy Wright, Michael Erde, Dr. William Thomas, Marc J. Lane, and Suzanne Roberts. A special thank you to Dan Amdur and Ellie Monty at Moving Station, and also to Mary Jo Zeller, Gloria Bersani, Pam and Jeff Smith at Gero Solutions, and to the Presto.com team—Joe Beninato, Peter Radsliff, Ray Stern, and Leah Davis.

To my Internet and media community, I sincerely thank you for helping me communicate the power of eldercare planning, and for consistently keeping caregiving issues in the limelight: Susan Dutcher and Andrew Goldstein of the *Today* show; NBC's Stuart Dan; Karen Petersen at *USA Today*; Barbara Buchholtz; Marja Mills; Sherren Leigh of *Today's Chicago Woman*; Diane Summers and Paul Clayton of KFUO-Radio; Chris Farrell of *Right on the Money*; Mike Schwanz, editor of *Solutions Benefits and Compensation Magazine*; Dave Baker and BenefitsLink.com; Susie Singer Carter and Tibesti.com; Virginia Morris; Sander Vanocur; Jacqueline Marcell; Beverly and Amy Roman at BR Anchor; Becky Bright at the *Wall Street Journal*; Karen Stevensen at Elderweb.com; Gregg Kroman at Get LTC.com; *Psychology Today*'s Carlin Flora; the Women Aloud team Melissa Walker, Mo, and Shana; Theresa Guiterrez and Karen Meyer at ABC7 Chicago; Walter and Susie Jacobson; CBS2 Chicago anchor Vince Gerasole; the team at Chicago's WGN-TV; the Wisdom Channel's Corinne Edwards; Todd Wineburner at WJBC, Bloomington, IL; Scott Slocum; the *Indianapolis Star*'s Shari Rudavsky; Mom Central's Stacy DeBroff; the team of the radio show *A Touch of Grey*; Carrington Cunnington at *Ladies Home Journal*; ABC News Now's Katie Escherich; Barbara Bedway; Laura Broadwell; Judi C. Randall; Toddi Gutner; Beatrix Parash of CBS's *The Early Show*; Pat Estess; Nancy Metcalf of *Consumer Reports*; *MORE* magazine's Susan Caminiti and Marisa Cohen; Kathy Ricketts at the *Daily Gazette*; Pam Kelley at the *Charlotte Observer*; the CareGuide.com team; Patricia Raskin, host of *Positive Living*; Phil Petersen at Raven Publishers; Francine Kaplan at *Pink* magazine; Kimberly-Clark's Kelly D. Burgess; Chris Courogen at *Patriot News*; the *Philadelphia Inquirer*'s Lini Kadaba; Cindi Dawson; Lynn Siprelle at Newhome maker.com; the American Society of Women Accountants' Kathleen Rakestraw; Patty Edmonds; Joanne Doxtater; *Your Money Live*, with Gregg Reenie; KFAB's Gary Sadlemyer; Mort Yulish at *Eldercare Network News*; Cathy Liebow; Linda Childers; Jane Haas; Liz Taylor; Bridget Malone; Carla Fried; Candy Purdom; Cindy Richards; Lisa Holton; Greg Daugherty; Kent Nurburn; Linda Lewis; Shira Levin at Mainstreet.com; and Norma Steinberg. To Wendy at Speaker's Platform, Jane Pasanen at Chelsea Forum, Rob Carsello at Speaker's Resource, and Jean Wilson at XA Events—thank you for keeping me busy on the speakers bureau circuit.

Thanks to the professional communicators who continually portray older people with respect and dignity: Dave Martino and Gavin Binzer and the team at Martino & Binzer; Sharon Brooks; Rob Adams and the SB&A team; GlynnDevins; Lori Bitter and the JWT Mature Market Group; Beth Wilbins at Forté Public Relations; Tammy Richards Public Relations; Stacey Foisy; Patty Jameson at Innisfree; the Ehlers Group; Jaime Buege of Blue Horse Public Relations; Libby Morgan; Ed Graziano; Christine Wirthwein; Jill O'Mahoney Stewart; Pam Bieri; Barrie Stefel; and Steve Mongelluzzo.

Thanks to my colleagues in the senior-housing profession who give special meaning to the word *community* and a loving home to thousands of older adults, especially to Joy Ricci; Matt Wilson; Lisa Cole; Maureen Wood; the Greystone team, especially Bruce Byers, John Spooner, and Nancy May; Kim Tramner; John Mulherin, Dan Hermann, Steve Johnson, and the Ziegler Capital Markets Group; Herbert J. Sims; Greenbrier Development, especially Mike Gilliam and Barry Johnson; the Franciscan Sisters of Chicago; Retirement Dynamics, especially Perry Aycock, Bobbie Sumner, and Bonnie Blair; Avery Rockefeller and the RLS team; Donna Scott at CRSA; Jean Awyll; David Ratchford, Jay Hibbard, Mike Wallace, and the Spectrum Consultants; Tim Parker and the University Village staff; Covenant Retirement Communities, especially Betty Olson, Moraine Byrne, and Tom Freudenstein; Sawgrass Partners; David Schless at the American Seniors Housing Association; Leslie Knight at the American Association of Homes and Services for the Aging; Don Gorsuch; Ed Kenny, Liz Bush, Joel Nelson, and the Life Care Services team; Mary and DeWayne McMullen; Josie Kingsley; Maureen Anderson and Nancy Carmen of New Life Management and Development; Jody Staszesky; Dennis Bozzi and Life Services Network; Sharon Baksa at Erickson Communities; Sunrise Senior Living, especially Nanci Wechsler and Kurt Conroy; Chris McKenzie at Ohio Presbyterian Retirement Services; Tom Slemmer at National Church Residences; David Smith at One on One Consulting; Ted Otto; Bob Ogle; Moore Diversified Services; Meredith Boyle; Patty Santiago; Monique Eliezer; Diane Baumgartner of the American Baptist Homes of the Midwest; Pam Claassen of the American Baptist Homes of the West; Lutheran Life Communities; Wynne Angell; Robert Synder; Steve Wright at Unicus; Susan Brecht; Sloan Bentley and the team at Seniority; Gerontological Services; Julie Stevens and the Classic Residence by Hyatt team; Gale Morgan at Mather LifeWays; Dan Gray; Third Age; Dixon Hughes; LarsenAllen; Cynthia Rozenberg at Kingston Regional Health Care; Patrick McShane of Masonic Health System; Dale Lilburn and the team at Plymouth Place; Ed Toy and David Ross at Lions Gate; Cathy Ritter and the team at Friendship Senior Options; Eileen Moore at Providence Point; Weitz Senior Living; Pacific Retirement Services; Glenn Brichacek at The Admiral at the Lake; FreemanWhite; Perkins Eastman; EGA; Bovis Lend Lease; Randalynn Kaye; Leslie Dominguez at Querencia at Barton Creek; Rita Vicary at Lutheran Senior Services; Walt Stroly; and the wondrous John Durso.

To my extended Italian family at the Joint Civic Committee of Italian Americans, thank you for helping me to keep my Italian heritage alive and thriving in the great city of Chicago and my mother's homeland, Lucca, Italy.

Thanks to my literary agent and dear friend, Joe Durepos, for his belief in me right from the start. To Elizabeth Rappoport and Lisa Hudson, whose commitment to my work began long before this edition of the book took flight—I am forever grateful for your trust and friendship. Thanks also to Brandi Bowles for getting this project off the ground. To Carrie Thornton and Heather Proulx at Random House—I am deeply honored for the opportunity, once again, to shed hope and light on the subject of eldercare.

Last, I am indebted to the thousands of caregivers and elders who have shared their joys, sorrows, and insights with me. You are always and forever in my thoughts and prayers.

ABOUT THE AUTHOR

Known as one of the leading experts on caregiving, Joy Loverde's proactive approach to elder-care has changed people's thinking about aging and feeling in better control of their future. Joy is a popular and seasoned keynote speaker and has presented to renowned organizations such as the National Institutes of Health and American Seniors Housing Association. Her work has been featured on the *Today* show, the CBS *Early Show*, and National Public Radio, and in the *Wall Street Journal, Consumer Reports*, and *USA Today*. Joy also serves as a consultant to professionals in the fast-growing eldercare industry and has served as a spokesperson for respected business leaders, including Energizer and Masterpiece Living. She lives in Chicago. Visit her website at ElderIndustry.com.